Developing Costimulatory Molecules for Immunotherapy of Diseases

Developing Costimulatory Molecules for Immunotherapy of Diseases

Manzoor Ahmad Mir
Department of Bioresources
University of Kashmir
Srinagar, India

and

College of Applied Medical Sciences
University of Majmaah
Kingdom of Saudi Arabia

ELSEVIER

AMSTERDAM • BOSTON • HEIDELBERG • LONDON
NEW YORK • OXFORD • PARIS • SAN DIEGO
SAN FRANCISCO • SINGAPORE • SYDNEY • TOKYO
Academic Press is an imprint of Elsevier

Academic Press is an imprint of Elsevier
32 Jamestown Road, London NW1 7BY, UK
525 B Street, Suite 1800, San Diego, CA 92101-4495, USA
225 Wyman Street, Waltham, MA 02451, USA
The Boulevard, Langford Lane, Kidlington, Oxford OX5 1GB, UK

ISBN: 978-0-12-802585-7

British Library Cataloguing-in-Publication Data
A catalogue record for this book is available from the British Library

Library of Congress Cataloging-in-Publication Data
A catalog record for this book is available from the Library of Congress

For information on all Academic Press publications
visit our website at http://store.elsevier.com/

Typeset by MPS Limited, Chennai, India
www.adi-mps.com

Dedicated to
My
Beloved Family
And
Teachers

Contents

About the Editor

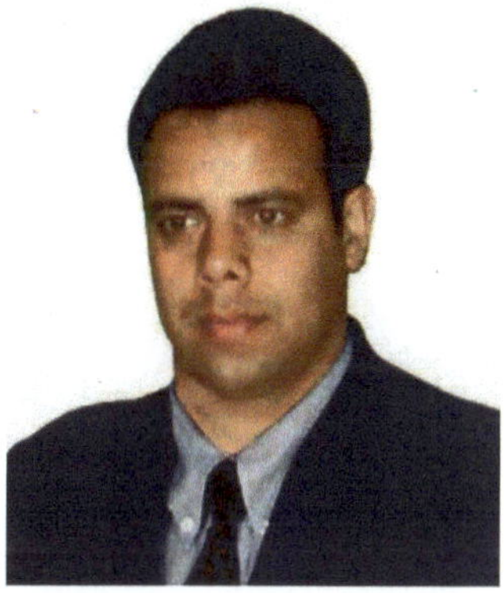

Dr. Manzoor completed his masters in life sciences with a gold medal and after qualifying with the prestigious JRF-NET-CSIR examination completed his PhD in immunopathology from IMTECH-JNU. His PhD work includes understanding the role of reverse costimulation in the survival of intracellular pathogens and cancer. His area of research includes costimulation biology and immunology of stroke. He is Assistant Professor at the Department of Bioresources, University of Kashmir, Srinagar, India, and presently working in the Stroke Research Chair on novel recombinational therapies for stroke as Research Scientist at the College of Applied Medical Sciences, Majmaah University, Kingdom of Saudi Arabia. He has several international research papers, review articles, and books to his credit. He is a member of many scientific societies across the globe. He has many courses to his credit besides a doctorate degree in immunology which includes PGDHE and PGDEE. Dr. Manzoor has already authored many books on costimulation immunotherapy and stroke biology.

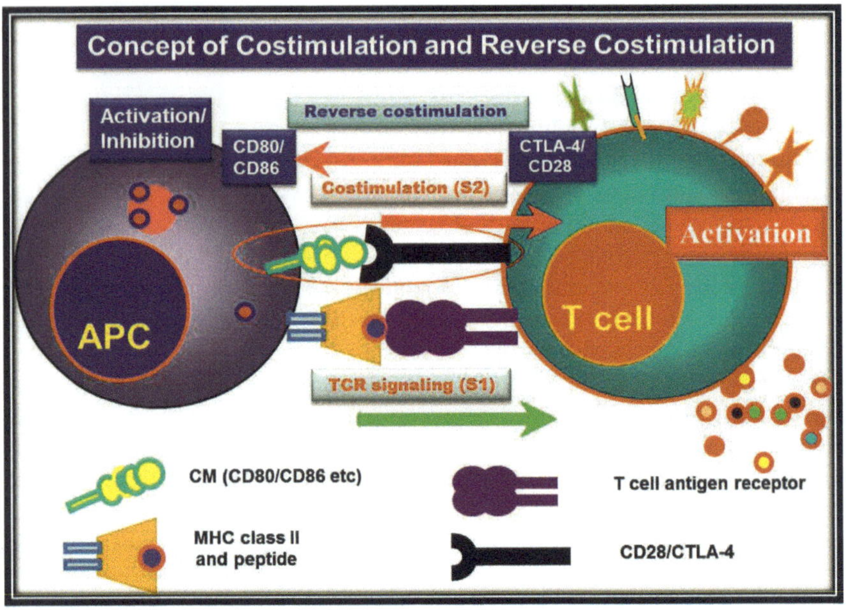

Concept of Costimulation and Reverse Costimulation
Activation/
Inhibition
Reverse costimulation
CD80/
CD86
CTLA-4/
CD28
Costimulation (S2)
Activation
APC
T cell
TCR signaling (S1)
CM (CD80/CD86 etc)
T cell antigen receptor
MHC class II
and peptide
CD28/CTLA-4

Preface

Considering the importance of complex roles played by CD28 and B7 costimulatory families in regulating the immune system, we predict that novel approaches targeting these families will yield new therapies for the treatment of inflammation, autoimmunity, transplantation, cancer, allergies, asthma, and other diseases. This book highlights the novel concept of reverse costimulation, which can be effectively exploited to develop immunotherapy either using humanized antibodies against CD80, CD86, and other costimulatory molecules or CD28 fusinogenic proteins for the treatment of cancer, especially relapse and refractory follicular lymphomas; infectious diseases like tuberculosis, typhoid, etc.; and transplantation therapeutics, inflammation, etc.

Therapeutic modalities targeting the B7 and CD28 costimulatory families of ligands and receptors are showing promise in the clinic. The encouraging results in targeting the B7/CD28/CTLA-4 pathway in the autoimmune diseases like psoriasis, multiple sclerosis, and rheumatoid arthritis underscore the importance of this costimulatory pathway, and validate the pathogenic contributions of T cells in the etiology of these diseases. This novel strategy of costimulation activation/inhibition can be effectively exploited to develop immunotherapy for the treatment of intracellular pathogens like *M. tuberculosis*, HIV, *L. donovani*, *T. cruzi*, etc. This strategy can also be used as an alternative strategy or in combination with the drugs. Because this approach is based on modulating the immune system of the hosts rather than targeting the pathogen, it significantly diminishes the chance of emergence of drug resistant strains of pathogens and if applied properly may overcome the rising menace of infectious diseases. To develop alternative or adjunct (with drugs) therapies using costimulatory molecules, an intensive effort has been undertaken in the last decade to understand how intracellular pathogens exploit costimulatory molecules, which are the tour de force of the immune system. The potent role of costimulatory molecules is aptly established in the optimum activation of T cells and APCs: cells that play a cardinal role in curbing the infections. Hence, immunotherapy involving costimulatory molecules can be a breakthrough strategy to treat various diseases, minimize side effects inflicted by drug therapies, and restrict the emergence of drug resistance.

This book highlights the novel concept of reverse costimulation, which can be effectively exploited to develop immunotherapy using either humanized antibodies against CD80, CD86, and other costimulatory molecules or CD28 fusinogenic proteins for the treatment of diseases like allergies, asthma, rheumatoid arthritis, multiple sclerosis, lupus nephritis and severe psoriasis vulgaris, tuberculosis, typhoid, therapeutic transplantation, cancer, and inflammation. Moreover the development of second and third generation CARs for the treatment of various cancers and viral infections is also discussed in Chapter 6 entitled "T cell Costimulation and Its Role in Diseases."

This book highlights the importance of complex roles played by CD28 and B7 costimulatory families in regulating the immune system. Despite the complex roles and interactions within the CD28 and B7 costimulatory families, the novel approaches targeting these families will yield new therapies for the treatment of inflammation, autoimmunity, transplantation, cancer, and infectious diseases. To translate this field into the clinic, it is urgent to develop novel methods to target the costimulatory pathway as currently understood and deeply comprehend the pathophysiology of the diseases involving costimulatory molecules.

Moreover no such book regarding developing costimulatory molecules for the treatment of diseases like allergy, asthma, lymphomas, cancer, autoimmunity, and transplantation was available to the best of my knowledge. Therefore it became imperative to pen a book with the concept of reverse costimulation immunotherapy in the treatment of diseases by developing various costimulatory molecules. Additionally up-to-date trends in the research like development of second and third generation CARs are included in this book with many tables and diagrams to make it more concise and readable. This book highlights mainly the following points:

- Describes the breakthrough strategy of immunotherapy involving costimulatory molecules to treat various diseases, minimizing side effects inflicted by drug therapies
- Contains many diagrams and tables highlighting costimulatory interactions
- Provides cutting-edge knowledge on costimulation and immunotherapy with relation to different diseases and their treatment
- Includes coverage of therapeutic and preventative methods
- Brings the basic science and clinical perspectives together in a single volume, facilitating translational possibilities
- Helps to integrate the value of costimulation immunotherapy outside of a cancer setting
- Brings out the development of second and third generation CARS for treatment of cancer and viral infections

The target audience will get up-to-date cutting-edge knowledge of costimulation and immunotherapy with relation to different diseases and their treatment. Moreover information is given on how the immune system is regulated by the costimulatory molecules and which costimulatory/coinhibitory pathways are important in disease control. This book highlights the regulation of the immune functioning by different costimulatory molecules and the treatment of lymphomas using reverse costimulation immunotherapy. Further, information is provided on how pathogens cause dreadful diseases and modulate the expression of various costimulatory molecules.

Acknowledgments

First I would like to thank Almighty for giving me strength, belief, and good health. It is under his grace that we all live, learn, and flourish.

Although it is difficult to thank everybody and interweave in words the genuine efforts made by the people directly or indirectly to make this book entitled *Developing Costimulatory Molecules for Immunotherapy of Diseases*, I would like to take this opportunity to pen down my appreciation for a number of people whose contribution in numerous ways immensely helped me to move toward my destination.

It gives me immense pleasure to express my sense of gratitude and respect to my mentors Dr. Javed N Agrewala, Prof Talat Ahmad, Prof Mohammad Afzal Zargar, Prof Inayetullah Tahir, Prof Raid Saleem Albaradie, and Prof Farooq Ahmad Malik whose constant support, utmost patience, invaluable advice, and guidance rekindled my interest for science from time to time. I will benefit for a long time from their sincerity, originality, and truthfulness which has nourished my intellectual maturity. I admire and respect them all for their sincerity, dedication, devotion, amazing memory, thorough knowledge, and constructive criticism.

The congenial company of Qazi Imtiyaz Sb, Raid, Fuzail, Faizan, and Aiman at Majmaah University and Tajamal, Reiaz, Altaf and Rffat, showkat at Kashmir University deserve a special mention. I am short of words to justify the care, affection, and untiring support showered by these very good friends.

I owe deepest gratitude to my parents Mohammad Abdullah Mir and Zoona Begum. A seed of loyalty, hard work, dedication, and sincerity sown in me by my parents played a crucial role in completion of this work. They have been a source of great strength throughout my life. I would like to thank other family members for continuous and unconditional support of all my undertakings, scholastic and otherwise. Without their affection, support, best wishes, love, and care this work would not have been completed.

I specially thank Mohammad Ashraf Malik and Posha Begum for their sincere and genuine efforts for making my entire stay pleasant here at the Kingdom of Saudi Arabia by taking care for all my liabilities way back at home.

Specifically I would like to cordially thank my Family (SM1319) i.e my wife Sumaira and son Aariz for their support and cooperation during the entire project. I thank everybody who was important to the successful realization of this book, as well as expressing my apology that I could not mention each and everyone personally.

Finally I would like to thank again the Prime Mover Almighty in whom I have great faith.

Manzoor Ahmad Mir

Chapter 1

Introduction to Costimulation and Costimulatory Molecules

INTRODUCTION

We live in an environment that contains a huge range of pathogenic microbes and toxic substances that threaten normal homeostasis and challenge the host by a very broad selection of pathogenic mechanisms. Pathogenic microbes possess a diverse collection of mechanisms by which they replicate, spread, and threaten normal host functions. The immune system must eliminate pathological microbes and toxic or allergenic proteins, and at the same time, it must avoid responses that produce excessive damage of self-tissues or that might eliminate beneficial, commensal microbes. It is not surprising, therefore, that the immune system uses a complex array of protective mechanisms to control and usually eliminate these organisms and toxins. A general feature of the immune system is that these mechanisms rely on detecting structural features of the pathogen or toxin that mark it as distinct from host cells. Such host–pathogen or host–toxin discrimination is essential to permit the host to eliminate the threat without damaging its own tissues.

Our immune system uses many mechanisms to combat infection by microbes. These mechanisms work together, and the fully integrated immune response draws elements from many effector systems in order to tailor a response to the specific invading pathogen. Activation of the immune system is dependent upon both innate and adaptive responses to environmental challenges such as infection. Activation of adaptive immune responses requires signals through antigen-specific T- and B-cell receptors (TCRs and BCRs, respectively). But this antigen-specific signal alone was not sufficient to drive the activation of naive T cells and led to the concept of two-signal model of T-cell activation, according to which productive T-cell activation requires a first signal provided by the interaction of antigenic peptide/major histocompatibility complex (MHC) with the TCR and a second, antigen-independent cosignal, the "costimulatory signal." The "first signal" delivered by the TCR mediates the specificity of a T-cell response via the recognition of specific epitopes of a given antigen presented in combination with

Developing Costimulatory Molecules for Immunotherapy of Diseases.
DOI: http://dx.doi.org/10.1016/B978-0-12-802585-7.00001-7

the MHC on antigen-presenting cells (APCs). However, activation of T cells by this receptor interaction alone fails to induce cytokine production and sustained proliferation, but rather results in T-cell apoptosis, or the induction of specific nonresponsiveness (anergy) to subsequent stimulation with the same antigen.[1] This gives rise to the concept of the two-signal model of T-cell activation (Figure 1.1). According to the two-signal model, T cells, to become fully activated, require additional signals delivered by the so-called costimulatory molecules. These molecules are transmembrane proteins that induce an intracellular signaling cascade via their cytoplasmic tail that modifies the TCR-mediated signal. Costimulatory molecules cannot activate T cells without concomitant TCR cross-linking. According to this definition, adhesion molecules such as intercellular adhesion molecule-1 are not costimulatory because they enhance T-cell activation merely by facilitating the contact between T cell and APC. Furthermore,

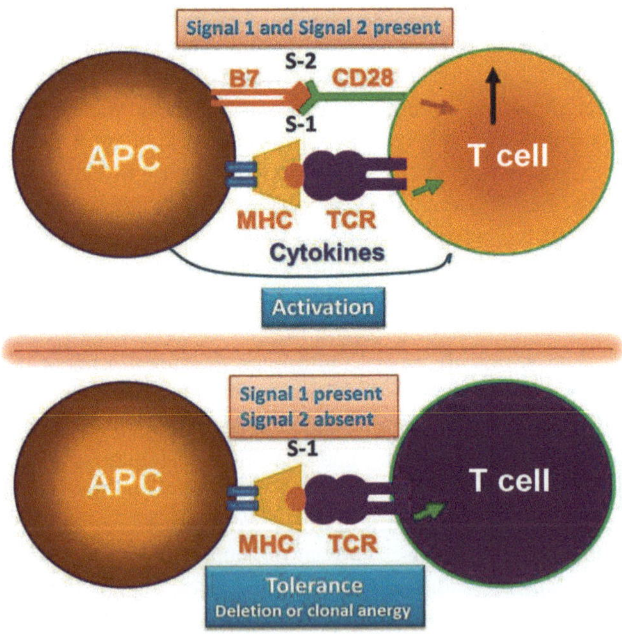

FIGURE 1.1 **Two-signal model of T-cell activation.** Two signals are needed for optimal activation of T cells. Signal 1, which is specific, is delivered through TCR on T cells and Signal 2, which is antigen independent and nonspecific, is delivered through costimulatory molecules present on APCs. Signal 2 is required for sustained T-cell proliferation, effector/memory cell generation, and prevention of anergy or apoptosis. If costimulatory signal is absent, the cell will undergo clonal anergy (unresponsiveness) or deletion. Expression of costimulatory molecules on professional APCs ensures that only pathogen-specific T cells are activated and minimizes the chances of acquired immune responses being mounted against self.

T-cell costimulation refers to a signal that is delivered to the T cell exclusively. In this respect, the CD40–CD40L interaction is also not considered as costimulatory, although this is an important receptor–ligand pair in T/B cooperation. The dependence of T-cell activation on this "second signal" delivered by costimulators adds a second line of regulation to antigen-specific T-cell responses that reaches far beyond a mere "on–off" command. With a growing number of both stimulatory and inhibitory costimulatory molecules being identified, the classic concept of costimulation as a two-signal event has changed. T cells simultaneously express an adjustable spectrum of costimulatory molecules. Today, T-cell costimulation is recognized as an integrating process of various positive and negative signals that determine the mode of T-cell activation.[2] The T-cell response to any given antigen involves the clonal expansion of a small number of T cells that share specificity but express unique TCRs. The integration of signals generated by these interactions determines the final outcome of encounters between T cells and APCs. The primary source of this costimulatory signal is interactions between the T-cell integral membrane protein CD28 and its ligands, B7-1 and B7-2, on the APC. Currently, the B7 family has seven members (B7-1, B7-2, inducible costimulator ligand (ICOS-L), programmed death ligand-1 (PD-L1), PD-L2, B7-H3, and B7-H4), whereas tumor necrosis factor (TNF) receptor (TNFR)/TNF family has six members (herpes virus entry mediator (HVEM), B- and T-lymphocyte attenuator (BTLA), CD70, CD30, 4-IBB-L, and OX40L) (Table 1.1 and Figure 1.2). The B7 family includes transmembrane or glycosylphosphatidylinositol-linked proteins characterized by extracellular IgV and IgC domains. B7-1 and B7-2 can engage either CD28 or cytotoxic T-lymphocyte antigen-4 (CTLA-4), resulting in complex positive and negative regulation of antigen receptor signaling.[3] ICOS-L is the only identified ligand for inducible costimulator (ICOS). Both PD-L1 and PD-L2 engage programmed death-1 (PD-1), although data suggest the existence of additional receptors for PD-L1 and PD-L2. Receptors for B7-H3 and B7-H4 have not been identified, although expression of these ligands modulates immune responses. The cell surface expression of B7 ligands is highly regulated, although, in general, ligands for costimulatory receptors are constitutively expressed on APCs, whereas ligands for coinhibitory receptors are expressed after induction by various inflammatory stimuli. The activation of a T cell is thus dictated by the integration of signals derived from the TCR, CD28, and CTLA-4. By regulating the expansion of individual T cells, CD28 and CTLA-4 could modulate the composition of a polyclonal antigen-specific T-cell response. The balance between activating signals generated by CD28 and inhibitory signals delivered by CTLA-4 determine the outcome of a T cell's interaction with an APC.

COSTIMULATORY MOLECULES

It is now well established that the optimum activation of T cells requires two distinct signals from APCs. The first signal is triggered by interaction

TABLE 1.1 Currently Known Costimulatory Molecules and Ligands

Expression	Superfamily	Costimulatory Molecule	Ligand	Signal Type
Constitutive	CD28/B7	CD28	B7-1, B7-2 (CD80, CD86)	Positive
	TNF/TNFR	CD27	CD70	Positive
	TNF/TNFR, CD28/B7	HVEM	LIGHT, BTLA	Positive
	TNF/TNFR, CD28/B7	BTLA	HVEM	Negative
Inducible	CD28/B7	ICOS	ICOSL	Positive
	TNF/TNFR	OX40 (CD134)	OX40L	Positive
	TNF/TNFR	4-1BB (CD137)	4-IBB-L	Positive
	TNF/TNFR	CD30	CD30L (CD153)	Positive
	CD2	SLAM (CD150)	SLAM (CD150)	Positive
	CD28/B7	CTLA-4 (CD152)	B7-1, B7-2 (CD80, CD86)	Negative
	CD28/B7	PD-1	PD-L1, PDL-2	Negative
	CD28/B7	Unknown	B7-H4	Negative
	CD28/B7	Unknown	B7-H3	Obscure

Note: TNF: tumor necrosis factor; R: receptor; HVEM: herpes virus entry mediator; LIGHT: homologous to lymphotoxin, inducible expression, competing for GpD of herpes virus, expressed on activated T lymphocytes; BLTA: B- and T-lymphocyte attenuator; ICOS: inducible costimulator; L: ligand; SLAM: signaling lymphocyte activation molecule; CTLA: cytotoxic T-lymphocyte antigen; PD: programmed death; B7-H4 and -H3: B7 homologues 4 and 3.

of antigen-specific TCR with the peptide MHC complex,[4] whereas the second nonspecific signal is delivered by the interaction of costimulatory molecules present on the surface of the APCs and their corresponding receptors on T cells.[5–8] The costimulatory signals are neither antigen specific nor MHC restricted, yet they are essential and critical for the development of effector functions. T-cell activation requires engagement of the TCR with the peptide–MHC complex presented on the cell surface of APCs.[9] In addition to this antigen-specific interaction, a second interaction involving costimulatory receptors (CD28, ICOS) on T cells and their respective ligands (B7-1/B7-2, ICOSL) on APCs is required for optimal T-cell activation.[10,11] Although these receptor–ligand pairs augment T-cell activation, interactions between T-cell costimulatory/inhibitory receptors CTLA-4 and PD-1 with their ligands, B7-1/B7-2 and PD-L1/PD-L2,

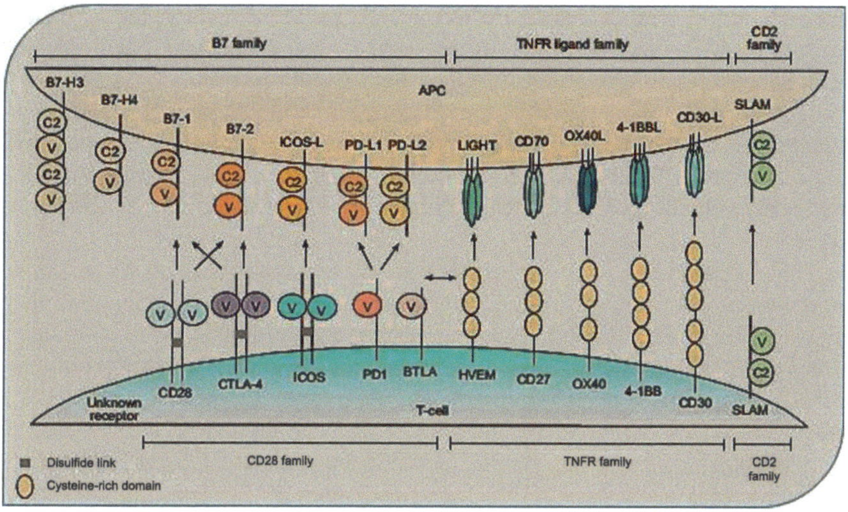

FIGURE 1.2 Currently known costimulatory molecules and their ligands. TNFR: tumor necrosis factor receptor; APC: antigen-presenting cell; B7-H3 and -H4: B7 homologues 3 and 4; ICOS: inducible costimulator; L: ligand; PD: programmed death; LIGHT: homologous to lymphotoxin, inducible expression, competing for GpD of herpes virus, expressed on activated T lymphocytes; V: Ig-like variable domain; C2: constant type-2 Ig-like domain; SLAM: signaling lymphocyte activation molecule; CTLA: cytotoxic T-lymphocyte antigen; BTLA: B- and T-lymphocyte attenuator; HVEM: herpes virus entry mediator.

respectively, lead to attenuation of the T-cell response.[12,13] The integration of signals delivered as a consequence of these interactions is essential for the initiation, modulation, and regulation of an effective T-cell response. The immunoregulatory potential of costimulation became clear when it was shown that TCR ligation in the absence of costimulatory signal can lead to anergy, deletion, or unresponsiveness in T cells.[14–17] This gave rise to two-signal model of T-cell costimulation.

Two-Signal Model of T-cell Activation

The basic concept that optimal and sustained activation of T cells, leading to proliferation, cytokine production, and effector functions, requires two signals has been known as "the two-signal model."[2] The first signal is delivered through the TCR after interaction with antigenic peptides presented on MHC molecules of APCs. This MHC–peptide–TCR signal is specific and determines which CD4+ T cells will respond to a particular antigen. The second signal is also accessory cell derived, but not antigen specific and has been termed as a costimulatory signal because, although essential, it does not by itself induce any response in T cells.[1,18,19] However, when a T cell has its receptor ligated and receives a costimulatory signal, the T cell proliferates and differentiates into an armed effector cell. These secondary, the so-called costimulatory, signals are critically required for the process of T-cell activation. Because landmark studies defined that T cells receiving a TCR signal without a costimulatory signal are tolerized *in vitro*, the investigation of T-cell costimulation has attracted intense interest. Early studies demonstrated that interrupting T-cell costimulation allows attenuation of the alloresponse, which is particularly difficult to modulate due to the clone size of alloreactive T cells.

The understanding of costimulation has since evolved substantially and now encompasses not only positive signals involved in T-cell activation but also negative signals that inhibit T-cell activation and promote T-cell tolerance. Moreover, the significance of costimulatory molecules in T-cell activation has gained considerable impetus following the observation that T cells that bind to antigens but do not receive costimulatory signals are thought to die or become anergic, a state of unresponsiveness, in which the cell cannot be activated even if it receives both the signals vital for its activation.[14,19,20] Thus, an encounter with the antigen can lead to two quite distinct outcomes, proliferation and differentiation into effector cells, or inactivation or death. Which outcome occurs is determined by the appropriate delivery of costimulatory signals through costimulatory molecules.[15] At present, several reports are available in the literature highlighting the potential role of a number of cell surface molecules necessary for the initiation of the differentiation events occurring during T cell–APC interaction. The various known costimulatory molecules expressed on the APC have both adhesive and costimulatory functions.

The known costimulatory molecules are CD80, CD86, CD40, B7-DC (PDL-2), B7H-3/B7H-4, CD70, OX40L, B7-H2/LICOS, B7-H1, and 4-1BBL. The recently discovered costimulatory molecules include the B7-DC (PDL-2), B7H-3, and B7H-4.[21] The exact mechanism of sequence of signals provided by these molecules in the activation and differentiation of cells on which they are present is not very well known. The best-characterized costimulatory pathway involves the CD28/CTLA-4 receptors present on T cells that bind to costimulatory molecules, CD80 and CD86.[12] CD28 is constitutively expressed on all T cells in mice and on 95% of CD4+ T cells and 50% of CD8+ T cells in humans. CD80 and CD86 are expressed mainly on APCs, including dendritic cells (DCs), macrophages, and B cells. The expression of CD80 and CD86 on APCs is enhanced by the presence of microbes and by cytokines that are produced in response to microbes. This regulated expression of B7 costimulators ensures that T cells respond best only when necessary, that is, when faced with pathogens. The interaction of CD80 and CD86 with CD28, in concert with T-cell–receptor signaling, promotes the expansion of antigen-stimulated T cells and their differentiation into effector and memory cells. CD28 is the major costimulatory receptor for naive T cells and is therefore important for initiating T-cell responses. CD28 signals enhance the production of interleukin-2 (IL-2) and other cytokines; upregulate cell survival genes (such as Bcl-xL); promote energy metabolism (glucose uptake and rate of glycolysis); and facilitate cell cycle progression.[22] One of the best-characterized costimulatory interactions is the binding of CD28/CTLA-4 on T cells with B7-1/B7-2 on APCs. CD28 and CTLA-4 are homologous receptors with approximately 30% sequence identity that belong to the immunoglobulin (Ig) superfamily and contain one membrane proximal IgV-like domain.[23,24] Furthermore, they are clustered in close proximity on chromosome 1C1 in mice and 2q33 in humans.[25,26] They are expressed as disulfide-linked homodimers and bind to the same ligands, B7-1 and B7-2. Although CTLA-4 is bivalent in nature, recent structural studies suggest that CD28 is monovalent.[27] Moreover, the expression pattern and the immunological roles of CD28 and CTLA-4 are vastly different. Although CD28 is constitutively expressed on both naive and activated T cells, CTLA-4 follows a more complex pattern of expression. In resting T cells, CTLA-4 is associated with the clathrin adaptor complex AP-1 and is present predominantly in intracellular vesicles. Upon T-cell activation, CTLA-4 is transported to the cell surface where it is again rapidly internalized by another clathrin adaptor complex AP-2.[28,29] The directional recruitment of CTLA-4 from intracellular vesicles to the immunological synapse is regulated by the TCR signal strength. Furthermore, CD28 has a slow turnover rate, whereas CTLA-4 has a rapid turnover with a half-life of 2 h.[30] As a consequence of these dynamic processes, only a small fraction of CTLA-4 is present on the cell surface, which seems to be sufficient to deliver the requisite signal for termination of T-cell activation. Functionally, the engagement of CD28 with B7 ligands delivers a positive signal to T cells that culminates in T-cell proliferation and cytokine production, and prevents induction of T-cell tolerance.[31,32] In contrast, the interaction of CTLA-4 with B7-1/B7-2 results in negative signaling, which leads to attenuation of T-cell activation and induction of T-cell anergy. Such processes are essential for regulating of a T-cell response and maintaining T-cell homeostasis.[33–35] The engagement of CD28 and CTLA-4 also indirectly delivers distinct signals to T cells through their different effects on DCs. The expression pattern of various known B7-CD28 family of costimulatory molecules along with their corresponding ligands is listed in Table 1.2 and described below in detail.

THE B7 FAMILY OF COSTIMULATORY LIGANDS

The B7:CD28 family of costimulatory molecules includes the costimulatory ligands present on the APCs and their corresponding receptors on the T cells. The B7 costimulatory ligands involve the CD80, CD86, ICOS-L, PDL-1 (B7-H1), PDL-2 (B7-DC), B7-H3, and B7-H4 (B7x/B7-S1) (Figure 1.3).[10,36,37] The receptors for the B7 family members present on T cells include the members of CD28 family such as CD28, CD152 (CTLA-4), ICOS, PD-1, and BTLA.[11,12] The functional characterization of all the costimulatory molecules

TABLE 1.2 Protein Expression of CD28 and B7 Superfamily Members

Costimulatory Ligands/Receptors	Type	Hematopoietic Cells	Nonhematopoietic Cells
Ligands	B7-1 (CD80)	Induced on T cells, B cells, myeloid cells, and macrophages	
	B7-2 (CD86)	Constitutive on B cells, DCs, monocytes/macrophages, and upregulated with activation	
	ICOSL	Induced on T cells, B cells, DCs, and monocytes/macrophages	Intestinal epithelial cells and muscle cells
	PDL-1	Constitutive on B cells, DCs, monocytes/macrophages, and upregulated with activation	Endothelial cells, Kuppfer cells, thymic, intestinal, and renal tubular epithelial cells, syncyciotrophoblasts, pancreatic islets, keratinocytes, and tumor cells (carcinomas, melanoma)
		Induced on T cells	
	PDL-2	Induced on monocytes/macrophages, and DCs	Small cell lung carcinoma, keratinocytes, endothelial cells, and thymic epithelial cells
	B7-H3	Induced on T cells, B cells, NK cells, DCs, and monocytes/macrophages	Osteoblasts
	B7-H4	Induced on T cells, B cells, DCs, and monocytes/macrophages	Tumor (lung, ovarian)
Receptors	CD28	Constitutive on T cells	
	CTLA-4	Induced on T cells	
	ICOS	Induced on T cells, B cells, and NK cells	
	PD-1	Induced on T cells, B cells, myeloid cells, and macrophages	

Note: ICOS: inducible costimulator; CTLA: cytotoxic T-lymphocyte antigen; PD: programmed death; B7-H3 and B7-H4: B7 homologues 3 and 4; NK: nuclear killer.

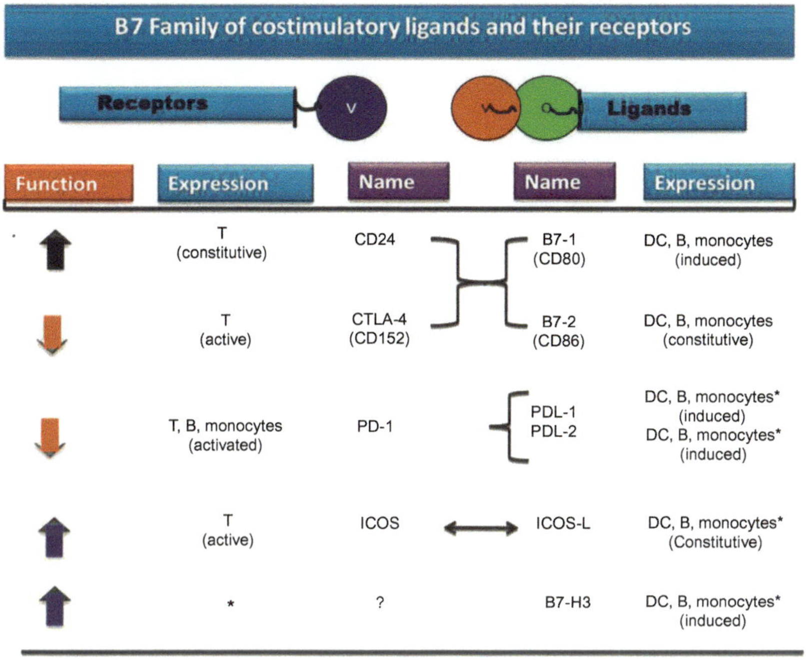

FIGURE 1.3 **Summary of B7 family ligands and their receptors.** The names of receptors and ligands are indicated, as well as a brief summary of predominant expression patterns for each. The conserved structure of a single IgV extracellular domain for receptors and IgV and IgC extracellular domains for ligands is depicted at the top. Function arrows summarize whether the pathway is thought predominantly to costimulate or inhibit the response of the receptor-bearing cell. Integration of signals through this family of costimulatory and inhibitory receptors and their ligands is critical for activation of immune responses and tolerance.

and their ligands is listed in Table 1.3. The discovery of new functions for the original B7 family members together with the identification of additional B7 and CD28 family members has revealed new ways in which the B7:CD28 family regulates T-cell activation and tolerance. The interaction between these molecules does not regulate T cells but also the cells on which these molecules are present, that is, APCs.[12]

Pathways in the B7:CD28 family have key roles in regulating T-cell activation and tolerance, and are thus promising therapeutic targets. In the B7 family, CD80 and CD86 are the best-defined and best-characterized costimulatory molecules present on APCs. T-cell activation is dependent upon signals delivered through the antigen-specific TCR and accessory receptors on the T cell. A primary costimulatory signal is delivered through the CD28 receptor after engagement with its ligands, CD80 or CD86, resulting in T-cell activation, whereas the engagement of CTLA-4 (CD152) with CD80 or CD86 ligands results in attenuation of T-cell responses. CD80/CD86:CD28/CD152

TABLE 1.3 Functional Characterization of Costimulatory Molecules

Functional Aspect	Characterization	Costimulatory Molecule
Expression pattern	Constitutive	CD28, CD27, HVEM, BTLA
	Inducible	ICOS, CTLA-4, PD-1, OX40, 4-IBB, CD80, SLAM, putative receptor for B7-H3 and B7-H4
T-cell modulation	Positive/ enhancement	CD28, ICOS, OX40, CD27, 4-IBB, CD30, HVEM, SLAM
	Negative/ Inhibition	CTLA-4, PD-1, BTLA-4, putative receptor for B7-H4
T-cell differentiation	Th1	4-IBB, SLAM, BTLA
	Th2	ICOS, OX40, CD30
	Treg	ICOS, CTLA-4, PD-1
T-cell function	T effector/helper	ICOS, CTLA-4, PD-1, OX40
	T memory	OX40, CD30, CD27
Location of action	Central	CD28, HVEM, CTLA-4
	Central or peripheral	ICOS, PD-1, OX40, 4-IBB

Note: HVEM: herpes virus entry mediator; BTLA: B- and T-lymphocyte attenuator; ICOS: inducible costimulator; CTLA: cytotoxic T-lymphocyte antigen; PD: programmed death; SLAM: signaling lymphocyte activation molecule; B7-H3 and B7-H4: B7 homologues 3 and 4; Th: T-helper cell; Treg: regulatory T cell.

interactions not only promote initial T-cell activation but also regulate self-tolerance by supporting CD4+ CD25+ regulatory T cell (Treg) homeostasis.[12]

The well-defined and best-characterized costimulatory ligands in T-cell activation are the two structurally related type I transmembrane glycoproteins CD80 and CD86 belonging to Ig superfamily. They share 25% sequence homology and have two Ig-like extracellular domains (one variable and one constant), in addition to transmembrane and short cytoplasmic domains. These proteins are expressed as monomers/dimers on professional APCs, namely, DC, activated B cell, and macrophage. CD80 expression is found on activated B and T cells and macrophages. CD86 is constitutively expressed on interdigitating DCs, Langerhans cells, peripheral blood DCs, memory B cells, and germinal center B cells. Both CD80 and CD86 are capable of binding the receptors, CD28 and CTLA-4. Both human and mouse CD80 and CD86 can bind to either human or mouse CD28 and CTLA-4. This suggests that there are conserved amino acids that form the critical binding sites. CD28 plays a role in activation, whereas CTLA-4 functions as an inhibitory receptor important for down-modulating the immune response.[3,13,38,39] These costimulatory

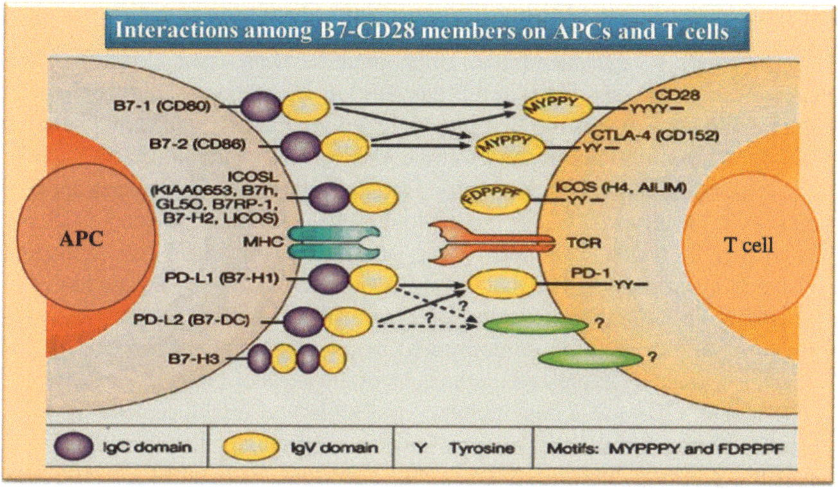

FIGURE 1.4 Schematic representation of the interactions among CD28 and B7 family members. Alternate names for receptors and ligands are shown in parentheses. IDO, indoleamine 2,3-dioxygenase.

molecules on APCs interact with their corresponding ligands on T cells and cause the inhibition/activation of the cell function depending upon the molecules involved and the intracellular domain of the molecules involved. For interactions of these molecules on APC and T cell, see Figure 1.4. Although CD86 is generally the first B7 molecule encountered, due to its constitutive expression on numerous APCs, there does not appear to be significant differences in the functions of CD80 and CD86. Rather, it depends on the type of APC encountered and its activation state.

The B7 and CD28 gene families have grown substantially with mining of the human genome sequence, and the pathways defined by these new members regulate the activation, inhibition, and fine-tuning of T-cell responses. A great surprise has been the abundance of inhibitory signals delivered by these new B7/CD28 family members. The newer CD28 family members, ICOS, PD-1, and BTLA are inducibly expressed on T cells and have important roles in controlling the balance between effector T cells and Tregs. PD-1 and BTLA are also expressed on B cells and APCs, and appear to have broader immunoregulatory functions, which necessitate cell-type specific analyses of their functions. The new B7 family members, ICOS ligand (B7h, GL50, B7RP-1, ligand of ICOS (LICOS), and B7-H2); PD-L1 (B7-H1); PD-L2 (B7-DC); B7-H3 and B7-H4 (B7x/B7-S1); B7S3; and BTNL2, can be expressed not only on professional APCs but also on nonhematopoietic cells. The nonhematopoietic cell expression of these B7 family members suggests that they may function to regulate T-cell activation and/or tolerance in nonlymphoid organs.

CD80 Costimulatory Molecule

CD80, a type-1 transmembrane glycoprotein, was first identified on Epstein–Barr virus-activated B-cell blasts, Burkitt's lymphomas, and B lymphoblastoid cell lines.[40] It was the first ligand to be identified for CD28 and later for CTLA-4.[41,42] Both the human and murine CD80 genes were cloned and shown to be the members of the Ig superfamily. Human and mouse CD80 shares approximately 44% identity.[43,44] CD80 has 10-fold higher affinities for both CD28 and CTLA-4 than for CD86. CD80 expression is found on activated B cells, activated T cells, and macrophages. The functional importance of CD80 molecule has been demonstrated in a number of studies of T-cell activation. The potent costimulatory role of CD80 has been demonstrated *in vivo* in transgenic mice in which CD80 was ectopically expressed on the cells of the islets of Langerhans.[45]

The role of CD80 as a costimulatory molecule was established by the ability of CD80-transfected cells to provide the costimulation to T cells. CD80 transfected Chinese hamster ovary cells, synergies with anti-CD3 antibody (Ab)-induced T-cell activation, ultimately leading to T-cell proliferation and the production of IL-2. The proliferation was enhanced in a CD28-dependent fashion because T-cell activation was blocked by anti-CD28 Ab.[46] In subsequent studies, CD80 was also shown to promote the breakdown of tolerance. Despite the apparent ability of CD80 to provide sufficient costimulation, it has been very difficult to demonstrate its function on normal APCs in mice. Anti-CD80 Ab minimally blocks a primary Mixed Lymphocyte Reaction (MLR), whereas human Cytotoxic T Lymphocyte Antigen 4 Immunoglobulin (hCTLA-4Ig) inhibits the response by 80%.[47] Additionally, the staining of either lipopolysaccharide (LPS)-activated B cells or whole spleen with hCTLA-4Ig was not inhibited by anti-CD80 Ab, which suggests the existence of an additional CTLA-4 ligand.[48,49] CD80 −/− mice are capable of mounting an immune response to nominal antigens and APCs isolated from these mice could be stained with labeled hCTLA-4Ig.[50] These observations led to the identification and eventual cloning of a second B7 family member, CD86.[50,51]

CD86 Costimulatory Molecule

CD86 is a 70-kDa glycoprotein made up of 329 amino acids, a transmembrane region, and a longer cytoplasmic domain than CD80.[50] CD86 is constitutively expressed on interdigitating DCs, Langerhans cells, peripheral blood DCs, memory B cells and germinal center B cells, and macrophages. CD86 is rapidly upregulated on B cells following activation by cross-linking of the Ig receptor or the addition of a variety of cytokines.[47] Additionally, CD86 is expressed at low levels on monocytes and is upregulated through interferon-γ (IFN-γ) stimulation. CD86 shows 25% identity with CD80 and are both coded on human chromosome 3q13.33q21. Similar to CD80 transfectant, CD86 transfectants augment T-cell proliferation and IL-2 production to suboptimal stimulation with anti-CD3 Ab or phorbol myristate acetate (PMA). This costimulation was inhibited by either hCTLA-4Ig or anti-CD28 Ab, but not by anti-CD80 Abs, demonstrating therefore that CD86 binds to both CD28 and CTLA-4.[50,52] A combination of both anti-CD80 and anti-CD86 Abs were the most effective at inhibiting the MLR. The role for both molecules in primary responses is further supported by the findings that a combination of anti-CD80 and anti-CD86 Abs can induce anergy.[53–55]

CD80 and CD86 Expression Kinetics

CD28 shares the ability to bind B7 family members with its homologue CTLA-4. However, B7 binds to CTLA-4 with up to 2500-fold higher avidity than to CD28.[23] Upon ligation to B7, CD28 and CTLA-4 deliver opposing signals for T-cell activation, with CD28 generating an activating costimulatory signal and CTLA-4 functioning to inhibit the response.[39] CD28 ligation enhances T-cell proliferation through multiple mechanisms, including increased production and stability of IL-2 mRNA and upregulation of antiapoptotic genes, such as Bcl-xL. In contrast, CTLA-4 signaling reduces the production of the growth factor IL-2[34] and cyclin D3, cyclin-dependent kinase (cdk)4, and cdk6, thus restricting T-cell expansion.[37,56] The expression of CD80 and CD86 is primarily limited to APCs; however, recently they have been shown to be expressed on T cells, but their functional significance is not very well understood. CD86 is constitutively expressed on some resting T cells, whereas CD80 is not present on resting T cells; however, both can be upregulated on T cells by different stimuli.[57] Resting B cells express no detectable CD80 and very low levels of CD86. Both CD80 and CD86 can be upregulated on B cells by LPS or Concovalin A (ConA). CD86 is expressed more rapidly than CD80 on B cells stimulated with LPS or anti-CD40 Ab.[58] CD80 is generally absent on unstimulated cells, whereas CD86 is constitutively expressed at moderate levels on DCs, macrophages, and monocytes.[51] CD80 and CD86 are rapidly upregulated by Granulocyte Maturing-Colony Stimulating Factor (GM-CSF), LPS, IFN-γ, and CD40 signaling on DCs and macrophages.[59,60] The induction of CD86 expression occurs within 6 h of stimulation, with maximal level of expression achieved between 18 and 24 h. In contrast, CD80 expression is not detected until 24 h poststimulation and does not reach maximal levels until 48–72 h.[47,48] Some microorganisms including *Mycobaterium leprae* inhibit B7 expression, whereas some including *Toxoplasma gondii* upregulate the CD86 expression.[61] CD80 expression is induced, while that of CD86 is upregulated when human monocytes encounter the viable *T. gondii* pathogen.[61,62] A number of cytokines have been shown to differentially regulate CD80 and CD86 expression. IL-4 is one of the most potent inducers of CD86 and, to a lesser extent, CD80 on B cells.[63,64] Incubation of small resting B cells with IL-4 upregulates CD86 expression within 6 h with maximal induction occurring by 24 h.[64] IFN-γ increases the expression of CD86 on B cells, peritoneal macrophages, and peripheral blood monocytes[49,64] but downregulates the expression of CD80 on peritoneal macrophages.[59] Interestingly, the engagement of Fc receptor downregulates both CD80 and CD86 on monocytes that have been activated with either IFN-γ or GM-CSF.[65] IL-10 blocks both CD80 and CD86 upregulation on peritoneal macrophages and downregulates CD86, but not CD80 on human DCs.[66,67] These results suggest that immunosuppressive properties of the IL-10 may, in part, be a result of its regulation of CD28/CTLA-4 ligands. Thus, the differences in the ability of the respective cytokines to regulate the level and temporal expression of CD80 and CD86 both qualitatively and quantitatively may result in the distinct effects during an immune response.

CD80 and CD86 Binding Kinetics to CD28 and CTLA-4

Recent evidence suggests that CD80 and CD86 have similar low avidities for CD28 and high avidities for CTLA-4.[10] Both these proteins have very fast on-and-off rates, but their binding kinetics to CD28 and CTLA-4 are distinct. CD80 is a more potent ligand for CTLA-4 based on its higher affinity and avidity. CD80, in contrast to CD86, binds two to three times more strongly to both CD28 and CTLA-4, with faster binding kinetics and slower dissociation constants. CD80 binds CTLA-4 and CD28 with equilibrium dissociation constants (K_d) of 0.2 and 4 μM, respectively (Figure 1.5), whereas CD86 exhibits 5–10-fold lower affinities with K_d of 2.6 and 20 μM for CTLA-4 and CD28, respectively.[10] Stoichiometrically, two B7 molecules, CD80 and CD86, bind to two sites on a CD28 or CTLA-4 homodimer. This stoichiometry and the different on/off rates for CD80 and CD86 suggest that the response to low concentration of B7 would not be linear. Although CD80 and CD86 bind to the same general region of CD28 and CTLA-4, the specific amino acids critical for CD80 or CD86 binding are different.[42] Interaction of CD80 or CD86 with CTLA-4 results in an inhibitory signal, in contrast to the positive signal generated after its interaction with CD28.

Different Oligomeric States of CD80 and CD86

Costimulatory ligands CD80 and CD86 expressed on the surface of APCs interact with their receptors CTLA-4 and CD28 on T cells. Although CD80 and CTLA-4 are homologous ligands having common receptors, they exhibit distinct biochemical features and roles in immune regulation. It was recently demonstrated that CD80 and CD86 adopt different oligomeric states on the cell surface. CD86 is present as a monomer on the cell surface, whereas CD80 exists as a mixed population of monomers and dimers with predominating dimers.[23,68,69] The point mutations made in the putative dimer interface of CD80 disrupt the dimeric state of the CD80 molecule and result in the generation of a population with enhanced monomers. This existence of the different oligomeric states of CD80 and CD86 indicates that

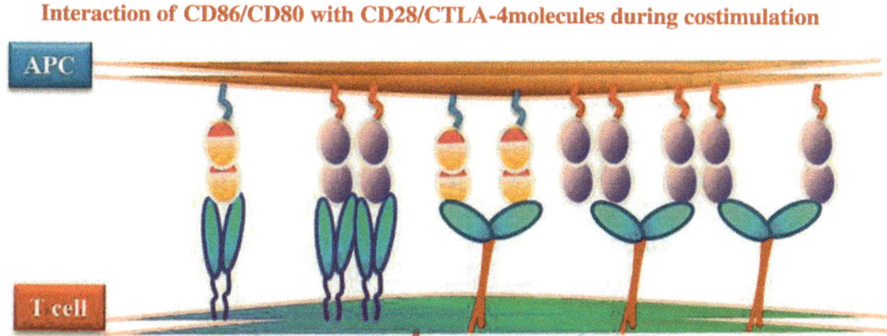

	CD86 / CD28	CD80 / CD28	CD86 / CTLA-4	CD80 / CTLA-4
K_d (μm)	20	4	2.6 22.4	0.2 1.4
K_{on} ($M^{-1}s^{-1} \times 10^6$)	≥1.4	≥0.66	1.96	≥2.15
K_{off} (s^{-1})	≥28	≥1.6	5.1	≥0.43

FIGURE 1.5 **Interaction of CD80/CD86 with CD28/CTLA-4.** The figure represents the interaction of CD80/CD86 with CTLA-4 and CD28. On the basis of expression, binding affinities, and crystal structure, it appears that CD80 shows better interaction with CTLA-4, and CD86 shows better interaction with CD28, thereby delivering bidirectional signaling, activating not only T cells but also APC. The association of CD80 with CTLA-4 is also considered better due to its faster association and slower dissociation (K_d) rates compared to CD28, which shows slower association and faster dissociation kinetics. The association of CD86 with CD28 is also considered better due to its faster association and slower dissociation rates compared to CTLA-4, which shows slower association and faster dissociation kinetics.

these molecules form costimulatory receptor–ligand complexes with distinct cell surface organizations, which may represent an important mechanistic determinant for the assembly and functional properties of signaling complexes at the T cell–APC interface.[10,68,69] This presence of different oligomeric states of CD80 and CD86 along with the different dissociation constants of CD80 and CD86 for CD28 and CTLA-4 may be the reasons why CD80 and CD86 behave differently and show different functional properties. CTLA-4 is only expressed by T cells after activation.

PD-L1/B7-H1 Costimulatory Molecule

B7-H1, also called PD-L1, is a recently identified member of B7 family of costimulatory molecules. B7-H1 shares approximately 20% amino acid identity with CD80 and 15% amino acid identity with CD86. Human and mouse B7-H1 (PD-L1) shares approximately 69% amino acid identity.[70–72] B7-H1 is a ligand for PD-1, a member of the CD28/CTLA-4 family.[73] B7-H1 is widely expressed on normal tissues (e.g., liver, lung, pancreas, heart) but not on resting peripheral blood cells. Expression on monocytes, macrophages, and DCs is upregulated with IFN-γ stimulation or upon activation. Experiments using TCR transgenic CD4+ or CD8+ T cells stimulated with APCs expressing PD-L1 show that both T-cell subsets are susceptible to this inhibitory pathway. However, CD8 + T cells may be more sensitive to modulation by the PD-1:PD-L pathway because of their intrinsic inability to produce significant levels of IL-2.[72,74] However, B7-H1 does not bind to CD28, CTLA-4, or ICOS.[3,73] The molecule can act as a T-cell costimulatory ligand during suboptimal TCR stimulation. As with B7-H2, both proliferation and IL-10 secretion are costimulated in the presence of immobilized B7-H1 or B7-H1-transfected COS cells, whereas IL-2 production is minimally enhanced. PD-L1 appears to have a strong inhibitory influence on autoreactive T cells in the islets, possibly by preventing cytokine secretion at the tissue site.[75,76] It has been shown to be an attractive target for the treatment of autoimmune diseases because it was found to be the main ligand restricting autoimmune diabetes in nonobese diabetic (NOD) mice.[77]

Interactions between the inhibitory receptor PD-1 and its ligands, PD-L1 and PD-L2, regulate both the induction and maintenance of peripheral T-cell tolerance.[78] In addition, PD-1 and PD-L1 exert critical inhibitory functions in the setting of persistent antigen expression, as in chronic viral infections and tumors.[79,80] Studies in the chronic lymphocytic choriomeningitis virus infection model provided the first indication that that this pathway contributes to T-cell dysfunction during chronic viral infection.[81] PD-1 is overexpressed on exhausted T cells, and immune function in these exhausted T cells is restored upon PD-1 or PD-L1 blockade. This observation has been extended to human immunodeficiency virus, Simian immunodeficiency virus, hepatitis B virus, and hepatitis C virus infections, and has led to new strategies for treating chronic viral infections.[82] High PD-L1 expression on tumor cells correlates with poor prognosis in a variety of human cancers, and PD-1 or PD-L1 blockade has been shown to mediate some tumor protection in mice. A humanized anti-PD-1 antibody is in clinical trials in cancer patients. Relatively little is known about PD-1 signaling. Riley[80] reviews the current understanding of signaling pathways altered by PD-1 and discusses distinct mechanisms by which PD-1 and CTLA-4 inhibit T cells. One key difference is that PD-1 engagement blocks induction of phosphatidylinositol 3-kinase activity, whereas CTLA-4 does not. The targeting of distinct signaling molecules by PD-1 and CTLA-4 suggests that approaches that block PD-1 and CTLA-4 signaling should be synergistic.

B7-H2/B7RP-1/LICOS Costimulatory Molecule

B7-H2, also known as B7RP-1, B7-H2, LICOS, and GL50, is another member of the growing B7 family of immune costimulatory proteins.[3] As with other B7 family members, B7-H2 is a type I transmembrane glycoprotein that is a member of the Ig superfamily. B7-H2 shares approximately 20–30% amino acid sequence identity with other members of the B7 family. Human and mouse B7-H2 shares approximately 49% amino acid sequence identity.[83,84] B7-H2 is expressed constitutively on resting B cells, DCs, and at low levels on monocytes, but IFN-γ stimulation upregulates expression on these cell types. The mechanisms of upregulation of B7-H2 expression appear to be distinct from those for CD80 and CD86.[85] B7-H2 expression could be regulated by inflammatory signals present in peripheral sites. It is the ligand for ICOS and does not bind to CD28, CTLA-4, or PD-1.[86] Consistent with a role of B7-H2 as a costimulatory ligand, T-cell proliferation in response to antigen presentation by B7-H2-transfected fibroblasts is significantly higher than that with untransfected fibroblasts, similar to that observed with CD86-transfected cells. B7-H2 costimulation of T cells, however, does not depend on either CD28 or CTLA-4 molecules because antagonism of B7-CD28 and B7-CTLA-4 interactions had no effect on costimulation by fibroblasts expressing B7-H2. Further, human B7-H2, which is also known as LICOS, shares 50% of its extracellular domain sequences with murine B7-H2 and can specifically bind *in vitro* to human ICOS. Exposure of mice to endotoxin induces the expression of B7-H2 mRNA in testes, kidney, and peritoneal tissues. Interestingly, *in vitro* differentiated DCs do not express B7-H2, even though they express CD80. As one additional functional test of the importance of B7-H2–ICOS interactions in the growth and differentiation of mature T cells, transgenic mice have been engineered to secrete a soluble form of the B7-H2 molecule into the bloodstream.[87] These animals develop a lymphoid hyperplasia by 12 weeks of age involving both the T-cell and B-cell compartments. Although it is difficult to ascertain whether this soluble B7-H2 molecule is acting as an agonist or an antagonist for ICOS in this system, the results do support a role for B7-H2–ICOS interactions in the regulation of T-cell homeostasis.

B7-DC/PD-L2 Costimulatory Molecule

PD-L2, also called B7-DC, is another recently identified member of the B7 family. It shares approximately 41% amino acid identity with PD-L1. Human and mouse PD-L2 shares approximately 72% amino acid identity. B7-H1 and PD-L2 are both ligands for PD-1, a member of the CD28/CTLA-4 family. PD-L2, like PD-L1, is widely expressed on normal tissues (e.g., liver, lung, pancreas, heart), but not on resting peripheral blood cells. Expression on monocytes, macrophages, and DCs is upregulated with IFN-γ stimulation. PD-L2 does not bind to CD28, CTLA-4, or ICOS[3,73] but has been shown to bind to PD-1 found on activated lymphocytes and has potent costimulatory property for naive T cells.[73] B7-DC costimulates T-cell proliferation more efficiently than CD80 and induces a distinct pattern of lymphokine secretion. In particular, B7-DC strongly costimulates IFN-γ but not IL-4 or IL-10 production from naive T cells. These properties of B7-DC may account for some of the unique activity of DCs, such as their ability to initiate potent T-helper-1 (Th1) responses.[73] It has been shown that B7-DC fusion protein costimulated higher levels of T-cell proliferation and IFN-γ expression than CD80 costimulation.

B7-H3 Costimulatory Molecule

B7-H3 is the recently identified member of the B7 family of immune costimulatory molecules. It is a type I Ig superfamily transmembrane glycoprotein that shares approximately 24% sequence identity with CD80, 26% with CD86, 28% with B7-H1, 29% with PD-L2, and 29% with B7-H2. Human and mouse B7-H3 shares 88% amino acid identity.[3] There are two isoforms of the human B7-H3 protein, which differ in the N-terminal sequence and, most importantly, differ in the number of extracellular Ig domains. It appears that the isoform with four, rather than two, Ig domains is most widely expressed in human tissues and has been designated as B7-H3b. This form is apparently the result of a gene duplication event that occurred in humans. The mouse homologue contains two extracellular Ig domains, as is usually observed in B7 family members.[88]

B7-H3 mRNA is not detectable in peripheral blood mononuclear cells, although it is found in various normal tissues such as the heart, kidney, testis, and colon, and in several tumor cell lines. However, the expression on DCs, monocytes, macrophages, and B and T cells can be induced and upregulated by LPS, cytokines (GM-CSF, IFN-γ) exposure, or a PMA/ionomycin combination.[12,88] LPS treatment stimulates B7-H3 expression on murine macrophages, DCs, and B cells.[89] Soluble B7-H3 protein binds a putative counter-receptor on activated T cells that is distinct from CD28, CTLA-4, ICOS, and PD-1. B7-H3 costimulates proliferation of both CD4+ and CD8+ T cells, enhances the induction of cytotoxic T cells, and selectively stimulates IFN-γ production in the presence of TCR signaling.[90] B7-H3 does not bind CD28, CTLA-4, ICOS, or PD-1. A recombinant B7-H3/Ig fusion protein can bind activated T cells. This suggests that a novel putative counter-receptor is present on activated T cells. This putative receptor has not been identified as of yet. Data obtained with the recombinant fusion protein demonstrates that B7-H3 can mediate T-cell proliferation and IFN-γ production. Collectively, the data suggest that B7-H3 plays a regulatory role after initial T-cell priming.[3]

Understanding of the function of the B7 family member B7-H3 is at an earlier stage. Dong and colleagues[78] and Chen and Yi[91] review data that support stimulatory and inhibitory functions for B7-H3, discuss recent work that has identified TLT-2 (triggering receptor expressed on myeloid cells-like transcript 2) as a receptor for B7-H3, and entertain the idea that additional receptor-mediating inhibitory responses for B7-H3 may exist. There is consensus that B7-H4 functions as a coinhibitory molecule, and Dong,[78] Chen,[91] and Allison[79] and their colleagues review the inhibitory functions of B7-H4 (B7x/B7S1). Yi and Chen[91] discuss new data that B7-H4 serves as an important negative regulator of innate immunity through inhibition of neutrophil growth. Functional studies of B7S3 and BTNL2 are limited but indicate that both can inhibit T-cell activation. Mutations in the human BTNL2 gene have been identified, which are linked with sarcoidosis, and polymorphisms strongly associated with several human autoimmune diseases,[92] suggesting that BTNL2 may serve to regulate tolerance or inflammation.

B7-H4 or B7x/B7S1 Costimulatory Molecule

B7-H4 is the newest member of the B7 family and is a negative regulator of T-cell responses. Mouse and human B7-H4 share 87% of amino acid identity, suggesting that there is an important evolutionary conserved function for this molecule. Human and mouse B7-H4 mRNAs are expressed broadly in both lymphoid and nonlymphoid organs. In mice, B7-H4 is expressed constitutively on B220+ B cells and can be induced in peritoneal macrophages and DCs. B7-H4Ig binds to a receptor on activated but not naive T cells. The receptor is distinct from CTLA-4, ICOS, and PD-1, and the receptor for B7-H3. Initially, it was implicated that B7-H4 is a ligand for BTLA, but later it was found that B7-H4Ig binds to wild type but not BTLA−/− cells.[12] Therefore, the receptor for the B7-H4 remains to be identified, and hence, B7-H4 is also an orphan ligand such as B7-H3. B7-H4 has been shown to negatively regulate T-cell activation. Its expression in nonlymphoid tissues suggests that it might mediate tolerance at the tissue level. In a mouse ovarian tumor model, macrophages treated with oligonucleotides to block B7-H4 expression reduced the growth of tumors. This blockade of B7-H4 enhances the activity of tumor-infiltrating T cells, thereby shifting the balance of immunity and immune evasion in favor of tumor destruction.[93,94] Hence, inhibiting the function of B7-H4 may be an effective strategy to boost antitumor immunity.

Recently, molecular homologues of CD28 and CTLA-4 receptors have been identified. ICOS is a CD28-like costimulatory receptor with a unique B7-like ligand such as B7RP-1, B7-H2, BH-2, and GL-50. PD-1 is an inhibitory receptor, with two B7-like ligands such as B7-H2 and B7DC. Additional members of B7 and CD28 gene families have been proposed. Integration of signals through this family of costimulatory and inhibitory receptors and their ligands is critical for activation of immune responses and tolerance.

CD28 Molecule

CD28 is the most effective and well-characterized T-cell costimulatory receptor discovered to date. The genes encoding CD28 costimulatory receptor are found on chromosome 1 in mice and chromosome 2 in humans. Mouse and human CD28 molecules share approximately 68% amino acid identity. It is a transmembrane cell surface glycoprotein belonging to Ig superfamily. It has a single Ig variable-like extracellular domain in addition to its transmembrane and cytoplasmic domains. CD28 is a 44-kDa, 212-amino acid, disulfide-linked homodimer receptor that is glycosylated at five different sites. Almost all murine T cells express CD28 and bind to the costimulatory ligands CD80 and CD86 to provide a costimulatory signal to T cells.[52] It is expressed on 95% of the resting CD4+ T cells and 50% of the resting CD8+ T cells in human peripheral blood. After MHC−peptide−TCR complex formation, the ligation of B7 to CD28 provides a critical costimulatory signal to the T cell, without which T cell would become either apoptotic or anergic.[39] CD28 ligation can alter the threshold level of TCR ligation required for activation, reduce the time needed to stimulate naive cells, and enhance the magnitude of the T-cell response.[95] CD28 ligation also induces the antiapoptotic gene BCL-xL; increases cytokine secretion, particularly IL-2; enhances cell adhesion; facilitates reorganization of the T-cell plasma membrane upon binding to an APC; prevents anergy induction; and supports germinal center formation.[96−98] Generally, CD28 engagement does not have a physiological effect in the absence of TCR signaling. The importance of the role of CD28-mediated costimulation has been demonstrated in a variety of model systems *in vitro* and *in vivo*.[99−102] Most importantly, in CD28 −/− mice, there was normal development of T cells. These mice showed profound, but selective defects in their immune responses. A putative role for CD28 in the differential regulation of Th1/Th2 CD4+ T-cell subsets was first suggested by studies using clones. Blocking CD28−B7 interactions greatly reduced IL-2 production and proliferation in Th1 cells, whereas Th2 cells remained unaffected.[103] After ligation, CD28 cell surface expression is downregulated, whereas that of CTLA-4 is upregulated. B7−CD28 interactions are also important in promoting T-cell tolerance because they have a critical role in the homeostasis of CD4+ CD25+ Tregs, which play an essential role in regulating self-tolerance. Hence, CD28 costimulation is necessary for the initiation of most T-cell responses, and blockade of CD28 signaling results in ineffective T-cell activation. This has therapeutic implications in that blockade of CD28 costimulation can be profoundly immunosuppressive, which prevents induction of pathogenic T-cell responses in autoimmune disease models and allows for prolonged acceptance of allograft in models of organ transplantation.

CTLA-4 Molecule

CTLA-4 (CD152) is also a member of the Ig gene superfamily present on T cells. The genes encoding CTLA-4 are closely linked on human chromosome 2 and mouse chromosome 1. Human and mouse CTLA-4 share approximately 76% amino acid identity.[104] Although CD28 and CTLA-4 share approximately 30% amino acid identity, there has been no evidence that they can exist as a heterodimer. There is only limited conservation between the cytoplasmic domains of the two molecules. Where the CD28 receptor has at least five known N-linked glycosylation sites, CTLA-4 appears to have only one N-linked glycosylation site.[105,106] CTLA-4 can be found on the surface of both CD4+ and CD8+ T cells within 24 h after activation but has not been detected by monoclonal antibodies (mAbs) in naive T cells.[107,108] In contrast to the stimulatory effects of CD28 ligation, CTLA-4 acts as an inhibitory receptor that is vital for down-modulation of the immune response. CTLA-4 could inhibit T-cell responses first by competing with CD28 binding to CD28 ligands because CTLA-4 has a markedly higher affinity for shared ligands CD80 and CD86 compared with CD28 (K_d 0.2–0.4 μm versus 4.0 μm) and a 40–100-fold higher avidity.[109,110] Second, CTLA-4 has a unique expression pattern. Unlike CD28, CTLA-4 is not expressed constitutively on the cell surface of naive T cells.[111] It is quickly upregulated upon TCR–CD28 engagement, with the biological effects of CTLA-4 cross-linking often being observed before the detection of protein. This appears to be because the majority of CTLA-4 is sequestered inside the cell, it traffics to the site of T cell–APC interaction and is quickly endocytosed into clathrin-coated pits.[112,113] The distinct affinities of CD28 and CTLA-4 for B7 ligands have led to the proposal of a model in which B7–CD28 and B7–CTLA-4 interactions predominate at distinct stages of an immune response. When B7 ligands are expressed at low levels on resting T cell, B7 molecules may preferentially be engaged by a high-affinity inhibitory receptor CTLA-4. When B7 ligands are upregulated and expressed at higher levels, the predominant interactions could be between CD28 and B7, enhancing T-cell proliferation and differentiation. Once CTLA-4 expression is upregulated following T-cell activation, the inhibitory B7-CTLA-4 interaction could once again predominate, leading to termination of T-cell activation.[114]

ICOS MOLECULE

ICOS is a costimulatory receptor homologous to CD28 and CTLA-4 costimulatory receptors found on activated, but not resting T cells. Mouse ICOS is a 47–57-kDa, disulfide-linked, N-glycosylated homodimer, whereas human ICOS is a 55–60-kDa, disulfide-linked, glycosylated homodimer found on activated T cells. ICOS gene is closely linked to the genes for CTLA-4 and CD28 on human chromosomes 2q23 and mouse chromosome 1. ICOS shares approximately 30–40% sequence similarity with CD28 and CTLA-4. The ICOS gene maps to the CD28/CTLA-4 locus, suggesting that these arose by gene duplication.[115,116] ICOS contains several conserved motifs found in CD28, including the extracellular Ig-V-like domain and the YXXM motif in the cytoplasmic tail.[97,117] However, ICOS does not have a conserved MYPPPY motif, which is necessary for CD28 and CTLA-4 binding to CD80/CD86 ligands.[24] ICOS is not constitutively expressed on naive T cells but is induced on CD4+ and CD8+ T cells following cell activation.[115–117] Triggering of ICOS significantly costimulates the proliferation of T cells but fails to substitute for CD28 ligation in the induction of IL-2 secretion. ICOS costimulation is equivalent to that mediated by CD28 for the production of the cytokines IL-4, IL-5, IFN-γ, and TNF-α, but shows greater induction of IL-10. ICOS costimulation also enhances CD40 ligand expression that leads to an increased polyclonal Ab secretion in T- and B-cell cocultures.[118] This indicates that the ICOS:ICOS-L pathway provides key positive signals that promote T-cell activation, differentiation, and effector responses and T-cell-dependent B-cell responses. Both CD28 and ICOS signaling upregulate Th1 as well as Th2 cytokines;[117,119] however, ICOS does not upregulate IL-2 production. Thus, ICOS stimulates T-cell effector functions but not T-cell expansion. The role of ICOS in stimulating IL-10 production may contribute to its role in regulating Treg, T-cell tolerance, and autoimmunity.[120,121] The function of ICOS during *in vivo* immune responses appears to depend on timing/stage of immune response as well as microenvironment because ICOS-L can be expressed on endothelial and epithelial cells as well as on professional APCs. Mutations in the ICOS gene result in impaired B-cell responses in both mice and humans.[118,122,123] Mice deficient in ICOS are resistant to collagen-induced arthritis,[124] and antibody blockade of ICOS-L also reduced disease severity in this model. This is consistent with the requirement of ICOS/ICOS-L signaling for productive B-cell responses, as collagen-induced arthritis is dependent on the development of pathogenic autoantibodies to collagen. Similarly, blockade of ICOS-L in NZB/NZW F1 mice, which spontaneously develop a lupus-like autoimmune syndrome characterized by autoantibodies to nuclear antigens, resulted in a delay in development of clinical signs of lupus nephritis. By contrast, ICOS-deficient mice were more susceptible to experimental autoimmune encephalomyelitis (EAE), a T-cell-mediated model of multiple sclerosis, and blockade of ICOS can either exacerbate or ameliorate EAE.[125] Blockade of ICOS in a diabetes model also augmented disease, and a role for ICOS in maintenance of regulatory T-cell function was proposed as a mechanism for this exacerbation.[120] These preclinical studies in arthritis and lupus models suggest that blockade of the ICOS pathway may be of greatest benefit in inflammatory or autoimmune diseases with a significant pathogenic B-cell component.

The ICOS/ICOS ligand pathway has critical roles in stimulating effector T-cell responses and T-dependent B-cell responses, and regulating T-cell tolerance.[78] Although CD28 and ICOS have overlapping functions in early T-cell activation, ICOS has emerged as an important receptor in the immune system to fine-tune T-cell effector functions. In addition, ICOS is important for generation of chemokine (CXC motif) receptor 5 (CXCR5)+ follicular helper T cells (TFH), a unique T-cell subset that regulates germinal center reactions and humoral immunity. Recent studies in ICOS −/− mice indicate that ICOS can regulate IL-21 production, which in turn regulates the expansion of T-helper type-17 (Th17) cells and TFH. ICOS also plays an important role in controlling IL-10-producing Tregs and peripheral T-cell tolerance. Grimbacher and colleagues[126] review the discovery of mutations in ICOS in patients with common variable immunodeficiency. Human ICOS deficiency leads to defective IL-10 and IL-17 production, impaired germinal center-affinity maturation, and isotype class switching, which result in profound hypogammaglobulinemia.

The Programmed Death-1

PD-1 is a 50–55-kDa, type I transmembrane receptor related to CD28 and CTLA-4, but it lacks the membrane proximal cysteine that allows these molecules to homodimerize, and hence, PD-1 is monomeric in nature.[72] PD-1 was identified in a T-cell line undergoing activation-induced cell death.[83,127] It lacks the MYPPPY motif, a sequence critical for CTLA-4 and CD28 binding to CD80 and CD86. PD-1 is constitutively expressed on a subset of CD4–CD8 thymocytes, immature B cells, and some peripheral T cells, and its expression can be induced on T cells, B cells, monocytes, and myeloid cells following activation.[128–131] The ligands of PD-1 are the B7 family members PD-L1 (B7-H1) and PD-L2 (B7-DC).[71,72,132] Resting B cells, monocytes, and DCs do not express either PD-L1 or PD-L2. The overall distribution of PD-L1 and PD-L2 transcript is similar in human and murine tissues, with a high level of expression in placenta, a low expression level in the spleen, lymph nodes, and thymus, and the absence of expression in brain tissue.[72,132] Expression of PD-L1 and PD-L2 in both lymphoid and nonlymphoid tissues suggests that the PD-L1/PD-L2 pathway may modulate immune responses in the secondary lymphoid organs as well as in peripheral sites. PD-1 coligation with the TCR complex that is induced by PD-1/PD-1 ligand interaction is also shown to inhibit proliferation and cytokine production of both CD4+ and CD8+ T cells. Costimulation with soluble anti-CD28 mAb can overcome PD-1-mediated inhibition by augmenting IL-2 production. The presence of ligands of PD-1, that is, PD-L1 and PD-L2 on parenchymal cells of the heart, lung, and kidney, suggests that the PD-1–PD-L system could provide unique negative signaling to help prevent autoimmune diseases.[130]

PD-1:PD-L1/PD-L2 has critical roles in regulating T-cell activation and tolerance. PD-1 and CTLA-4 have important nonredundant inhibitory functions. CTLA-4 appears to have a more central role in the lymphoid organs, whereas PD-1 has an important role in regulating inflammatory responses in peripheral tissues. PD-1, a receptor for PD-L1 and PD-L2, functions as a negative regulator of immune responses.[133] PD-L1 and PD-L2 are expressed in nonlymphoid cells and tissues in both normal and inflammatory conditions, suggesting that these ligands regulate immune responses in nonimmune peripheral sites. PD-1-deficient mice develop autoimmune disorders, including lupus-like arthritis in the C57BL/6 background and dilated cardiomyopathy in Balb/c mice,[130] which emphasizes the negative regulatory function of PD-1. Administration of antagonistic anti-PD-1 antibodies in EAE in the NOD model of type I diabetes and in a model of graft versus host disease results in accelerated and more severe disease development.[77,134] In all cases, worsening of disease was associated with increased IFN-γ production, suggesting that the PD-1/PD-L pathway is a negative regulator of this cytokine *in vivo*. PD-1 blockade in tumor models enhances effector T-cell function and impairs metastasis in B16 melanoma and CT26 colon cancer models.[135] Thus, development of agonistic and antagonistic anti-PD-1 antibodies is an approach for the treatment of autoimmune disorders and cancer, respectively. Although antagonistic antibodies have been identified for PD-1, agonistic antibodies for coinhibitory receptors such as PD-1 and CTLA-4 have yet to be reported.

CD40 Costimulatory Molecule

CD40 is an approximately 50-kDa, type I transmembrane glycoprotein belonging to the TNFR superfamily. It is expressed on a variety of cells, including B cells, follicular DCs, activated monocytes, macrophages, endothelial cells, vascular smooth muscle cells, and several tumor cell lines.[136–139] Recent studies have indicated that CD40–CD154 interaction can upregulate costimulatory molecules, activate APCs, and influence T-cell priming and T-cell-mediated effector functions. This interaction can activate macrophages, natural killer (NK) cells, and endothelial cells, as well as participate in the pathogenic processing of chronic inflammatory diseases, such as autoimmune diabetes, graft rejection, atherosclerosis, and cancer.[140,141] During a normal T-cell response, CD40 on DC is engaged by CD40L, which is transiently expressed on activated CD4+ T cells. CD40 molecules are therefore cross-linked, which induces DC maturation and enables them to efficiently present Ag to T cells.[142] CD40L–CD40 interaction is of great significance in induction of immune responses because mice and humans that lack CD40 or CD40L (CD154) genes have reduced Ab production and Ig class switching and are unable to mount effective responses against infectious agents. However, novel and recent data provide ample evidence that the functions of the CD40 molecule may extend well beyond their role in humoral immune response. CD40 signaling in macrophages induces the activity against an intracellular pathogen independently of IFN-γ and reactive nitrogen intermediates. In BCG-infected DCs, it was shown that CD40 stimulation not only promotes their ability to secrete IL-12 but increases the release of other inflammatory mediators such as IL-1α, IL-1β, and IL-6.[143] This shows that CD40 stimulation may potentiate the development of inflammatory responses, which play a critical role in antimycobacterial immunity.

CD40L/CD154 Costimulatory Molecule

CD40 ligand (CD40L), also known as CD154, TNFSF5, TRAP, or gp39, is a 260-amino acid, type II transmembrane glycoprotein belonging to the TNF superfamily. Murine CD40L consists of a 22-amino acid cytoplasmic domain, a 24-amino acid transmembrane domain, and 214-amino acid extracellular domains bearing a single glycosylation site. CD40L is expressed predominantly on activated CD4 + T lymphocytes and some other types of cells such as NK cells, mast cells, basophils, and eosinophils.[138,144,145] Murine CD40L shares 78% amino acid sequence identity with human CD40L. Both forms of CD40L, that is, membrane bound and soluble, induce similar effects on B cells. Although all monomeric, dimeric, and trimeric forms of soluble CD40L can bind to CD40, the soluble trimeric form of CD40L has the most potent biological activity through oligomerization of cell surface CD40, a common feature of TNFR family members. Expression of CD154 was detectable 4 h after activation, peaked between 6 and 8 h, and returned to near resting levels between 24 and 48 h. The CD154–CD40 interaction regulates the activation of APCs by upregulating the expression of other costimulatory molecules and by inducing the production of cytokines. Recent studies have suggested that CD40–CD154 interactions regulate the production of IL-12 by DCs and macrophages. IL-12 is required for the development of Th1 type of response. Further, the role of anti-CD154 Ab in the prevention of Th1-cell-mediated autoimmune diseases is also reported.[146] CD40L mediates a range of activities on B cells, including induction of activation-associated surface antigen, entry into cell cycle, isotype switching, Ig secretion, and memory generation. CD40–CD40L interaction also plays important roles in monocyte activation and DC maturation.

PATHWAYS IN THE TNFR/TNF FAMILY

TNFR family members can recruit TNFR-associated factor (TRAF) adapter proteins and activate the nuclear factor κ-B signaling pathway, making them fundamentally distinct from costimulators such as CD28 or ICOS. CD40 and its ligand, CD154, were the first costimulatory molecules to be identified as members of the TNFR/TNF superfamily and are crucial for the functions of B cells and DCs. CD40 signals into DCs and B cells as well as other cell types, including tumor cells. Noelle and colleagues[147] discuss downstream signaling pathways initiated by CD40 through TRAF proteins and the essential functions of CD4–CD40L interactions in controlling humoral, cellular, and tumor immunity.[79]

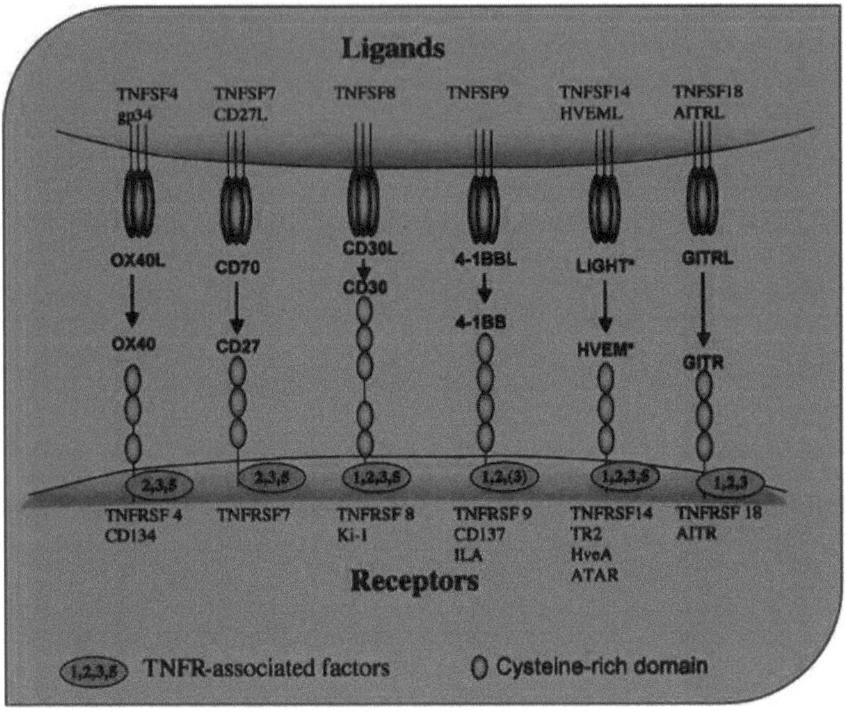

FIGURE 1.6 **Summary of TNFR/TNF family ligands and their receptors.** The names of receptors and ligands are indicated, as well as a brief summary of predominant expression patterns for each. The TNFR family costimulatory members such as OX40, CD27, CD30, 4-IBB, HVEM, and GITR are type I transmembrane proteins characterized by cysteine-rich motifs in their extracellular domains. The ligands for the costimulatory TNFR family members contain TRAF2-binding motifs consisting of the major conserved motif (P/S/A/T)x (Q/E)E or the minor motif PxQxxD. TRAF trimers are recruited to TNFRs upon receptor ligation. Remember TRAF3 association is observed with human but not mouse 4-IBB.

Studies of the CD27/CD70, CD30/CD30L, OX40/OX40L, 4-1BB/4-1BBL, glucocorticoid-induced TNF receptor (GITR)/GITR ligand, and HVEM/lymphotoxin-like have revealed that these molecules exhibit inducible expression, compete with herpes simplex virus glycoprotein D for HVEM, which is a receptor expressed by T lymphocytes (LIGHT) pathways, and indicate that these TNFR/TNF family members can provide important costimulatory signals. With the exception of CD27, which is constitutively expressed on naive T cells, the other TNFRs are expressed only upon T-cell activation. In addition, memory T cells and Tregs constitutively express certain family members. All the members of TNFR/TNF costimulatory molecules are depicted in Figures 1.2 and 1.6. These expression patterns have suggested that the TNFR/TNF family may be important in controlling effector and memory responses.

Recent work indicates that OX40/OX40L and 4-1BB/4-1BBL interactions have key roles in regulating the balance between effector and Treg responses. As reviewed by Croft et al.,[148] OX40 promotes effector T-cell expansion and survival, as well as the generation, reactivation, and maintenance of memory T cells. OX40 also blocks natural Treg activity and antagonizes the generation of inducible Tregs. Thus, OX40 can promote effector and memory T-cell responses directly by stimulating these cells and indirectly by inhibiting Tregs. OX40 has become an attractive therapeutic target; OX40 blockade can attenuate autoimmunity and inflammation, whereas stimulating OX40 can enhance antitumor immunity. As reviewed by Watts and colleagues,[149] the major role of 4-1BB is for survival of activated and memory T cells, with preferential effects on CD8+ T cells.

However, when other costimulatory signals are limiting, 4-1BB signals can cooperate with TCR-induced signals to enhance proliferation and development of effector function, perhaps by allowing T cells to survive through rounds of division. In addition, 4-1BB can exert immunosuppressive effects in some settings. Agonistic anti-4-1BB mAbs can not only expand CD8+ T cells but also inhibit humoral immunity and ameliorate autoimmunity. 4-1BB is expressed on Tregs, and ligation of 4-1BB on Tregs can enhance their expansion and possibly their suppressive function. 4-1BB also can induce IFN-c and CD8+ T-cell-dependent suppression. Further work is needed to understand how 4-1BB controls the balance between effector and regulatory cell function. This is a clinically relevant issue, as agonistic anti-4-1BB mAbs are in clinical trials.

The CD27/CD70 pathway is also important for generation of effector and memory T-cell responses and promotes proliferation and survival of activated T cells.[150] The potency of costimulation by CD27/CD70 interactions is illustrated by the development of immunopathology in transgenic mice that constitutively express CD70 or CD27. These findings give impetus to studies examining the impact of CD70/CD27 interactions during chronic antigen stimulation, such as chronic virus infection and autoimmunity. HVEM sits at a pivot point, connecting the TNFR and Ig superfamilies with a complicated molecular cross talk among its receptors: LIGHT, LTa, CD160, and BTLA. LIGHT can influence T-cell activation both directly and indirectly by engaging receptors expressed on T cells and other cell types. The binding of LIGHT or LTa to HVEM delivers a costimulatory signal,[151] whereas the binding of BTLA or CD160 to HVEM delivers a coinhibitory signal.[152] Thus, HVEM is a bidirectional switch regulating T-cell activation in a costimulatory or coinhibitory fashion depending upon which ligand is engaged. LIGHT or LTa1b2 binding to lymphotoxin-bR, which is expressed by DCs and stromal cells in lymph nodes and other tissues, induces chemokine production by stromal cells resulting in the development of lymphoid structures and DC expansion. Thus, LIGHT has the capacity to serve as both a costimulatory ligand for T cells and a stromal activator to induce chemokine production and lymphoid recruitment. For these reasons, it has become an attractive target for immunotherapy, and methods for intratumoral delivery of LIGHT are being studied. Freeman and Cai[152] discuss the inhibitory consequences of HVEM interactions with CD160 and BTLA, and provide insight into how engagement of HVEM can lead to stimulatory or inhibitory outcomes. HVEM has distinct domains for binding its stimulatory ligand LIGHT and its coinhibitory ligands CD160 and BTLA. Therapies targeting the cysteine-rich domain-1 of HVEM to block BTLA and CD160 binding are being developed to enhance immune responses and vaccination.

4-1BB/4-1BBL

4-1BB (CD137) is another costimulatory receptor expressed on activated T cells (CD4+, CD8+, and NKT), activated NK cells, DCs, eosinophils, and mast cells. 4-1BB is a member of the TNFR superfamily that is inducibly expressed on T cells following stimulation through the TCR complex.[153–155] The ligand of 4-1BB (4-1BBL or CD137L), a member of the TNF family, is expressed on activated macrophages, DCs, and B cells.[156,157] When coupled to a strong signal through the TCR, engagement of 4-1BB can induce IL-2 production independently of CD28 ligation.[158] Early studies also demonstrated that ligation of 4-1BB by either cell surface 4-1BBL or specific antibodies provides a costimulatory signal particularly to CD8+ T cells, enhancing proliferation, cytokine production, and particularly survival.[159–161] More recent data point to the role of 4-1BB engagement in augmenting rather than initiating T-cell response and in sustaining effector functions.[162] *In vivo*, the first use of anti-4-1BB antibodies as an antitumor therapy was reported by Melero et al.,[163] who demonstrated the therapeutic potential of this strategy to promote rejection of P815 mastocytoma and Ag104A sarcoma tumors.[163] Further studies using either 4-1BB agonistic antibodies or gene-modified tumor cells expressing 4-1BBL confirmed their efficacy to expand tumor-reactive T cells, suppress tumor growth, and in some cases induce regression of preestablished tumor in different tumor models.[164–166] CD8+ T cells constitute the main effector subset involved in tumor rejection following treatment by 4-1BB mAb because CD4+ T cells, NK, and NKT cells were not required for the antitumor effects.[167] Interestingly, several reports in rodent models have shown synergistic effects of agonistic anti-4-1BB mAb in combination with anti-TNF-related apoptosis-inducing ligand and CD40 mAbs,[168] with intratumoral introduction of the IL-12 gene,[169] or with chemotherapy or radiotherapy.[170,171] These observations provide a guide for developing combination studies in the clinic. An unusual feature of anti-4-1BB mAb therapy is the almost paradoxical observation that, although improved immunity is seen in tumor settings, diminished pathology has been observed in autoimmune models. Fu and colleagues[172] showed that same agonist antibody to 4-1BB used to promote antitumor immunity resulted in ameliorating both the incidence and the severity of EAE. Many other studies have confirmed the beneficial effects of anti-4-1BB mAB in various autoimmune disease models, including rheumatoid arthritis, EAE, and systemic lupus erythematosis.[173] In a transplantation model, anti-4-1BB also was shown to inhibit rejection of intestinal allografts in mice.[174] Although a complete understanding of these differential effects is lacking, the promotion of Tregs development and activity is believed to play a role.[175] Additional potential explanations for immune suppression in some settings include the apparent ability to delete CD4+ T cells, retard B-cell function, and upregulate indoleamine-2,3-dioxygenase and IFN-γ.[166,173] Together these results suggest that the possibility of both immune-potentiating and immune-suppressive effects of 4-1BB engagement should be taken into consideration and monitored in clinical/translational studies in patients. A human antihuman 4-1BB mAB (BMS-663513) is currently under investigation by Bristol-Myers Squibb in a number of phase I and II trials in patients with metastatic or locally advanced solid tumors.[165,176]

OX40/OX40L

OX40, also known as CD134, is another costimulatory molecule of the TNFR superfamily that was identified in 1987[177] and that is expressed mainly on activated CD4+ but also CD8+ T cells. Its ligand OX40L is mainly expressed on professional APCs such as DCs, B cells, and macrophages, particularly after stimulation with TLR ligands or CD40L.[178–180] OX40L also has been observed on T cells and endothelial cells.[181,182] OX40 functions as a late costimulatory receptor and artificial engagement by OX40L stimulates proliferation, cytokine secretion, and survival of T cells, in part by increasing the expression of antiapoptotic molecules of the Bcl-2 family.[183] Several systems have shown that OX40 expression is not dependent on CD28 but that CD28 can augment the level of OX40 expression,[183,184] suggesting that the two molecules cooperate in a sequential manner. Therefore, a model was proposed whereby OX40 signals act in a temporal manner after CD28 signals, supporting continued survival and proliferation of effector.[185] Interestingly, recent data have also shown that OX40 ligation may suppress the function and generation of CD4+ Foxp3+ Tregs.[186,187] *In vivo*, OX40L transduction of tumor cells and engagement of OX40 by an agonist Ab or an OX40-Ig chimeric protein has been shown to increase tumor immunity against different murine tumor models, including B16 melanoma and hepatic colon metastases.[164] Interestingly, it was shown that agonistic anti-OX40 mAb given in combination with agonistic anti-4-1BB and intratumoral injection of an adenovirus expressing IL-12 showed a synergistic effect to induce long-term survival of mice bearing large chemically induced colon carcinoma.[188]

The first phase I clinical trial using a murine antihuman OX40 mAb has been initiated in patients with advanced cancer. This trial is essentially a proof of concept, as neutralizing human antimouse antibodies are expected to be limiting, and a humanized or fully human antibody should be pursued. A humanized OX40 agonist was recently developed that could be tested in future clinical studies.[189]

HVEM/LIGHT

HVEM is another member of the TNFR superfamily but in contrast to others is expressed by both resting and activated T cells. The principal ligand for HVEM is the TNF superfamily member 14 (LIGHT/TNFSF14), and ligation by LIGHT acts as a positive costimulatory signal. LIGHT expression is induced on activated T cells themselves, but also by NK cells, monocytes, and DCs.[164] In addition to its binding to HVEM, LIGHT also can bind the LT-β receptor, which can be expressed by stromal cell populations in lymph nodes and other tissues, including the tumor microenvironment. Evidence supporting the costimulatory effect of LIGHT came from experiments, showing that blocking of LIGHT inhibits early T-cell proliferation and cytokine secretion in an allogeneic mixed lymphocyte reaction.[190–192] However, *in vivo* experiments suggest that a major impact of LIGHT is through induction of chemokine production by stromal cells that results in recruitment of T cells and DCs, leading to the generation of lymph node-like structures. Transgenic mice expressing LIGHT driven by the CD2 promoter show an increased number of activated T cells, higher proportions of effector and memory T cells, and signs of autoimmunity.[193,194] Transgenic mice expressing LIGHT driven by the rat insulin promoter develop autoimmune diabetes mellitus, with pancreatic islets showing a lymph node-like morphology.[195] LIGHT knockout mice also have been generated. These mice show defective expansion of superantigen-reactive CD8+ T cells and defective CTL generation after peptide priming *in vivo*,[196,197] which supports a positive immunoregulatory role.

The attractive properties of LIGHT to serve as both a costimulatory ligand for T cells and a stromal cell activator to induce chemokine production and lymphoid recruitment made it attractive to consider for intratumoral application. Introduction of a LIGHT cDNA in P815 tumor cells induced regression of established tumors with the maximal therapeutic effect requiring both CD4+ and CD8+ T cells. The antitumor effect of LIGHT was shown to be CD28 independent in this model.[198] Introduction of LIGHT in Ag104 sarcoma cells expressing the alloantigen Ld has been shown to promote direct antigen presentation, *in vivo* chemokine production, T-cell recruitment, and tumor rejection.[199] LIGHT also appears to promote recruitment of NK cells into tumor sites, which may participate in a bridge to adaptive immunity.[200] There is growing interest to bring therapies involving LIGHT forward into the clinic. As the maximal impact is expected to be at the level of altering the tumor microenvironment, strategies for intratumoral targeting would be desirable. Along these lines, an adenoviral vector encoding LIGHT injected intratumorally was shown to promote T-cell recruitment, control of the injected tumor, and elimination of noninjected metastases in mice.[201] Another potential strategy for clinical translation would be *in vivo* electroporation directly into tumor metastases, as has recently been reported using an IL-12 cDNA in patients with melanoma.[202]

ICOS, GITR, and CD27/CD70

Other receptors that have been described as having positive costimulatory functions and could be attractive to consider for augmenting antitumor immunity include ICOS, a member of the B7 family, and GITR, and CD27, members of the TNFR superfamily. ICOS and GITR are mainly expressed by activated CD4+ and CD8+ T cells but constitutive expression by CD25+ CD4+ Foxp3+ Tregs has also been demonstrated.[203] CD27 is expressed on naive CD4+ and CD8+ T cells, and also by NK cells. The ligands for these receptors, GITR ligand (GITRL), CD27 ligand (CD70), and ICOS ligand (B7h or LICOS), are predominantly expressed on populations of APCs (B cells, macrophages, and DCs).[164,185] Interestingly, recent studies have confirmed the critical role for CD70 expression on activated DCs to promote optimal T-cell activation *in vivo*. Transgenic expression of CD70 on DCs enabled T-cell priming *in vivo* in the absence of adjuvant,[204] which argues that it is perhaps one of the most critical of the costimulatory ligands for adaptive immunity. Animal models targeting these additional costimulatory pathways in the tumor context are under evaluation but earlier in their development. B7h expression on tumor cells was demonstrated to promote regression in the Sa1/N fibrosarcoma and J558 plasmocytoma models via a CD8-dependent mechanism.[205,206] Like for B7-1 and B7-2, this strategy was ineffective when weakly immunogenic tumors were investigated.[207] Other studies have shown that CD27/CD70 can enhance tumor rejection, with CD70 transfection enhancing both NK-dependent and T-cell-dependent mechanisms of tumor elimination.[208–210] The administration of an anti-GITR agonistic antibody (clone DTA-1) also has been shown to induce the rejection of several murine syngeneic tumors through an IFN-γ-dependent mechanism and without obvious autoimmune manifestations.[211,212] Anti-GITR mAb promoted the activation of effector CD4+ and CD8+ T cells, and altered the intratumoral ratio of Tregs/T effectors. More recently, observations made by Zhou et al.[213] have suggested that the antitumor effects of anti-GITR antibody were mainly driven by its positive costimulatory signal in effector CD4+ T cells rather than by its possible effect to abrogate the suppressive functions of Tregs.

SUMMARY

The modern concept of costimulation has shed new light on the mechanisms involved in the regulation of T-cell activation and differentiation. The identification of several new costimulatory molecules and their receptors supports the idea of fine-tuning T-cell functions via a multitude of simultaneously or consecutively expressed T-cell molecules. The joint action of various costimulatory receptors on T cells adds not only to the complexity of this mechanism but also to the availability of ligands on different cell types and in different organs. The identification of the orphan ligands B7 homologues 3 and 4 shows that there may be more costimulatory molecules to be identified. Table 1.3 categorizes the currently known costimulatory molecules that were introduced in this chapter according to functional aspects. With a growing insight into costimulatory mechanisms, a vast array of potential targets for the modulation and redirection of T-cell responses becomes available. Accordingly, many experimental studies using animal models have explored the efficacy of targeting costimulatory molecules for the inhibition, or even prevention of, the development of the different diseases.

Among these, allergen-induced sensitization and airway disease are of the most interest, because they are clearly mediated by misled T-cell responses against common environmental antigens. Most of the aforementioned molecules have been studied in murine models of allergic airway inflammation. Chapter 2 will give, therefore, an overview on these studies in murine models as well as discuss preliminary data in the human system. Finally, Chapter 3 will discuss the utilization and feasibility of costimulatory molecules for novel treatment strategies of allergic airway disease.

In sum, our understanding of costimulation has evolved significantly from the two-signal model for T-cell activation. There are both stimulatory and inhibitory second signals, and the inhibitory signals play important roles in the induction and maintenance of T-cell tolerance. In addition, we now realize that costimulatory pathways not only regulate the initial activation of naive T cells but also control effector, memory, and Tregs. These pathways may control tolerance by preventing effector T-cell responses and by promoting/maintaining Tregs. Costimulatory and coinhibitory molecules can be expressed on nonhematopoietic cells as well as professional APCs, and expression on parenchymal cells may regulate T-cell responses in specific microenvironments. Although costimulatory molecules are generally viewed through their effects on T cells, many receptor ligand interactions may lead to bidirectional signaling with important consequences for the non-T-cell partner. Thus, molecular definition of T-cell costimulatory pathways is providing insights into the exquisite regulation of T-cell activation and tolerance. Cosignaling pathways are major regulators of the critical balance between tolerance and immune responses to pathogens that are effective with an acceptable level of tissue damage. Therefore, understanding the relationships between these costimulatory ligands and their receptors in different immune effector pathways will surely help us in improving immunomodulatory therapeutics, development of improved vaccines, and avoidance of unintended tissue injury.

REFERENCES

1. Mueller DL, Jenkins MK, Schwartz RH. Clonal expansion versus functional clonal inactivation: a costimulatory signalling pathway determines the outcome of T cell antigen receptor occupancy. *Annu Rev Immunol* 1989;**7**:445–80.
2. Bretscher P, Cohn M. A theory of self-nonself discrimination. *Science* 1970;**169**:1042–9.
3. Sharpe AH, Freeman GJ. The B7-CD28 superfamily. *Nat Rev Immunol* 2002;**2**:116–26.
4. Janeway Jr. CA. The priming of helper T cells. *Semin Immunol* 1989;**1**(1):13–20.
5. Jenkins MK. The ups and downs of T cell costimulation. *Immunity* 1994;**1**:443–6.
6. Janeway Jr. CA, Bottomly K. Signals and signs for lymphocyte responses. *Cell* 1994; **76**:275–85.
7. Dubey C, Croft M, Swain SL. Costimulatory requirements of naive CD4+ T cells. ICAM-1 or B7-1 can costimulate naive CD4 T cell activation but both are required for optimum response. *J Immunol* 1995;**155**:45–57.
8. Dubey C, Croft M, Swain SL. Naive and effector CD4 T cells differ in their requirements for T cell receptor versus costimulatory signals. *J Immunol* 1996;**157**:3280–9.
9. Bromley SK, Iaboni A, Davis SJ, Whitty A, Green JM, et al. The immunological synapse and CD28–CD80 interactions. *Nat Immunol* 2001;**2**:1159–66.
10. Carreno BM, Collins M. The B7 family of ligands and its receptors: new pathways for costimulation and inhibition of immune responses. *Annu Rev Immunol* 2002;**20**:29–53.
11. Collins M, Ling V, Carreno BM. The B7 family of immune-regulatory ligands. *Genome Biol* 2005;**6**:223.
12. Greenwald RJ, Freeman GJ, Sharpe AH. The B7 family revisited. *Annu Rev Immunol* 2005; **23**:515–48.
13. Greenwald RJ, Latchman YE, Sharpe AH. Negative co-receptors on lymphocytes. *Curr Opin Immunol* 2002;**14**:391–6.
14. Schwartz RH. A cell culture model for T lymphocyte clonal anergy. *Science* 1990; **248**:1349–56.
15. Kroczek RA, Mages HW, Hutloff A. Emerging paradigms of T-cell co-stimulation. *Curr Opin Immunol* 2004;**16**:321–7.
16. Jenkins MK, Pardoll DM, Mizuguchi J, Chused TM, Schwartz RH. Molecular events in the induction of a nonresponsive state in interleukin 2-producing helper T-lymphocyte clones. *Proc Natl Acad Sci USA* 1987;**84**:5409–13.
17. Jenkins MK, Schwartz RH. Antigen presentation by chemically modified splenocytes induces antigen-specific T cell unresponsiveness *in vitro* and *in vivo*. *J Exp Med* 1987; **165**:302–19.
18. Mueller DL. Do tolerant T cells exist? *Nature* 1989;**339**:513–14.
19. Mueller DL, Jenkins MK, Schwartz RH. An accessory cell-derived costimulatory signal acts independently of protein kinase C activation to allow T cell proliferation and prevent the induction of unresponsiveness. *J Immunol* 1989;**142**:2617–28.
20. Harding FA, McArthur JG, Gross JA, Raulet DH, Allison JP. CD28-mediated signalling co-stimulates murine T cells and prevents induction of anergy in T-cell clones. *Nature* 1992;**356**:607–9.
21. Rietz C, Chen L. New B7 family members with positive and negative costimulatory function. *Am J Transplant* 2004;**4**:8–14.
22. Sharpe AH, Abbas AK. T-cell costimulation—biology, therapeutic potential, and challenges. *N Engl J Med* 2006;**355**:973–5.

23. Greene JL, Leytze GM, Emswiler J, Peach R, Bajorath J, et al. Covalent dimerization of CD28/CTLA-4 and oligomerization of CD80/CD86 regulate T cell costimulatory interactions. *J Biol Chem* 1996;**271**:6762–71.
24. Greene JL, Leytze GM, Emswiler J, Peach R, Bajorath J, et al. Complementarity determining region 1[CDR1]-and CDR3-analogous regions in CTLA-4 and CD28 determine the binding to B7-1. *J Exp Med* 1994;**180**:2049–58.
25. Harper K, Balzano C, Rouvier E, Mattéi MG, Luciani MF, Golstein P. CTLA-4 and CD28 activated lymphocyte molecules are closely related in both mouse and human as to sequence, message expression, gene structure, and chromosomal location. *J Immunol* 1991;**147**:1037–44.
26. Ling V, Wu PW, Finnerty HF, Agostino MJ, Graham JR, Chen S, et al. Assembly and annotation of human chromosome 2q33 sequence containing the CD28, CTLA4, and ICOS gene cluster: analysis by computational, comparative, and microarray approaches. *Genomics* 2001;**78**:155–68.
27. Evans EJ, Esnouf RM, Manso-Sancho R, Gilbert RJ, James JR, Yu C, et al. Crystal structure of a soluble CD28–Fab complex. *Nat Immunol* 2005;**6**:271–9.
28. Bradshaw JD, Lu P, Leytze G, Rodgers J, Schieven GL, Bennett KL, et al. Interaction of the cytoplasmic tail of CTLA-4 [CD152] with a clathrin-associated protein is negatively regulated by tyrosine phosphorylation. *Biochemistry* 1997;**36**:15975–82.
29. Schneider H, Martin M, Agarraberes FA, Yin L, Rapoport I, Kirchhausen T, et al. Cytolytic T lymphocyte-associated antigen-4 and the TCR zeta/CD3 complex, but not CD28, interact with clathrin adaptor complexes AP-1 and AP-2. *J Immunol* 1999;**163**:1868–79.
30. Egen JG, Allison JP. Cytotoxic T lymphocyte antigen-4 accumulation in the immunological synapse is regulated by TCR signal strength. *Immunity* 2002;**16**:23–35.
31. Linsley PS1, Brady W, Grosmaire L, Aruffo A, Damle NK, Ledbetter JA. Binding of the B cell activation antigen B7 to CD28 costimulates T cell proliferation and interleukin 2 mRNA accumulation. *J Exp Med* 1991;**173**:721–30.
32. Thompson CB, Lindsten T, Ledbetter JA, Kunkel SL, Young HA, Emerson SG, et al. CD28 activation pathway regulates the production of multiple T-cell-derived lymphokines/cytokines. *Proc Natl Acad Sci USA* 1989;**86**:1333–7.
33. Tivol EA, Borriello F, Schweitzer NA, Lynch WP, Bluestone JA, et al. Loss of CTLA-4 leads to massive lymphoproliferation and fatal multiorgan tissue destruction, revealing a critical negative regulatory role of CTLA-4. *Immunity* 1995;**3**:541–7.
34. Walunas TL, Lenschow DJ, Bakker CY, Linsley PS, Freeman GJ, Green JM, et al. CTLA-4 can function as a negative regulator of T cell activation. *Immunity* 1994;**1**:405–13.
35. Waterhouse P, Penninger JM, Timms E, Wakeham A, Shahinian A, Lee KP, et al. Lymphoproliferative disorders with early lethality in mice deficient in CTLA-4. *Science* 1995;**270**:985–8.
36. Hansen JD, Pasquier LD, Lefranc MP, Lopez V, Benmansour A, Boudinot P. The B7 family of immunoregulatory receptors: a comparative and evolutionary perspective. *Mol Immunol* 2009;**46**:457–72.
37. Zang X, Allison JP. The B7 family and cancer therapy: costimulation and coinhibition. *Clin Cancer Res* 2007;**13**:5271–9.
38. Abbas AK, Sharpe AH. T-cell stimulation: an abundance of B7s. *Nat Med* 1999;**5**:1345–6.
39. Alegre ML, Frauwirth KA, Thompson CB. T-cell regulation by CD28 and CTLA-4. *Nat Rev Immunol* 2001;**1**:220–8.

40. Yokochi T, Holly RD, Clark EA. B lymphoblast antigen (BB-1) expressed on Epstein–Barr virus-activated B cell blasts, B lymphoblastoid cell lines, and Burkitt's lymphomas. *J Immunol* 1982;**128**:823–7.
41. Linsley PS, Clark EA, Ledbetter JA. T-cell antigen CD28 mediates adhesion with B cells by interacting with activation antigen B7/BB-1. *Proc Natl Acad Sci USA* 1990;**87**:5031–5.
42. Linsley PS, Peach R, Gladstone P, Bajorath J. Extending the B7 (CD80) gene family. *Protein Sci* 1994;**3**:1341–3.
43. Freeman GJ, Freedman AS, Segil JM, Lee G, Whitman JF, Nadler LM. B7, a new member of the Ig superfamily with unique expression on activated and neoplastic B cells. *J Immunol* 1989;**143**:2714–22.
44. Freeman GJ, Gray GS, Gimmi CD, Lombard DB, Zhou LJ. Structure, expression, and T cell costimulatory activity of the murine homologue of the human B lymphocyte activation antigen B7. *J Exp Med* 1991;**174**:625–31.
45. Guerder S, Picarella DE, Linsley PS, Flavell RA. Costimulator B7-1 confers antigen-presenting-cell function to parenchymal tissue and in conjunction with tumor necrosis factor alpha leads to autoimmunity in transgenic mice. *Proc Natl Acad Sci USA* 1994;**91**:5138–42.
46. Gimmi CD, Freeman GJ, Gribben JG, Sugita K, Freedman AS, et al. B-cell surface antigen B7 provides a costimulatory signal that induces T cells to proliferate and secrete interleukin 2. *Proc Natl Acad Sci USA* 1991;**88**:6575–9.
47. Lenschow DJ, Su GH, Zuckerman LA, Nabavi N, Jellis CL, et al. Expression and functional significance of an additional ligand for CTLA-4. *Proc Natl Acad Sci USA* 1993;**90**:11054–8.
48. Hathcock KS, Laszlo G, Dickler HB, Bradshaw J, Linsley P, Hodes RJ. Identification of an alternative CTLA-4 ligand costimulatory for T cell activation. *Science* 1993;**262**:905–7.
49. Hathcock KS, Laszlo G, Pucillo C, Linsley P, Hodes RJ. Comparative analysis of B7-1 and B7-2 costimulatory ligands: expression and function. *J Exp Med* 1994;**180**:631–40.
50. Freeman GJ, Borriello F, Hodes RJ, Reiser H, Hathcock KS, Laszlo G, et al. Uncovering of functional alternative CTLA-4 counter-receptor in B7-deficient mice. *Science* 1993;**262**:907–9.
51. Azuma M, Ito D, Yagita H, Okumura K, Phillips JH, Lanier LL, et al. B70 antigen is a second ligand for CTLA-4 and CD28. *Nature* 1993;**366**:76–9.
52. Greenfield EA, Nguyen KA, Kuchroo VK. CD28/B7 costimulation: a review. *Crit Rev Immunol* 1998;**18**:389–418.
53. Chen C, Gault A, Shen L, Nabavi N. Molecular cloning and expression of early T cell costimulatory molecule-1 and its characterization as B7-2 molecule. *J Immunol* 1994;**152**:4929–36.
54. Chen C, Nabavi N. In vitro induction of T cell anergy by blocking B7 and early T cell costimulatory molecule ETC-1/B7-2. *Immunity* 1994;**1**:147–54.
55. Lenschow DJ, Ho SC, Sattar H, Rhee L, Gray G, Nabavi N, et al. Differential effects of anti-B7-1 and anti-B7-2 monoclonal antibody treatment on the development of diabetes in the nonobese diabetic mouse. *J Exp Med* 1995;**181**:1145–55.
56. Lindsten T, Lee KP, Harris ES, Petryniak B, Craighead N, Reynolds PJ, et al. Characterization of CTLA-4 structure and expression on human T cells. *J Immunol* 1993;**151**:3489–99.
57. Taylor PA, Lees CJ, Fournier S, Allison JP, Sharpe AH, Blazar BR. B7 expression on T cells down-regulates immune responses through CTLA-4 ligation via T-T interactions [corrections]. *J Immunol* 2004;**172**:34–9.
58. Lenschow DJ, Sperling AI, Cooke MP, Freeman G, Rhee L. Differential up-regulation of the B7-1 and B7-2 costimulatory molecules after Ig receptor engagement by antigen. *J Immunol* 1994;**153**:1990–7.

59. Freedman AS, Freeman GJ, Rhynhart K, Nadler LM. Selective induction of B7/BB-1 on interferon-gamma stimulated monocytes: a potential mechanism for amplification of T cell activation through the CD28 pathway. *Cell Immunol* 1991;**137**:429–37.
60. Inaba K, Steinman RM. Resting and sensitized T lymphocytes exhibit distinct stimulatory (antigen-presenting cell) requirements for growth and lymphokine release. *J Exp Med* 1984;**160**:1717–35.
61. Subauste CS, de Waal Malefyt R, Fuh F. Role of CD80 (B7.1) and CD86 (B7.2) in the immune response to an intracellular pathogen. *J Immunol* 1998;**160**:1831–40.
62. Costello RT, Mallet F, Sainty D, Maraninchi D, Gastaut JA, Olive D. Regulation of CD80/B7-1 and CD86/B7-2 molecule expression in human primary acute myeloid leukemia and their role in allogenic immune recognition. *Eur J Immunol* 1998;**28**:90–103.
63. Valle A, Aubry JP, Durand I, Banchereau J. IL-4 and IL-2 upregulate the expression of antigen B7, the B cell counterstructure to T cell CD28: an amplification mechanism for T-B cell interactions. *Int Immunol* 1991;**3**:229–35.
64. Stack RM, Lenschow DJ, Gray GS, Bluestone JA, Fitch FW. IL-4 treatment of small splenic B cells induces costimulatory molecules B7-1 and B7-2. *J Immunol* 1994;**152**:5723–33.
65. Barcy S, Wettendorff M, Leo O, Urbain J, Kruger M, Ceuppens JL, et al. FcR cross-linking on monocytes results in impaired T cell stimulatory capacity. *Int Immunol* 1995;**7**:179–89.
66. Buelens C, Willems F, Delvaux A, Pierard G, Delville JP, Velu T, et al. Interleukin-10 differentially regulates B7-1 (CD80) and B7-2 (CD86) expression on human peripheral blood dendritic cells. *Eur J Immunol* 1995;**25**:2668–72.
67. Willems F, Marchant A, Delville JP, Gerard C, Delvaux A, Velu T, et al. Interleukin-10 inhibits B7 and intercellular adhesion molecule-1 expression on human monocytes. *Eur J Immunol* 1994;**24**:1007–9.
68. Bhatia S, Edidin M, Almo SC, Nathenson SG. Different cell surface oligomeric states of B7-1 and B7-2: implications for signaling. *Proc Natl Acad Sci USA* 2005;**102**:15569–74.
69. Bhatia S, Edidin M, Almo SC, Nathenson SG. B7-1 and B7-2: similar costimulatory ligands with different biochemical, oligomeric and signaling properties. *Immunol Lett* 2006;**104**:70–5.
70. Tamura H, Dong H, Zhu G, Sica GL, Flies DB, Tamada K, et al. B7-H1 costimulation preferentially enhances CD28-independent T-helper cell function. *Blood* 2001;**97**:1809–16.
71. Dong H, Zhu G, Tamada K, Chen L. B7-H1, a third member of the B7 family, co-stimulates T-cell proliferation and interleukin-10 secretion. *Nat Med* 1999;**5**:1365–9.
72. Freeman GJ, Long AJ, Iwai Y, Bourque K, Chernova T, Nishimura H, et al. Engagement of the PD-1 immunoinhibitory receptor by a novel B7 family member leads to negative regulation of lymphocyte activation. *J Exp Med* 2000;**192**:1027–34.
73. Tseng SY, Otsuji M, Gorski K, Huang X, Slansky JE, Pai SI, et al. B7-DC, a new dendritic cell molecule with potent costimulatory properties for T cells. *J Exp Med* 2001;**193**:839–46.
74. Carter L, Fouser LA, Jussif J, Fitz L, Deng B, Wood CR. PD-1:PD-L inhibitory pathway affects both CD4(+) and CD8(+) T cells and is overcome by IL-2. *Eur J Immunol* 2002;**32**:634–43.
75. Martin-Orozco N, Dong C. New battlefields for costimulation. *J Exp Med* 2006;**203**:817–20.

76. Martin-Orozco N, Wang YH, Yagita H, Dong C. Cutting edge: programmed death (PD) ligand-1/PD-1 interaction is required for CD8+ T cell tolerance to tissue antigens. *J Immunol* 2006;**177**:8291–5.
77. Ansari MJ, Salama AD, Chitnis T, Smith RN, Yagita H. The programmed death-1 (PD-1) pathway regulates autoimmune diabetes in nonobese diabetic (NOD) mice. *J Exp Med* 2003;**198**:63–9.
78. Nurieva RI, Liu X, Dong C. Yin-Yang of costimulation: crucial controls of immune tolerance and function. *Immunol Rev* 2009;**229**:88–100.
79. Pentcheva-Hoang T, Corse E, Allison JP. Negative regulators of T-cell activation: potential targets for therapeutic intervention in cancer, autoimmune disease, and persistent infections. *Immunol Rev* 2009;**229**:67–87.
80. Riley JL. PD-1 signaling in primary T cells. *Immunol Rev* 2009;**229**:114–25.
81. Barber DL, et al. Restoring function in exhausted CD8 T cells during chronic viral infection. *Nature* 2006;**439**:682–7.
82. Sharpe AH, Wherry EJ, Ahmed R, Freeman GJ. The function of programmed cell death 1 and its ligands in regulating autoimmunity and infection. *Nat Immunol* 2007;**8**:239–45.
83. Wang L, Mo HM, Wang QH, Jiang ZW, Cheng YL, Liu WQ, et al. Up-expression of PD-1–PD-L induced by immunization with SEA and SMWA of *Schistosoma japonicum* in mice. *Chinese Journal of Parasitology and Parasitic Diseases* 2008;**26**:170–3.
84. Wang S, Zhu G, Chapoval AI, Dong H, Tamada K, Ni J, et al. Costimulation of T cells by B7-H2, a B7-like molecule that binds ICOS. *Blood* 2000;**96**:2808–13.
85. Aicher A, Hayden-Ledbetter M, Brady WA, Pezzutto A, Richter G, et al. Characterization of human inducible costimulator ligand expression and function. *J Immunol* 2000;**164**: 4689–96.
86. Brodie D, Collins AV, Iaboni A, Fennelly JA, Sparks LM, et al. LICOS, a primordial costimulatory ligand? *Curr Biol* 2000;**10**:333–6.
87. Yoshinaga SK, Whoriskey JS, Khare SD, Sarmiento U, et al. T-cell costimulation through B7RP-1 and ICOS. *Nature* 1999;**402**:827–32.
88. Sun M, Richards S, Prasad DV, Mai XM, Rudensky A, Dong C. Characterization of mouse and human B7-H3 genes. *J Immunol* 2002;**168**:6294–7.
89. Suh WK, Gajewska BU, Okada H, Gronski MA, Bertram EM, Dawicki W, et al. The B7 family member B7-H3 preferentially down-regulates T helper type 1-mediated immune responses. *Nat Immunol* 2003;**4**:899–906.
90. Chapoval AI, Ni J, Lau JS, Wilcox RA, Flies DB, Liu D. B7-H3: a costimulatory molecule for T cell activation and IFN-gamma production. *Nat Immunol* 2001;**2**:269–74.
91. Yi KH, Chen L. Fine tuning the immune response through B7-H3 and B7-H4. *Immunol Rev* 2009;**229**:145–51.
92. Valentonyte R, et al. Sarcoidosis is associated with a truncating splice site mutation in BTNL2. *Nat Genet* 2005;**37**:357–64.
93. Kryczek I, Wei S, Zou L, Zhu G, Mottram P, Xu H, et al. Cutting edge: induction of B7-H4 on APCs through IL-10—novel suppressive mode for regulatory T cells. *J Immunol* 2006;**77**:40–4.
94. Kryczek I, Zou L, Rodriguez P, Zhu G, Wei S, Mottram P, et al. B7-H4 expression identifies a novel suppressive macrophage population in human ovarian carcinoma. *J Exp Med* 2006;**203**:871–81.
95. Viola A, Lanzavecchia A. T cell activation determined by T cell receptor number and tunable thresholds. *Science* 1996;**273**:104–6.

96. Lenschow DJ, Herold KC, Rhee L, Patel B, Koons A, et al. CD28/B7 regulation of Th1 and Th2 subsets in the development of autoimmune diabetes. *Immunity* 1996;**5**:285–93.
97. Lanzavecchia A. Three signals and a master switch in the regulation of T-cell immunity. *Cold Spring Harb Symp Quant Biol* 1999;**64**:253–7.
98. Lanzavecchia A, Lezzi G, Viola A. From TCR engagement to T cell activation: a kinetic view of T cell behavior. *Cell* 1999;**96**:1–4.
99. Hurwitz AA, Kwon ED, van Elsas A. Costimulatory wars: the tumor menace. *Curr Opin Immunol* 2000;**12**:589–96.
100. McAdam AJ, Schweitzer AN, Sharpe AH. The role of B7 costimulation in activation and differentiation of CD4+ and CD8+ T cells. *Immunol Rev* 1998;**65**:231–47.
101. McAdam AJ, Chang TT, Lumelsky AE, Greenfield EA, et al. Mouse inducible costimulatory molecule (ICOS) expression is enhanced by CD28 costimulation and regulates differentiation of CD4+ T cells. *J Immunol* 2000;**165**:5035–40.
102. van Elsas A, Hurwitz AA, Allison JP. Combination immunotherapy of B16 melanoma using anti-cytotoxic T lymphocyte-associated antigen 4 (CTLA-4) and granulocyte/macrophage colony-stimulating factor (GM-CSF)-producing vaccines induces rejection of subcutaneous and metastatic tumors accompanied by autoimmune depigmentation. *J Exp Med* 1999;**190**:355–66.
103. McKnight AJ, Perez VL, Shea CM, Gray GS, Abbas AK. Costimulator dependence of lymphokine secretion by naive and activated CD4+ T lymphocytes from TCR transgenic mice. *J Immunol* 1994;**152**:5220–5.
104. Dariavach P, Mattei MG, Golstein P, Lefranc MP. Human Ig superfamily CTLA-4 gene: chromosomal localization and identity of protein sequence between murine and human CTLA-4 cytoplasmic domains. *Eur J Immunol* 1988;**18**:1901–5.
105. Ward SG. CD28: a signalling perspective. *Biochem J* 1996;**318**:361–77.
106. Schwartz RH. Costimulation of T lymphocytes: the role of CD28, CTLA-4, and B7/BB1 in interleukin-2 production and immunotherapy. *Cell* 1992;**71**:1065–8.
107. Lindsten T, Lee KP, Harris ES, Petryniak B, Craighead N, Reynolds PJ, et al. Characterization of CTLA-4 structure and expression on human T cells. *J Immunol* 1993;**151**:3489–99.
108. Freeman GJ, Borriello F, Hodes RJ, Reiser H, Hathcock KS, Laszlo G, et al. Uncovering of functional alternative CTLA-4 counter-receptor in B7-deficient mice. *Science* 1993;**262**:907–9.
109. Ikemizu S, Gilbert RJ, Fennelly JA, Collins AV, Harlos K, et al. Structure and dimerization of a soluble form of B7-1. *Immunity* 1993;**12**:51–60.
110. Bhatia S, Sun K, Almo SC, Nathenson SG, Hodes RJ. Dynamic equilibrium of B7-1 dimers and monomers differentially affects immunological synapse formation and T cell activation in response to TCR/CD28 stimulation. *J Immunol* 2010;**184**(4):1821–8.
111. Fecteau S, Basadonna GP, Freitas A, Ariyan C, Sayegh MH, Rothstein DM. CTLA-4 up-regulation plays a role in tolerance mediated by CD45. *Nat Immunol* 2001;**2**:58–63.
112. Chambers CA. The expanding world of costimulation: the two-signal model revisited. *Trends Immunol* 2001;**22**:217–23.
113. Chambers CA, Kuhns MS, Egen JG, Allison JP. CTLA-4-mediated inhibition in regulation of T cell responses: mechanisms and manipulation in tumor immunotherapy. *Annu Rev Immunol* 2001;**19**:565–94.
114. Greenwald RJ, Boussiotis VA, Lorsbach RB, Abbas AK, Sharpe AH. CTLA-4 regulates induction of anergy *in vivo*. *Immunity* 2001;**14**:145–55.

115. Coyle AJ, Lehar S, Lloyd C, Tian J, Delaney T, Manning S, et al. The CD28-related molecule ICOS is required for effective T cell-dependent immune responses. *Immunity* 2000;**13**:95–105.
116. Mages HW, Hutloff A, Heuck C, Buchner K, Himmelbauer H, et al. Molecular cloning and characterization of murine ICOS and identification of B7h as ICOS ligand. *Eur J Immunol* 2000;**30**:1040–7.
117. Hutloff A, Dittrich AM, Beier KC, Eljaschewitsch B, Kraft R, et al. ICOS is an inducible T-cell co-stimulator structurally and functionally related to CD28. *Nature* 1999;**397**: 263–6.
118. McAdam AJ, Greenwald RJ, Levin MA, Chernova T, et al. ICOS is critical for CD40-mediated antibody class switching. *Nature* 2001;**409**:102–5.
119. Kopf M, Coyle AJ, Schmitz N, Barner M, Oxenius A, Gallimore A, et al. Inducible costimulator protein (ICOS) controls T helper cell subset polarization after virus and parasite infection. *J Exp Med* 2000;**192**:53–61.
120. Herman AE, Freeman GJ, Mathis D, Benoist C. CD4+CD25+ T regulatory cells dependent on ICOS promote regulation of effector cells in the prediabetic lesion. *J Exp Med* 2004;**199**:1479–89.
121. Akbari O, Freeman GJ, Meyer EH, Greenfield EA, Chang TT, et al. Antigen-specific regulatory T cells develop via the ICOS-ICOS-ligand pathway and inhibit allergen-induced airway hyperreactivity. *Nat Med* 2002;**8**:1024–32.
122. Tafuri A, Shahinian A, et al. ICOS is essential for effective T-helper-cell responses. *Nature* 2001;**409**:105–9.
123. Grimbacher B, Hutloff A, et al. Homozygous loss of ICOS is associated with adult-onset common variable immunodeficiency. *Nat Immunol* 2003;**4**:261–8.
124. Nurieva RI, Treuting P, et al. Inducible costimulator is essential for collagen-induced arthritis. *J Clin Invest* 2003;**111**:701–6.
125. Rottman JB, Smith T, et al. The costimulatory molecule ICOS plays an important role in the immunopathogenesis of EAE. *Nat Immunol* 2001;**2**:605–11.
126. Yong PFK, Salzer U, Grimbacher B. The role of costimulation in antibody deficiencies: ICOS and common variable immunodeficiency. *Immunol Rev* 2009;**229**:101–13.
127. Ishida Y, Agata Y, Shibahara K, Honjo T. Induced expression of PD-1, a novel member of the immunoglobulin gene superfamily, upon programmed cell death. *EMBO J* 1992; **1**:3887–95.
128. Agata Y, Kawasaki A, Nishimura H, Ishida Y, Tsubata T, Yagita H, et al. Expression of the PD-1 antigen on the surface of stimulated mouse T and B lymphocytes. *Int Immunol* 1996;**8**:765–72.
129. Nishimura H, Agata Y, Kawasaki A, Sato M, Imamura S, Minato N, et al. Developmentally regulated expression of the PD-1 protein on the surface of double-negative (CD4− CD8−) thymocytes. *Int Immunol* 1996;**8**:773–80.
130. Nishimura H, Honjo T. PD-1: an inhibitory immunoreceptor involved in peripheral tolerance. *Trends Immunol* 2001;**22**:265–8.
131. Nishimura H, Minato N, Nakano T, Honjo T. Immunological studies on PD-1 deficient mice: implication of PD-1 as a negative regulator for B cell responses. *Int Immunol* 1998;**10**:1563–72.
132. Latchman Y, Wood CR, Chernova T, Chaudhary D, Borde M, et al. PD-L2 is a second ligand for PD-1 and inhibits T cell activation. *Nat Immunol* 2001;**2**:261–8.
133. Khoury SJ, Sayegh MH. The roles of the new negative T cell costimulatory pathways in regulating autoimmunity. *Immunity* 2004;**20**:529–38.

134. Blazar BR, Carreno BM, et al. Blockade of programmed death-1 engagement accelerates graft-versus-host disease lethality by an IFN-gamma-dependent mechanism. *J Immunol* 2003;**171**:1272–7.
135. Iwai Y, Terawaki S, Honjo T. PD-1 blockade inhibits hematogenous spread of poorly immunogenic tumor cells by enhanced recruitment of effector T cells. *Int Immunol* 2005;**17**:133–44.
136. Grewal IS, Flavell RA. The role of CD40 ligand in costimulation and T-cell activation. *Immunol Rev* 1996;**153**:85–106.
137. Grewal IS, Flavell RA. A central role of CD40 ligand in the regulation of CD4+ T-cell responses. *Immunol Today* 1996;**17**:410–14.
138. Grewal IS, Flavell RA. The CD40 ligand. At the center of the immune universe? *Immunol Res* 1997;**16**:59–70.
139. Grewal IS, Flavell RA. CD40 and CD154 in cell-mediated immunity. *Annu Rev Immunol* 1998;**16**:111–35.
140. Xu Y, Song G. The role of CD40-CD154 interaction in cell immunoregulation. *J Biomed Sci* 2004;**11**:426–38.
141. Qi CJ, Zheng L, Zhou X, Tao Y, Ge Y, Zhuang YM, et al. Cross-linking of CD40 using anti-CD40 antibody, 5C11, has different effects on XG2 multiple myeloma cells. *Immunol Lett* 2004;**93**:151–8.
142. Schoenberger SP, Toes RE, van der Voort EI, Offringa R, Melief CJ. T-cell help for cytotoxic T lymphocytes is mediated by CD40–CD40L interactions. *Nature* 1998;**393**:480–3.
143. Demangel C, Palendira U, Feng CG, Heath AW, Bean AG, Britton WJ. Stimulation of dendritic cells via CD40 enhances immune responses to *Mycobacterium tuberculosis* infection. *Infect Immun* 2001;**69**:2456–61.
144. Armitage RJ, Fanslow WC, Strockbine L, Sato TA, Clifford KN, et al. Molecular and biological characterization of a murine ligand for CD40. *Nature* 1992;**357**:80–2.
145. Noelle RJ, Roy M, Shepherd DM, Stamenkovic I, Ledbetter JA, Aruffo A. A 39-kDa protein on activated helper T cells binds CD40 and transduces the signal for cognate activation of B cells. *Proc Natl Acad Sci USA* 1992;**89**:6550–4.
146. Stuber E, Strober W, Neurath M. Blocking the CD40L–CD40 interaction *in vivo* specifically prevents the priming of T helper 1 cells through the inhibition of interleukin 12 secretion. *J Exp Med* 1996;**183**:693–8.
147. Elgueta R, Benson MJ, de Vries VC, Wasiuk A, Guo Y, Noelle RJ. Molecular mechanism and function of CD40/CD40L engagement in the immune system. *Immunol Rev* 2009;**229**: 152–72.
148. Croft M, So T, Duan W, Soroosh P. The significance of OX40 and OX40L to T-cell biology and immune disease. *Immunol Rev* 2009;**229**:173–91.
149. Wang C, Lin GHY, McPherson AJ, Watts TH. Immune regulation by 4-1BB and 4-1BBL: complexities and challenges. *Immunol Rev* 2009;**229**:192–215.
150. Nolte MA, van Olffen RW, Van Gisbergen KPJM, van Lier RAW. Timing and tuning of CD27-CD70 interactions: the impact of signal strength in setting the balance between adaptive responses and immunopathology. *Immunol Rev* 2009;**229**:216–31.
151. Wang Y, Zhu M, Miller M, Fu YX. Immunoregulation by tumor necrosis factor superfamily member LIGHT. *Immunol Rev* 2009;**229**:232–43.
152. Cai G, Freeman GJ. The CD160, BTLA, LIGHT/HVEM pathway: a bidirectional switch regulating T-cell activation. *Immunol Rev* 2009;**229**:244–58.
153. Kwon BS, Weissman SM. cDNA sequences of two inducible T-cell genes. *Proc Natl Acad Sci USA* 1989;**86**(6):1963–7.

154. Pollok KE, et al. Inducible T cell antigen 4-1BB. Analysis of expression and function. *J Immunol* 1993;**150**(3):771–81.
155. Schwarz H, Valbracht J, Tuckwell J, von Kempis J, Lotz M. ILA, the human 4-1BB homologue, is inducible in lymphoid and other cell lineages. *Blood* 1995;**85**(4):1043–52.
156. Goodwin RG, et al. Molecular cloning of a ligand for the inducible T cell gene 4-1BB: a member of an emerging family of cytokines with homology to tumor necrosis factor. *Eur J Immunol* 1993;**23**(10):2631–41.
157. Vinay DS, Kwon BS. Role of 4-1BB in immune responses. *Semin Immunol* 1998;**10**(6):481–9.
158. Saoulli K, et al. CD28-independent, TRAF2-dependent costimulation of resting T cells by 4-1BB ligand. *J Exp Med* 1998;**187**(11):1849–62.
159. Gramaglia I, Cooper D, Miner KT, Kwon BS, Croft M. Co-stimulation of antigen-specific CD4 T cells by 4-1BB ligand. *Eur J Immunol* 2000;**30**(2):392–402.
160. Shuford WW, et al. 4-1BB costimulatory signals preferentially induce CD8 + T cell proliferation and lead to the amplification *in vivo* of cytotoxic T cell responses. *J Exp Med* 1997;**186**(1):47–55.
161. Lee HW, Park SJ, Choi BK, Kim HH, Nam KO, Kwon BS. 4-1BB promotes the survival of CD8+ T lymphocytes by increasing expression of Bcl-xL and Bfl-1. *J Immunol* 2002;**169**(9):4882–8.
162. Pulle G, Vidric M, Watts TH. IL-15-dependent induction of 4-1BB promotes antigen-independent CD8 memory T cell survival. *J Immunol* 2006;**176**(5):2739–48.
163. Melero I, et al. Monoclonal antibodies against the 4-1BB T-cell activation molecule eradicate established tumors. *Nat Med* 1997;**3**(6):682–5.
164. Watts TH. TNF/TNFR family members in costimulation of T cell responses. *Annu Rev Immunol* 2005;**23**:23–68.
165. Lynch DH. The promise of 4-1BB (CD137)-mediated immunomodulation and the immunotherapy of cancer. *Immunol Rev* 2008;**222**:277–86.
166. Lee SW, Croft M. 4-1BB as a therapeutic target for human disease. In: Grewal IS, editor. *Therapeutic targets of the TNF superfamily*. Bothell, WA: Landes Bioscience; 2009. pp. 120–9
167. Miller RE, et al. 4-1BB-specific monoclonal antibody promotes the generation of tumor-specific immune responses by direct activation of CD8 T cells in a CD40-dependent manner. *J Immunol* 2002;**169**(4):1792–800.
168. Uno T, et al. Eradication of established tumors in mice by a combination antibody-based therapy. *Nat Med* 2006;**12**(6):693–8.
169. Xu DP, Sauter BV, Huang TG, Meseck M, Woo SL, Chen SH. The systemic administration of Ig-4-1BB ligand in combination with IL-12 gene transfer eradicates hepatic colon carcinoma. *Gene Ther* 2005;**12**(20):1526–33.
170. McMillin DW, Hewes B, Gangadharan B, Archer DR, Mittler RS, Spencer HT. Complete regression of large solid tumors using engineered drug-resistant hematopoietic cells and anti-CD137 immunotherapy. *Hum Gene Ther* 2006;**17**(8):798–806.
171. Shi W, Siemann DW. Augmented antitumor effects of radiation therapy by 4-1BB antibody (BMS-469492) treatment. *Anticancer Res* 2006;**26**(5A):3445–53.
172. Sun Y, et al. Administration of agonistic anti-4-1BB monoclonal antibody leads to the amelioration of experimental autoimmune encephalomyelitis. *J Immunol* 2002;**168**(3):1457–65.
173. Vinay DS, Cha K, Kwon BS. Dual immunoregulatory pathways of 4-1BB signaling. *J Mol Med* 2006;**84**(9):726–36.

174. Wang J, et al. Role of 4-1BB in allograft rejection mediated by CD8+ T cells. *Am J Transplant* 2003;**3**(5):543–51.
175. So T, Lee SW, Croft M. Immune regulation and control of regulatory T cells by OX40 and 4-1BB. *Cytokine Growth Factor Rev* 2008;**19**(3–4):253–62.
176. Sznol MHF, et al. Phase I study of BMS-663513, a fully human anti-CD137 agonist monoclonal antibody, in patients (pts) with advanced cancer (CA). *J Clin Oncol* 2008;**26** (Suppl). [abstract 3007].
177. Paterson DJ, et al. Antigens of activated rat T lymphocytes including a molecule of 50,000 Mr detected only on CD4 positive T blasts. *Mol Immunol* 1987;**24**(12):1281–90.
178. Stuber E, Neurath M, Calderhead D, Fell HP, Strober W. Cross-linking of OX40 ligand, a member of the TNF/NGF cytokine family, induces proliferation and differentiation in murine splenic B cells. *Immunity* 1995;**2**(5):507–21.
179. Ohshima Y, Tanaka Y, Tozawa H, Takahashi Y, Maliszewski C, Delespesse G. Expression and function of OX40 ligand on human dendritic cells. *J Immunol* 1997;**159**(8): 3838–48.
180. Murata K, et al. Impairment of antigen-presenting cell function in mice lacking expression of OX40 ligand. *J Exp Med* 2000;**191**(2):365–74.
181. Wang HC, Klein JR. Multiple levels of activation of murine CD8(+) intraepithelial lymphocytes defined by OX40 (CD134) expression: effects on cell-mediated cytotoxicity, IFN-gamma, and IL-10 regulation. *J Immunol* 2001;**167**(12):6717–23.
182. Imura A, et al. The human OX40/gp34 system directly mediates adhesion of activated T cells to vascular endothelial cells. *J Exp Med* 1996;**183**(5):2185–95.
183. Rogers PR, Song J, Gramaglia I, Killeen N, Croft M. OX40 promotes Bcl-xL and Bcl-2 expression and is essential for long-term survival of CD4 T cells. *Immunity* 2001;**15** (3):445–55.
184. Walker LS, et al. Compromised OX40 function in CD28-deficient mice is linked with failure to develop CXC chemokine receptor 5-positive CD4 cells and germinal centers. *J Exp Med* 1999;**190**(8):1115–22.
185. Croft M. Costimulation of T cells by OX40, 4-1BB, and CD27. *Cytokine Growth Factor Rev* 2003;**14**(3–4):265–73.
186. Vu MD, et al. OX40 costimulation turns off Foxp3+ Tregs. *Blood* 2007;**110**(7):2501–10.
187. So T, Croft M. Cutting edge: OX40 inhibits TGF-beta- and antigen-driven conversion of naïve CD4 T cells into CD25+ Foxp3+ T cells. *J Immunol* 2007;**179**(3):1427–30.
188. Pan PY, Zang Y, Weber K, Meseck ML, Chen SH. OX40 ligation enhances primary and memory cytotoxic T lymphocyte responses in an immunotherapy for hepatic colon metastases. *Mol Ther* 2002;**6**(4):528–36.
189. Morris NP, et al. Development and characterization of recombinant human Fc:OX40L fusion protein linked via a coiled-coil trimerization domain. *Mol Immunol* 2007;**44**(12): 3112–21.
190. Harrop JA, et al. Antibodies to TR2 (herpesvirus entry mediator), a new member of the TNF receptor superfamily, block T cell proliferation, expression of activation markers, and production of cytokines. *J Immunol* 1998;**161**(4):1786–94.
191. Scheu S, Alferink J, Potzel T, Barchet W, Kalinke U, Pfeffer K. Targeted disruption of LIGHT causes defects in costimulatory T cell activation and reveals cooperation with lymphotoxin beta in mesenteric lymph node genesis. *J Exp Med* 2002;**195**(12):1613–24.
192. Kwon BS, et al. A newly identified member of the tumor necrosis factor receptor superfamily with a wide tissue distribution and involvement in lymphocyte activation. *J Biol Chem* 1997;**272**(22):14272–6.

193. Shaikh RB, et al. Constitutive expression of LIGHT on T cells leads to lymphocyte activation, inflammation, and tissue destruction. *J Immunol* 2001;**167**(11):6330–7.
194. Wang J, et al. The regulation of T cell homeostasis and autoimmunity by T cell-derived LIGHT. *J Clin Invest* 2001;**108**(12):1771–80.
195. Lee Y, et al. Recruitment and activation of naive T cells in the islets by lymphotoxin beta receptor dependent tertiary lymphoid structure. *Immunity* 2006;**25**(3):499–509.
196. Tamada K, et al. Cutting edge: selective impairment of CD8+ T cell function in mice lacking the TNF superfamily member LIGHT. *J Immunol* 2002;**168**(10):4832–5.
197. Tamada K, et al. Blockade of LIGHT/LTbeta and CD40 signaling induces allospecific T cell anergy, preventing graft-versus-host disease. *J Clin Invest* 2002;**109**(4):549–57.
198. Tamada K, et al. Modulation of T-cell-mediated immunity in tumor and graft-versus-host disease models through the LIGHT co-stimulatory pathway. *Nat Med* 2000;**6**(3):283–9.
199. Yu P, et al. Priming of naive T cells inside tumors leads to eradication of established tumors. *Nat Immunol* 2004;**5**(2):141–9.
200. Fan Z, et al. NK-cell activation by LIGHT triggers tumor-specific CD8+ T-cell immunity to reject established tumors. *Blood* 2006;**107**(4):1342–51.
201. Yu P, et al. Targeting the primary tumor to generate CTL for the effective eradication of spontaneous metastases. *J Immunol* 2007;**179**(3):1960–8.
202. Daud AI, et al. Phase I trial of interleukin-12 plasmid electroporation in patients with metastatic melanoma. *J Clin Oncol* 2008;**26**(36):5896–903.
203. McHugh RS, et al. CD4(+)CD25(+) immunoregulatory T cells: gene expression analysis reveals a functional role for the glucocorticoid-induced TNF receptor. *Immunity* 2002;**16**(2):311–23.
204. Keller AM, Schildknecht A, Xiao Y, van den Broek M, Borst J. Expression of costimulatory ligand CD70 on steady-state dendritic cells breaks CD8+ T cell tolerance and permits effective immunity. *Immunity* 2008;**29**(6):934–46.
205. Liu X, et al. B7H costimulates clonal expansion of, and cognate destruction of tumor cells by, CD8(+) T lymphocytes *in vivo*. *J Exp Med* 2001;**194**(9):1339–48.
206. Wallin JJ, Liang L, Bakardjiev A, Sha WC. Enhancement of CD8+ T cell responses by ICOS/B7h costimulation. *J Immunol* 2001;**167**(1):132–9.
207. Ara G, et al. Potent activity of soluble B7RP-1-Fc in therapy of murine tumors in syngeneic hosts. *Int J Cancer* 2003;**103**(4):501–7.
208. Couderc B, et al. Enhancement of antitumor immunity by expression of CD70 (CD27 ligand) or CD154 (CD40 ligand) costimulatory molecules in tumor cells. *Cancer Gene Ther* 1998;**5**(3):163–75.
209. Nieland JD, Graus YF, Dortmans YE, Kremers BL, Kruisbeek AM. CD40 and CD70 co-stimulate a potent *in vivo* antitumor T cell response. *J Immunother* 1998;**21**(3):225–36.
210. Lorenz MG, Kantor JA, Schlom J, Hodge JW. Anti-tumor immunity elicited by a recombinant vaccinia virus expressing CD70 (CD27L). *Hum Gene Ther* 1999;**10**(7):1095–103.
211. Cohen AD, et al. Agonist anti-GITR antibody enhances vaccine-induced CD8(+) T-cell responses and tumor immunity. *Cancer Res* 2006;**66**(9):4904–12.
212. Ko K, et al. Treatment of advanced tumors with agonistic anti-GITR mAb and its effects on tumor-infiltrating Foxp3 + CD25+ CD4+ regulatory T cells. *J Exp Med* 2005;**202**(7):885–91.
213. Zhou P, L'Italien L, Hodges D, Schebye XM. Pivotal roles of CD4+ effector T cells in mediating agonistic anti-GITR mAb-induced-immune activation and tumor immunity in CT26 tumors. *J Immunol* 2007;**179**(11):7365–75.
214. Hancock WW, Sayegh MH, Zheng XG, Peach R, Linsley PS, Turka LA. Costimulatory function and expression of CD40 ligand, CD80, and CD86 in vascularized murine cardiac allograft rejection. *Proc Natl Acad Sci USA* 1996;**93**:13967–72.

Chapter 2

Concept of Reverse Costimulation and Its Role in Diseases

INTRODUCTION

The development of immune response, especially in case of naive T cells, needs at least two distinct signals for full activation to proliferate and differentiate. The first signal is provided by the specific antigen [major histocompatibility complex (MHC)−peptide complex] recognition by the T-cell receptor (TCR) and the second signal is provided by the costimulatory molecules. This requirement for the second signal explains why adaptive immune responses are stimulated by microbes but not by most self-antigens, which are not normally recognized by the innate immune system and therefore do not elicit adaptive immune responses. The second signal, which is not delivered via TCR and is not antigen specific, has been termed as costimulatory signal because, although essential, it does not by itself induce any response in T cells. However, when a T cell has its receptor ligated and receives a costimulatory signal, the T cell will proliferate and differentiate into an effector cell. Moreover, T cells that bind antigen but do not receive a costimulatory signal are thought to die or to become anergic, a state in which the cell cannot be activated even if it receives both of the signals required to activate a T cell.[1−4] Thus, an encounter with antigen can lead to two quite distinct outcomes: proliferation and differentiation into effector cells, or inactivation or death, which outcome occurs is determined by the appropriate delivery of costimulatory signals.

Because the original proposal of a two-signal model (Figure 2.1) for lymphocyte activation, it has become firmly established that costimulatory signals mediated primarily via the conventional CD28-B7 and CD154/CD40 pathways, are necessary for full T-cell activation and play a crucial role in mediating allograft rejection, immune tolerance, infections, and so on. In several transplantation

Developing Costimulatory Molecules for Immunotherapy of Diseases.
DOI: http://dx.doi.org/10.1016/B978-0-12-802585-7.00002-9

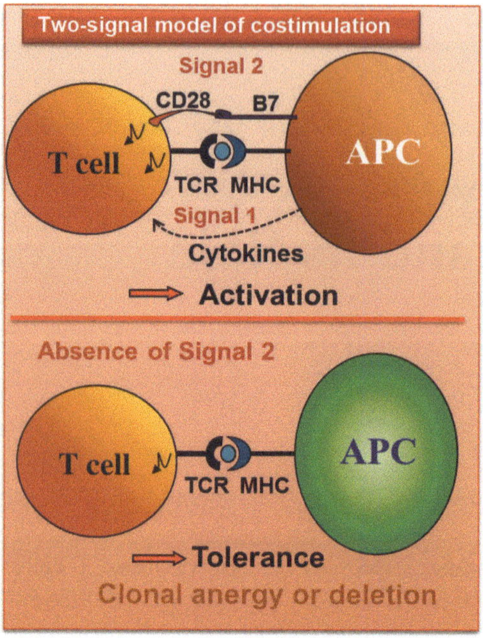

FIGURE 2.1 **Two-signal model of T-cell activation.** Two signals are needed for optimal activation of T cells. Signal 1 which is specific is delivered through TCR on T cells and Signal 2 which is antigen independent and nonspecific is delivered through costimulatory molecules present on APCs. Signal 2 is required for sustained T-cell proliferation, effector/memory cell generation, and prevention of anergy or apoptosis. If costimulatory signal is absent, the cell will undergo clonal anergy (unresponsiveness) or deletion. Expression of costimulatory molecules on professional APCs ensures that only pathogen-specific T cells are activated and minimize the chances of acquired immune responses being mounted against self.

models, CD28-B7 or CD154-CD40 blockade has been shown to prevent acute rejection, induce long-term allograft survival, and prevent the development and progression of chronic rejection. With the continuous discovery of new costimulatory molecules on antigen-presenting cells (APCs) and their receptors on T cells, the story is very much an evolving one. However, to date, CD80 and CD86 remain the best-defined costimulatory molecules on APCs, which provide the second signals for activation of naive T cells. The question remains: Can CD80 and CD80 deliver bidirectional costimulation?

CONCEPT OF BIDIRECTIONAL COSTIMULATION

The best-defined costimulatory molecules to date are two structurally related proteins, CD80 (B7-1) and CD86 (B7-2). These two B7 ligands, CD80 and CD86, can augment immune responses by binding to CD28 and downregulate responses by binding to CTLA-4. It has been suggested that CD86 participates in initiating immune response, whereas CD80 may be more important in sustaining or regulating immune responses (Table 2.1). The upregulation of CTLA-4 on activated T cells parallels the kinetics of CD80 expression. This property, together with the higher avidities of CD80 ligands for CTLA-4 than those of CD28, has raised the possibility that CD80/CTLA-4 interactions predominate late to terminate immune responses.[5–7] Although both of these B7 ligands play a major role in providing costimulation to T cells by binding to CD28,

TABLE 2.1 B7 Family of Costimulatory Molecules, Their Expression Patterns, and Functions

Ligand	Expression	Receptor	Function
B71 [CD80]	DCs, activated macrophages, and B cells	CD28/ CTLA-4	Activation of naive T cells, T-cell proliferation, IL-2 production, T-cell survival/inhibition of T-cell responses
B72 [CD86]	DCs, activated macrophages, and B cells	CD28/ CTLA-4	Activation of naive T cells, T-cell proliferation, IL-2 production, T-cell survival/inhibition of T-cell responses
B7-H1 [PD-L1]	DCs, monocytes, macrophages, B cells, activated T cells, endothelial cells, and tumor cells	?	Effector T-cell functions, T-cell proliferation, cytokine [IL-10, IFN-γ] production, apoptosis of CTLs, DCs, and monocytes, inhibition of T-cell responses
B7-DC [PD-L2]	DCs, monocytes, macrophages, B cells, activated T cells, endothelial cells, and tumor cells	PD-1	Effector T-cell functions, T-cell proliferation, cytokine [IL-10, IFN-γ] production, apoptosis of CTLs, DCs, and monocytes, inhibition of T-cell responses, regulation of DC biology
B7-H2 [B7-H2, B7RP-1, GL50, LICOS]	DCs, monocytes, Langerhan's cells, B cells, fibroblasts, endothelial cells, etc.	ICOS	Effector T-cell function, T-cell proliferation, Ig isotype class switching, cytokine [IFN-γ, IL-10, IL-4] production
B7-H3	Induced on DCs and monocytes	? [orphan ligand]	T-cell proliferation, IFN-γ production, enhancement of CTL activity
B7-H4	Induced on T cells, B-cells, DCs, and macrophages	BTLA [?]	Inhibition of T-cell proliferation, cytokine production, cell cycle arrest

Note: DC: dendritic cells; IFN-γ: interferon-γ; PD-1: programmed death-1; IL: interleukin; CTL: cytotoxic T lymphocyte.

which leads to their proliferation, cytokine production, and development of effector functions. The binding to CTLA-4 provides the inhibitory signals required for downregulation of the immune response.[8] The ability of APCs to deliver the costimulatory signal to T cells by B7 molecules is very well

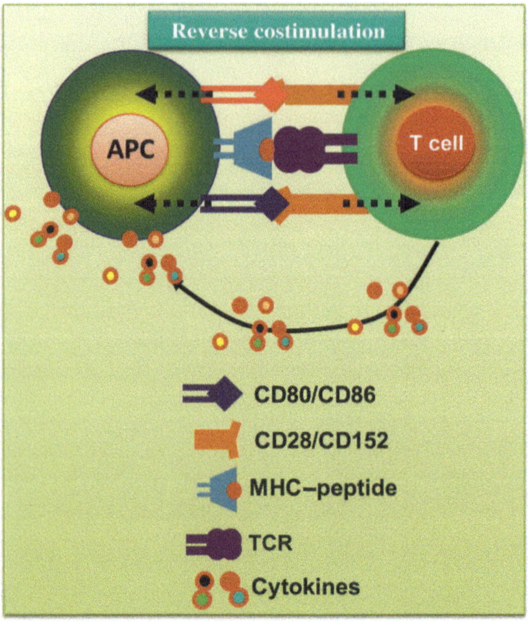

FIGURE 2.2 **CD80/CD86 deliver bidirectional signaling for the activation of T cell and APC.** Cognate association between T cell and APC leads to interaction between MHC and peptide with TCR and CD80/86 with CD28/CD152. This steers toward the activation and differentiation of T cell. Activated T cell secretes cytokines that ultimately help in the activation and differentiation of APC. The arrows shown in the diagram depict that there occurs as well an alternative pathway of bidirectional signaling through costimulatory molecules CD80/CD86 and CD28/CD152 that activate both T cell and APC.

established.[9–11] However, despite the fact that both CD80 and CD86 play a major role in providing costimulation to T cells, these molecules can also serve as counter-receptors that transduce signals to APCs upon engagement with CD28/CD152 (Figure 2.2). CD80 and CD86 could also serve as counter-receptors that transduce distinct signal to the APCs upon engagement by CD28 or CTLA-4. The intracellular domains of CD80 and CD86 are quite distinct and could mediate differential signal transduction. Such signaling could influence the ability of APCs to function as effector cells.[12–14] However, whether the engagement of CD80 and CD86 molecules with CD28 and CD152 affects the function of the APC has been poorly documented until recently.[15,16] There was indirect evidence suggesting that CD28/CD152/B7 signaling pathways may affect B-cell responses and immunoglobulin (Ig) synthesis.[14–16] Studies done with CD80 − /− and CD86 −/− mice do indicate the role of CD80 and CD86 in delivering bidirectional costimulation. Mice lacking CD80 and CD86 were found to be profoundly deficient in their ability to generate *in vivo* germinal center formation, Ig class switching, memory formation, and affinity maturation through somatic hypermutation.[15–18] Thus, a role of CD80 and CD86 in the activation of B cells is plausible and needs to be systematically addressed.

However, for the first time Suvas et al.[19] from our lab gave a concept of bidirectional costimulation and demonstrated that costimulation through CD80 specifically inhibits the proliferation and IgG secretion by lipopolysaccharide (LPS)-stimulated B cells and B-cell lymphoma by upregulating the expression of proapoptotic molecules caspase-3, caspase-8, Fas, FasL, Bak, and Bax, and downregulating the levels of antiapoptotic molecule Bcl-x(L).[19] In contrast, costimulation through CD86 augmented the level of antiapoptotic molecules Bcl-w and Bcl-x(L), and decreased the levels of caspase-8. Thus, the costimulatory signals not only influence the activation of T cells, but can also affect the activity of B cells by reverse costimulation. CD80 has been shown to be involved in bidirectional costimulation. Signaling through anti-CD80 Ab in LPS-activated B cells declined the proliferation and production of IgG1 and IgG2a antibodies (Abs). Signaling through CD80 molecule retarded the growth of B cells and mainly augmented the levels of proapoptotic molecules, that is, caspase-3, caspase-8, Fas, FasL, Bak, and Bax, and downregulated the expression of Bcl-x(L) and Bfl-1, which suggests that CD80 signaling induces apoptosis by upregulating proapoptotic molecules and therefore restricting their proliferation.[19] These findings clearly establish that CD80 signaling not only costimulates T cells on ligation with CD28/CD152 but can also influence B cells through bidirectional costimulation. Signaling through CD86 molecule has been shown to play an important role in the bidirectional costimulation of B cells. Cross-linking of CD86 on LPS-activated B cells not only enhanced the proliferation and production of IgG1 and IgG2a Abs but also increased the expression of antiapoptotic molecules Bcl-w and Bcl-x(L) and downregulated the expression of proapoptotic molecules such as caspase-8, thereby promoting their survival by enhancing the expression of antiapoptotic proteins.[19]

After the report published by Suvas et al.,[19] many groups have endorsed the concept of bidirectional costimulation. Schmidt et al.[20] has shown that targeting death receptor-6 on B cells can enhance B-cell expansion, survival, and humoral responses. Consistent with this, increased nuclear levels and activity of nuclear factor kappa-B (NF-κB) transcription factor, c-Rel, and elevated Bcl-x(L) expression were observed.[21] Nguyen et al. have shown that cross-linking B7-DC with the monoclonal antibody (mAb) directly potentates dendritic cell (DC) function by enhancing antigen uptake and DC presentation of MHC−peptide complexes, promoting DC survival, and increasing secretion of interleukin (IL)-12p70.[17,20] Radhakrishnan et al.[21] have demonstrated that B7-DC cross-linking restores antigen uptake and augments APC function by matured DCs. Lumsden et al. have shown that CD80/86 and CD40 are required on B cells for T-dependent Ab responses.[17] Mukherjee et al. have shown that CD80 and CD86 expression on mouse CD4 + T lymphocytes enhance their cell cycle progression and survival.[22] Grohmann et al. have shown that upon recognition of CTLA-4 on T cells by B7 expressed on APCs, both molecules could become activated, leading to changes in the functional state not only of T cell but also of the APCs.[23] NF-κB, a family of transcription factors, consists of five major subunits, namely, NF-κB (P105/P50), NF-κB2 (P100/P52), Rel-A (P65), Rel-B, and C-Rel, that form various homo- and heterodimeric complexes.[24,25] CD86 cross-linking on IL-4 and CD40L-activated B cells increased the rate and level of IgG1 transcription, nuclear localization of NF-κB p50 subunit, and phosphorylation of Rel-A (p65) and IκBα. It also increased octamer-binding transcription factor 2 (oct-2) expression and binding to the 3′Ig H enhancer. These results were not observed in CD86−/− B cells.[25] All these results clearly establish that CD86 does not only costimulate T cells but can also deliver reverse signals into B cells and modulate their activity. NF-κB remains sequestered in the cytoplasm of the resting cell in a complex with IκB proteins. Upon activation of the classical NF-κB pathway, IκB proteins are phosphorylated, polyubiquinylated, and degraded within the proteasome, which causes the release of NF-κB dimmers that translocate to the nucleus and regulate gene activity. Recent reports indicate that CD86 stimulation on a B cell activates the classical NF-κB pathway, which leads to a protein kinase C-3 (PKC-3)-independent phosphorylation and degradation of IκBα and subsequent nuclear localization of P50/P65. CD86 is also reported to increase the phosphorylation of P65 in a PKC-dependent manner.[26] It has been reported that cross-linking CD40 on B cells rapidly activates NF-κB.[27]

REVERSE COSTIMULATION OF APCS

Many studies since then have shown the significance of CD80 and CD86 in influencing the activity of B cells, stem cells, DCs, and macrophages. Recently, many reports have appeared in literature highlighting the role of bidirectional signaling (reverse costimulation) through different costimulatory molecules into APCs and in particular DCs. Reverse signaling through CD80, CD86, B7-DC, CD40L, and OX40 has been shown to regulate the immune functions of DCs. It has been shown that cross-linking of B7-DC, a member of B7 family on DC, modulates its biology by increasing survival, antigen presentation, IL-12p70 production, and migration to draining lymph nodes.[19–21,28] This indicates that B7-DC can deliver directly to DCs. As we know, DCs has two states: the immature DCs that perform sentinel functions, sampling for antigen, and danger signals, and the mature DCs that perform enhanced APC functions but are no longer capable of acquiring the antigen. However, recently a new DC activation phenotype has been achieved when mature DCs were cross-linked with B7-DC. This B7-DC cross-linking restored the antigen-acquiring function of immature DCs and augmented APC function of matured DCs.[22] During a normal T-cell response, CD40 on DC is engaged by CD40L, which is transiently expressed on activated CD4+ Th cells. CD40 molecules are thereby cross-linked, which induce DC maturation and enable them to efficiently present antigen to T cells. Agonistic ligation of anti-CD40 Ab effectively helps the Th cells in DC maturation. Hence, the ligation of CD40 induces maturation of DCs and could be a useful target for vaccines.[29] Ligation of CD40 on DCs promotes upregulation of the costimulatory molecules CD80 and CD86,[30] IL-12 secretion, and release of chemokines such as IL-8, macrophage inflammatory protein (MIP)-1α, and MIP-1β.[31,32] DCs also up-regulate OX40L, another member of the tumor necrosis factor (TNF) super family in response to CD40 ligation. OX40L binding to OX40 costimulatory molecule enhances production of cytokines such as TNF-α, IL-12, IL-1, and IL-6 by DCs, and also induces the expression of costimulatory molecules.[32,33]

Very recently, it has been shown that CD28 induces immunostimulatory signals in DC via CD80 and CD86. Logue and Sha have indicated that CD28-B7 bidirectional signaling is a two-way street to activation of DC.[34] Bidirectional signaling along the B7-CTLA-4 coreceptor pathway enables reciprocal stimulation of T cells and DCs. Binding of CD28 to CD80/CD86 ligands leads to enhanced production of IL-6 by DCs.[23] However, binding of CD152 to CD80/CD86 augments the secretion of interferon-γ (IFN-γ), which in turn upregulates the expression of the enzyme indolamine 2,3-dioxygenase (IDO) in DCs, resulting in tryptophan catabolism and suppression of T-cell proliferation.[23] Further, ligation of CD86 leads to antiapoptotic signals.[35] It has been shown that CD86 is recruited to lipid rafts upon T-cell–DC interaction. In this bidirectional interaction between CD28 on a T cell and CD86 on the DC, naive CD4 + T cells receive their costimulatory signal and the DCs appear to respond by reorganizing their CD86 to lipid rafts.[36,37] Although the functional significance of CD86 response remains to be determined, the fact that the ligation and recruitment of CD86 to lipid rafts are required for the appearance of phosphorylated serines in rafts supports the idea that this is a mutually beneficial interaction that modulates not only T cell but also DC signaling. These findings on DCs also further confirm the interaction between CD80/CD86 and CD28/CD152 that delivers a bidirectional costimulation, which activates both T cells and DCs.

ROLE OF CD80 AND CD86 IN THE COSTIMULATION OF B CELLS

Although many costimulatory molecules, such as CD80, CD86, CD40, heat-stable antigen, intercellular adhesion molecule, vascular cell adhesion molecule, B7-DC/programmed death ligand-2 (PD-L2), B7-H1/programmed death ligand-1 (PD-L1), are known to be expressed on the surface of APCs. However, the best-defined costimulatory molecules are two structurally related proteins known as CD80 (B7-1) and CD86 (B7-2). Both CD80 and CD86 have their ligands, CD28 and CTLA-4, expressed on T cells (Table 2.2). It has been established recently that CD80 and CD86 play a role in the activation of APCs.[19] Stimulation via CD86 in B cells can modulate their proliferation, IgG secretion and expression of proapoptotic and antiapoptotic molecules, nuclear localization of NF-κB (p50) subunit, and phosphorylation of v-rel reticuloendotheliosis viral oncogene homolog A (Rel-A) (p65) and IκBα; and increase oct-2 expression.[18,25–27] We have investigated the impact of CD80 and CD86 on B cells.[19] Signaling in LPS-stimulated B cells was delivered through CD80 and CD86 molecules by their respective Abs. Exciting features observed during the study were that cross-linking of CD86 enhanced the proliferation and

TABLE 2.2 Characteristics of CD80 and CD86 Costimulatory Molecules

Characteristic	CD80 (B7-1)	CD86 (B7-2)
Expression	B cell, macrophage, DC	B cell, macrophage, DC
Kinetics of expression	Induced slowly and expressed for a longer duration (4–5 days)	Expression is modulated rapidly but stays for short duration (48 h)
Ligand	CD28, CD152	CD28, CD152
CD152 association	Faster association and slower dissociation rates	Faster association and dissociation rates
CD152 binding affinity	high	low
Sequence Identity	25%	25%
Structure	Dimer	Monomer
Location	Transmembrane	Transmembrane
Antibody blockade	Enhances immune response	Attenuates immune response

production of IgG1 and IgG2a Abs. In contrast, anti-CD80 Ab could reduce the proliferation and production of IgG1 and IgG2a Abs. Importantly, anti-CD80 Ab could also retard the growth of B cells and upregulate the expression of proapoptotic molecules (Figure 2.3). The involvement of Fas and FasL expression in B cells in inducing apoptosis was demonstrated by flow cytometry. In addition, the association of CD80 and CD86 molecules in the regulation of the activation of pro- and antiapoptotic molecules [Fas, FasL, FADD, FAP, FAF, TRAIL (Fas2L), TNFR (p55), TRADD, RIP, Bcl-w, Bfl-1, Bcl-x(L), Bak, Bax, Bcl-2, Bad, caspase-3, caspase-8] was examined by ribonuclease protection assay in B cells.[26] We observed that signaling through CD80 molecule mainly augmented the levels of proapoptotic molecules, that is, caspase-3, caspase-8, Fas, FasL, Bak, and Bax, and downregulated the expression of Bcl-x(L) and Bfl-1 (Figures 2.4). This suggests that CD80 signaling induces apoptosis via mechanisms involving proapoptotic molecules rendering the cells more vulnerable to apoptosis and therefore restricting their proliferation. In contrast, signaling through CD86 increased the expression of antiapoptotic molecules Bcl-w and Bcl-x(L) and downregulated the expression of caspase-8 (Figures. 2.4). Thus, there may be a possibility that ligation of CD86 on B cells may promote their survival by increasing the expression of antiapoptotic proteins. It is worth mentioning here that we demonstrated the role of CD80 and CD86 not only in

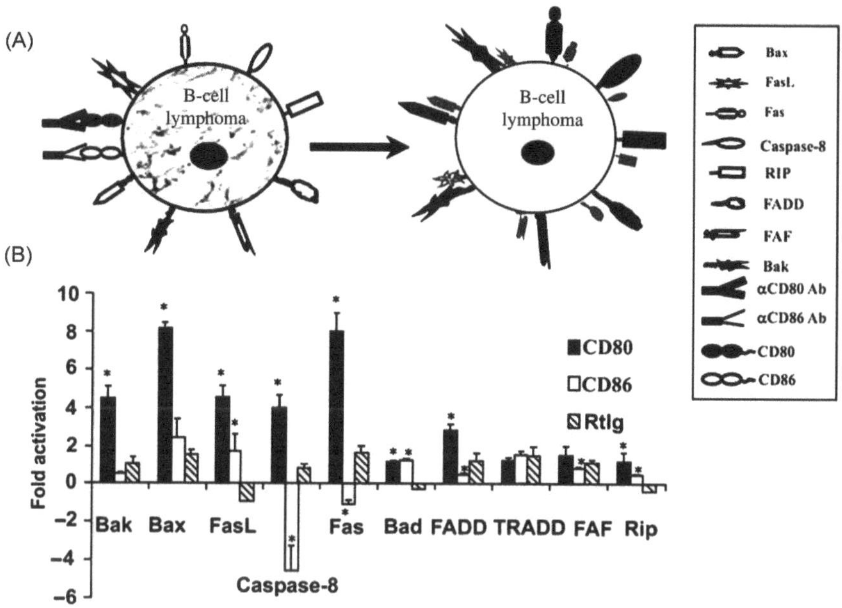

FIGURE 2.3 **Modulation of the expression of proapoptotic molecules by CD80 and CD86 signaling.** (A) The normal expression of proapoptotic molecules (open symbols) on B-cell lymphoma. Signaling through CD80 significantly upregulates Fas, FasL, caspase-8, Bak, Bax, and FADD (solid symbols) and triggering through CD86 downregulates caspase-8 (gray color symbols). (B) The WEHI-279 cells were cultured with anti-CD80 Ab, anti-CD86 Ab, and RtIg, and cross-linked with anti-RtIg Ab. Total RNA was extracted from the cells by the guanidinium isothiocyanate-phenol-chloroform method using Trizol reagent. The expression was determined using the RiboQuant multiprobe RNase protection assay system. The figure depicts the summary of results of Suvas et al.[19] The resulting resolved bands were imaged using a phosphor imager. The normalized quantity for each band was obtained by dividing with L32 housekeeping gene control. The old change was calculated by dividing the value of normalized quantity of the experimental samples with that of cells cultured with medium alone and is expressed as mean ± SD obtained from two experiments. "*" indicates that $P < 0.001$ employing Student's t test.

case of B cells isolated from mouse splenocytes but also for B-cell lymphomas.[19] Because B-cell lymphomas (WEHI-279 and A20) are 100% B cells, this finding therefore rules out any involvement of cytokines secreted by contaminating T cells in activating B cells. After our report,[19] many reports in literature started accumulating which demonstrate the role of CD80 and CD86 in bidirectional signaling of APCs.[25–28,34,38–44] CD86 cross-linking studies on CD40 ligand and IL-4-activated B cells have shown that there is increase in the rate and level of IgG1 transcription, nuclear localization of NF-κB p50 subunit, and phosphorylation of Rel-A (p65) and IκBα. It also increased oct-2 expression and binding to the 3′Ig H enhancer. These effects do not occur in CD86−/− B cells.[25,26,41,42] It has also been demonstrated that increased expression of Bcl-x(L)

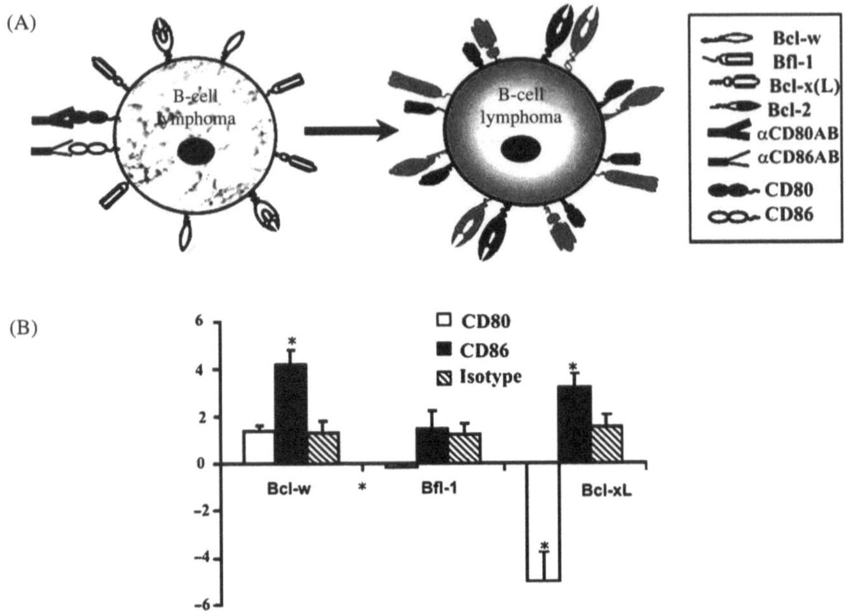

FIGURE 2.4 **Modulation of the expression of antiapoptotic molecules by CD80 and CD86 signaling.** (A) The normal expression of antiapoptotic molecules (open symbols) on B-cell lymphoma. Signaling through CD80 significantly downregulates Bcl-x(L) and Bfl-1 (solid symbols) and triggering through CD86 upregulates Bcl-w and Bcl-x(L) (gray color symbols). (B) The WEHI-279 cells were cultured for 72 h with anti-CD80 Ab, anti-CD86 Ab, and RtIg, and cross-linked with anti-RtIg Ab. Total RNA was extracted from the cells by the guanidinium isothiocyanate-phenol-chloroform method using Trizol reagent. The expression was determined using the RiboQuant multiprobe RNase protection assay system. The figure depicts the summary of results of Suvas et al.[19] The resulting resolved bands were imaged using a phosphor imager. The normalized quantity for each band was obtained by dividing with L32 housekeeping gene control. The -fold change was calculated by dividing the value of normalized quantity of the experimental samples with that of cells cultured with medium alone and are expressed as mean ± SD obtained from two experiments. "*" indicates that $P < 0.001$ employing Student's *t* test.

but not Bcl-2 can prevent the apoptosis in B-cell lymphoma. Moreover, signaling through CD40 upregulated Bcl-x(L) and Bfl-1, and protected B-cell lymphoma from apoptosis.[45,46] Thus, this finding accurately establishes that CD80 and CD86 not only costimulate T cells on ligation with CD28/CD152 but can also influence B cells through bidirectional costimulation, consequently not only modulating the activity of T cells but also of B cells.

ROLE OF BIDIRECTIONAL COSTIMULATION IN THE ACTIVATION OF DCS

Many studies have now established the role of reverse costimulation through CD80/CD86 and B7-DC costimulatory molecules in the modulation of activity of DCs. It has been shown that CD86 is recruited to lipid rafts upon T-cell–DC interaction. In this bidirectional interaction between CD28 on a T cell and CD86 on the DC, naive CD4+ T cells receive their costimulatory signal and the DCs appear to respond by reorganizing their CD86 to lipid rafts.[36,37] Although the functional significance of CD86 response remains to be determined, the fact that the ligation and recruitment of CD86 to lipid rafts are required for the appearance of phosphorylated serines in rafts supports the idea that this is a mutually beneficial interaction that modulates not only T cell but also DC signaling. Cross-linking of B7-DC, a member of B7 family on DCs, modulates the DC biology by increasing their survival, antigen presentation, IL-12p70 production, and migration to lymph nodes.[28,43,44] These findings on DCs further confirm the interaction between CD80/CD86 and CD28/CD152 that delivers a bidirectional costimulation, which activates both T cells and APCs. Logue and Sha have indicated that CD28-B7 bidirectional signaling is a two-way street to activation of DC. Engagement of B7 molecules on DCs by the CTLA-4–immunoglobulin (CTLA-4–Ig) fusion protein or by CTLA-4 expressed on regulatory T cells induces expression of the T-cell–tolerogenic enzyme IDO in DCs, which catabolizes tryptophan and leads to inhibition of T-cell function.[23,47] In an unexpected twist to those studies, in this issue of *Nature Immunology*, Orabona et al.[38] have revisited those experiments using CD28-Ig to engage B7 molecules on DCs and report notably different effector outcomes for treated DCs3. CD28-Ig treatment, in contrast to CTLA-4–Ig treatment, leads to production of IL-6 from DCs that squelches the previously described IFN-γ-driven immunosuppressive pathway of tryptophan catabolism in DCs. Engagement of B7 molecules on DCs by CD28-Ig thus results in activated DCs, whereas engagement of B7 molecules on DCs by CTLA-4–Ig results in tolerogenic DCs. Induction of tolerogenic IDO in DCs by CTLA-4–Ig treatment involves multiple steps. Engagement of B7 molecules by CTLA-4–Ig leads to the activation of several intracellular signaling pathways in DCs: the transcription factor NF-κB, the kinase p38 mitogen-activated protein kinase (MAPK), and the transcriptional activator STAT1. These activated DCs secrete IFN-γ, which, in an autocrine or paracrine way, promotes the subsequent expression of IDO by DCs.[23] IFN-γ does not seem to be absolutely required for IDO expression, as IFN-γ receptor-deficient DCs can still upregulate IDO in response to CTLA-4–Ig treatment. IDO expression by DCs promotes tolerance by catabolizing tryptophan, leading to a local decrease in tryptophan and an increase in catabolic by-products that inhibit T-cell proliferation and may also induce apoptotic death. In contrast to results with CTLA-4–Ig treatment, Orabona et al.[38] report that DCs treated with CD28-Ig secrete IL-6, in addition to IFN-γ, and do not undergo upregulation of IDO expression (Figure 2.5). This failure to induce the IDO immunosuppressive pathway by CD28-Ig treatment does not seem to be due to inadequate engagement of B7 molecules on DCs, but instead depends

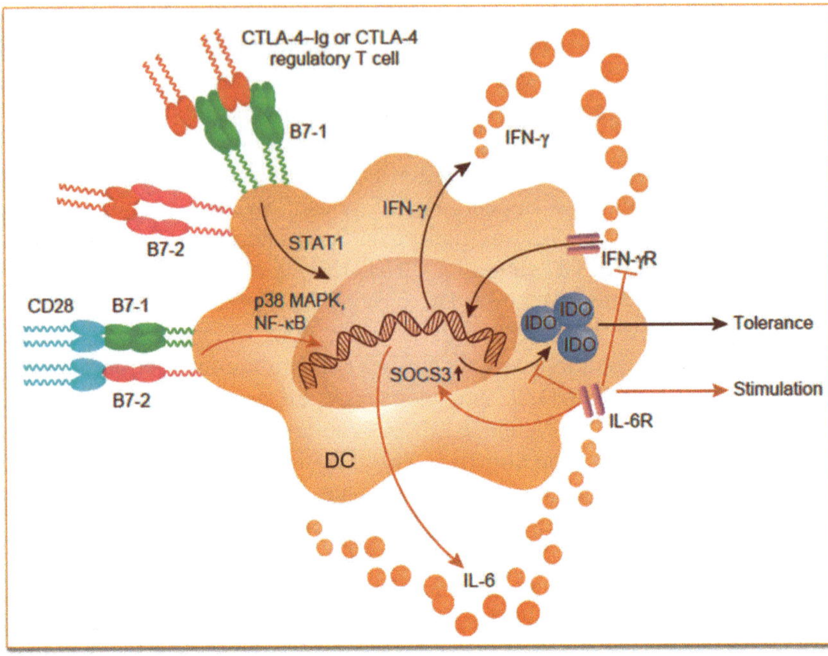

FIGURE 2.5 **Distinct effector responses in DCs treated with CTLA-4–Ig and CD28-Ig.** CTLA-4–Ig engagement of B7 molecules on DCs leads to activation of STAT1, p38 MAPK, and NF-κB, which stimulates the DC to produce IFN-γ. In an autocrine or paracrine way, IFN-γ promotes upregulation of IDO, an enzyme that catabolizes tryptophan and leads to potent inhibition of T-cell responses. CD28-Ig engagement of B7 molecules on DCs, however, results in concomitant secretion of both IL-6 and IFN-γ. IL-6, in an autocrine or paracrine way, inhibits the IFN-γ-driven upregulation of IDO through downregulation of the IFN-γ receptor (IFN-γR) and upregulation of suppressor of cytokine signaling-3 (SOCS-3). IL-6 effects are thus dominant in CD28-Ig-treated DCs and lead to DCs capable of enhanced cell-mediated immunity. IL-6R, IL-6 receptor.

critically on IL-6 secretion. Blockade of IL-6 signaling restores IDO expression in CD28-Ig-treated DCs, indicating that IL-6 effects are dominant over IFN-γ effects in CD28-Ig-treated DCs. The basis for the unique induction of IL-6 secretion in DCs treated with CD28-Ig but not those treated with CTLA-4–Ig is unclear, as both fusion proteins activate MAPK and NF-κB pathways, albeit with different kinetics. The three different *in vivo* models used by Orabona et al.[38] demonstrate the potential for CD28-Ig to be used as an adjuvant. This adjuvant activity is clearly demonstrated, as CD28-Ig conditioning of DCs results in enhanced reactivity in a skin test assay using poorly immunogenic peptides and also allows a normally nonprotective DCs pulsed with hyphae to become protective in an infectious model using *Candida albicans*. This adjuvant effect of CD28-Ig is further demonstrated in a tumor model in which CD28-Ig injection allows for the eradication of a poorly immunogenic tumor through the enhancement of the antitumor cytotoxic T lymphocyte (CTL) response and reduction of regulatory T-cell-suppressive activity. As with the *in vitro* studies of CD28-Ig, the *in vivo* adjuvant activity of CD28-Ig in all three models seems to depend critically on IL-6 signaling. These data suggest that CD28-Ig treatment could be a valuable tool to enhance immune responses during vaccination or to induce antitumor immune responses. In addition to the potential clinical implications for using CD28-Ig therapeutically, the findings by Orabona et al.[38] raise several intriguing questions. Does the adjuvant effect of CD28 as a fusion protein also extend to bidirectional activation of DCs by T cells expressing endogenous CD28? The original observation of CTLA-4–Ig inhibition of DCs has since been extended to endogenous regulation in studies, demonstrating that regulatory T cells, which have high constitutive CTLA-4 expression, can activate IDO expression on DCs through a CTLA-4-dependent mechanism.[47] Orabona et al.[38] found that IL-6 was also secreted when CD28 expressed on the surface of Jurkat cells was used to stimulate DCs, suggesting that the stimulatory effects of CD28 could also be relevant to natural cellular interactions between T cells and DCs. Although it is clear that engagement of B7 molecules leads to alterations in DC function, the most proximal signaling events elicited by CD28-Ig and CTLA-4–Ig treatment remain murky. In contrast to CD28 and CTLA-4, whose function as receptors is better understood, the cytoplasmic tails of B7 molecules have so far yielded very few insights into potential biochemical signaling mechanisms at the level of modification or association with other signaling molecules. The need to address this issue is emphasized by the demonstration in the article of Orabona et al.[38] that engagement of B7 molecules on DCs by CD28 and CTLA-4 fusion proteins can lead to notable functional differences in DCs.

Studies have begun to demonstrate previously unrecognized structural and biophysical differences between CD28 and CTLA-4, as well as between B7-1 and B7-2, that may underlie functional differences mediated by these costimulatory molecules.[48] In addition to the approximately 20-fold higher affinity of CTLA-4 versus CD28 for B7 molecules, it is now recognized that although both CD28 and CTLA-4 are structurally dimers, dimeric CD28 can bind only one B7 molecule, whereas CTLA-4 can bind two B7 molecules.[49] It is unclear whether these differences in valency and affinity of B7 binding underlie the functional differences observed by Orabona et al.[38] between CTLA-4–Ig and CD28-Ig treatment. B7-1 and B7-2 can also exert an unexpected degree of control over localization of CD28 and CTLA-4 during immunological synapse formation. Because B7-1 is a dimer, whereas B7-2 is a monomer, CTLA-4 will preferentially form extensive arrays with B7-1 but not with B7-2.[50–52] These affinity differences between CD28 and CTLA-4 binding to B7-1 and B7-2 allow selective recruitment of CTLA-4 to the immunological synapse to be mediated principally by B7-1 and selective recruitment of CD28 to the immunological synapse to be mediated by B7-2.[53] In sum, the cell-extrinsic adjuvant effect of CD28-Ig on DCs reported by Orabona et al.[38] provides an unexpected symmetry to the cell-intrinsic stimulatory effect of CD28 on T cells and indicates that CD28 and CTLA-4 as ligands of B7 molecules can signal DCs to initiate distinct effector responses. The potential for costimulatory molecules to exert both cell-intrinsic and cell-extrinsic regulation of effector responses is likely to also be relevant to newer members of the CD28–B7 family costimulatory molecules.[54] Cross-linking of the B7 family member PD-L2 on DCs, for example, has also been shown to activate the immune function of DCs.[28] Furthermore, the broader expression of more recently discovered CD28–B7 costimulatory molecules, such as the inhibitory PD-1 receptor expressed on activated T and B cells, suggests the potential for previously unknown immune regulation through bidirectional signaling. Further, it has been shown that CD28 induces immunostimulatory signals in DC via CD80 and CD86. Bidirectional signaling along the B7–CTLA-4 coreceptor pathway enables reciprocal stimulation of T cells and DCs. Binding of CD28 to CD80/CD86 ligands lead to enhanced production of IL-6 by DCs.[38,55] However, binding of CD152 to CD80/CD86 augments the secretion of IFN-γ, which in turn up-regulates the expression of the enzyme IDO in DCs, resulting in tryptophan catabolism and suppression of T-cell proliferation.[23,56,57]

ROLE OF REVERSE COSTIMULATION ON MACROPHAGES

We have investigated the impact of costimulation on macrophages. In this study, we have attempted to analyze the distinct role of CD80, CD86, and CD40 costimulatory molecules in the activation of macrophages and their influence on the survival of intracellular pathogens. The following five major findings have emerged from this study: (1) Costimulation through CD80, CD86, and CD40 augmented the release of nitric oxide (NO), IL-1, IL-6, and TNF-α; (2) CD80, CD86, and CD40 worked synergistically with IFN-γ in the production of NO, IL-1, IL-6, TNF-α, and IL-12; (3) CD80 and CD86 modulated the expression of CD14, CD206, CD80, CD86, MHC-I, and MHC-II molecules; (4) triggering of CD86 and CD40 but not CD80 increased the uptake of soluble and particulate antigens; and (5) engagement of mainly CD80 reduced the survival of intracellular pathogens.[58] The enhanced secretion of NO by macrophages on costimulation by CD86 molecule will help in the eradication of intracellular infections. Augmented release of NO by macrophages is known to be beneficial in case of many intracellular infections. These results further substantiate our earlier findings[19] and are now endorsed by other groups as well; the finding that signals delivered through CD80 and CD86 can affect the function of APCs. Because B7-1/B7-2 activates the induction of TNF-α as well as reactive oxygen species and bactericidal activity in macrophages, anti-B7-1/anti-B7-2 mAb treatment can be used to tailor immune responses to induce cytotoxicity against intracellular pathogens that reside inside the macrophages.[58] This approach may be limited not only to *Mycobacterium tuberculosis* but also to other infections, including AIDS, leishmania, and malaria. This novel strategy can also be effectively exploited to develop immunotherapy using humanized Abs against B7-1 and B7-2 or CD28 fusinogenic proteins for the treatment of intracellular pathogens because this approach is based on modulating the immune system of the host rather than targeting the pathogen; hence, it diminishes the chances of emergence of drug-resistant strains of bacteria. Our results have important implications for the efforts to establish a vaccine against intracellular pathogens, such as *M. tuberculosis* and *Salmonella typhimurium*, because they suggest that vectors that induce/upregulate the expression of costimulatory ligands on APCs such as macrophages (which are also the host for *M. tuberculosis*) will help to generate a protective IFN-γ-dependent immune response, which is desired in tuberculosis.

In another study, the functional significance of costimulatory interactions between decidual macrophages (DMs) and T cells with a particular focus on B7-H1:PD-1 signaling was investigated. It was observed that human DMs suppress IFN-γ production by T cells through costimulatory B7-H1:PD-1 signaling in early pregnancy.[59] On analysis, the expression profile of B7 ligands on human DMs revealed that B7-H1 was present on DMs isolated from early but not term pregnancies. B7-H1 was not expressed on the peripheral monocytes (PMs) of pregnant women. In response to IFN-γ, B7-H1 expression was induced on PMs and was enhanced on DMs, suggesting that this cytokine might be a key factor in the control of B7-H1 expression in the decidua. The majority of decidual T cells were noted to exhibit robust expression of PD-1, whereas the expression was limited to a small subpopulation of circulating T cells. Functional assays demonstrated that DMs are able to suppress T-cell IFN-γ production via B7-H1–PD-1 interactions. This suppressive property was not observed for PMs, which lack B7-H1. B7-H1 on DMs may function as a key regulator of local IFN-γ production and therefore contribute to the development of appropriate maternal immune responses to the fetus in early pregnancy.[59]

In another study, it was observed that there was early induction of suppressor of cytokine signaling-1 (SOCS-1), and the downregulation of toll-like receptors (TLRs) 7 and 9 induces tolerance in costimulated macrophages.[60] In this study, mouse macrophages were simultaneously stimulated with the TLR7 agonist, gardiquimod, and the TLR9 agonist, CpG ODN 1826, to examine the mechanism and effector functions of macrophage tolerance. Compared with individual stimulation, the costimulation of both TLRs reduced the secretion of TNF-α and IL-6 through the delayed activation of the NF-κB pathway; notably, IL-10 remained unchanged in costimulated macrophages. This tolerance reflected the early induction of SOCS-1, according to the detection of elevated TNF-α secretion and restored NF-κB signaling in response to the small interference RNA-mediated abrogation of SOCS-1 signaling. In addition, the restimulation of each TLRs using the same ligand significantly reduced the expression of both TLRs in endosomes. These findings revealed that the costimulation of TLR7 and TLR9 induced macrophage tolerance via SOCS-1, and the restimulation of each receptor or both TLR7 and TLR9 downregulated TLR expression through a negative feedback mechanism that protects the host from excessive inflammatory responses. Moreover, the insufficient and impaired immune response in chronic viral infection might also reflect the repeated and simultaneous stimulation of those endosomal TLRs.[60]

APPLICATION OF REVERSE COSTIMULATION IN DISEASES

Many reports on *in vivo* studies reveal the distinct role of CD80 and CD86 in diseases. We have for the first time reported that signals delivered via CD80 into B-cell lymphomas restrict their growth by modulating the expression of antiapoptotic molecules.[19] Thus, providing a novel insight into the mechanism where triggering through CD80 could control the growth of lymphomas. These observations constitute a rationale for development of a therapy using anti-CD80 Ab for cancer cells that express CD80 molecule. Interestingly, after our report, clinical studies evaluated anti-CD80 Ab as a targeted therapy for lymphomas with promising results.[61,62] Reverse costimulation has been used in CD80-positive hematologic malignancies [e.g., diffuse large B-cell non-Hodgkin's lymphoma (NHL), chronic lymphocytic leukemia, Hodgkin's disease, and multiple myeloma] and has showed promising results.[61,62] CD80 and CD86 have been shown to have differential effects on the development of spontaneous autoimmune diabetes in nonobese diabetic mice. Ab neutralization of CD80 has been shown to exacerbate diabetes, whereas neutralization of CD86 was shown to abrogate the development of diabetes.[63] Differential effects of signaling by CD80 and CD86 have also been demonstrated in other autoimmune models, including lupus nephritis in the Murphy Roths large (MRL)-lpr/lpr mice and experimental autoimmune encephalomyelitis (EAE). The animals lacking CD86 showed diminished renal Ig deposition and attenuated pathology, but CD80-deficient animals developed more severe nephritis.[64,65] Recently, a novel regulatory role for CD80-mediated intracellular signals in CD4+ T cells has been shown to have important implications in the relapse of EAE.[26] It has been established that *in vivo* blockade of CD86 costimulation could suppress maternal immune attack to the fetus.[66] Further, cross-linking of CD80 on the surface of neural stem cells *in vitro* enhances apoptosis.[40] Besides this, CD80 and CD86 have been implicated to have opposing roles in regulation of xenotransplantation rejection, where CD80 drives cell-mediated rejection (CMR) and attenuates acute vascular rejection (AVR), whereas CD86 drives AVR. Remarkably, indefinite xenograft survival can be achieved by suppressing AVR with CD86 neutralization in combination of cyclosporine A therapy, which inhibits CMR.[67] An important question arises in the studies using Abs, whether the influence of anti-CD80 and CD86 Abs arises due to obstruction of the interaction of T cells with APCs or due to signaling delivered by Abs. It is evident from the recently published work that triggering through CD80 can *vis-à-vis* deliver signals as well.[16,19,61,62]

Based on the pleiotropic activities of the CD28/CD152–CD80/CD86 pathway mentioned above, it can thus be exploited for the potential clinical usefulness in immune intervention in diseases such as autoimmunity, transplant rejection, and allergy, and in the elimination of tumors that evade immune surveillance.[67–72] Hence, the interest lies in understanding the therapeutic manipulation of these costimulatory molecules. These molecules may provide a means to either promote immune responses against cancer or reduce graft rejection and autoimmunity. CD80/CD86 signaling/blockade by CTLA-4–Ig has been studied in clinical trials as treatment for severe psoriasis vulgaris, rheumatoid arthritis, multiple sclerosis, lupus nephritis, and renal transplantation.[71,72] Importantly, the experimental data showing distinct functions of CD80 and CD86 in regulating the immune response in various disease models underscore the need to design tailor-made therapeutic strategies for humans for preventing transplant rejection and treatment of autoimmune diseases. Some of the studies done recently have established the therapeutic potential of Abs against CD80 and CD86.[19,61,62,72] However, it is imperative to evaluate their clinical significance in other diseases as well. In the case of autoimmune diseases and allergy, it will be worth studying the role of signaling through CD80/CD86 in promoting clonal deletion of highly pathogenic auto-reactive B and T cells (Figure 2.6).

REVERSE COSTIMULATION THROUGH CD80 (B7-1)

CD80 is a costimulatory molecule known for its role in T-cell activation and also in regulating the activity of normal and malignant B cells.[19] Surface CD80 is expressed transiently on activated B cells, macrophages, and DCs. Surprisingly, CD80 is downregulated on most of the cancer cells, and the loss of CD80 alone is sufficient to allow them to escape the attack of the immune system and to impart anergy and apoptosis in tumor-infiltrating T cells.[73] In the absence of costimulation, recognition of antigens by T cells may not cause any response, even if tumor cells express MHC molecules and tumor-specific antigens (Figure 2.7). Hence, most human malignancies that lack CD80 expression have been suggested to evade immune surveillance and therefore contribute for failure of immune recognition.[74] However, follicular lymphomas express CD80 and therefore could potentially be targeted by CD80 immunotherapies. Lack of either CD80 or MHC-I must be sufficient to allow tumor cells to evade immune response, but it has been shown in some tumors that high expression of MHC-I and absence of costimulatory molecules render them resistant to lysis by CTLs (Figure 2.7A). It has been shown that high expression of MHC-I but lack of CD80 does not

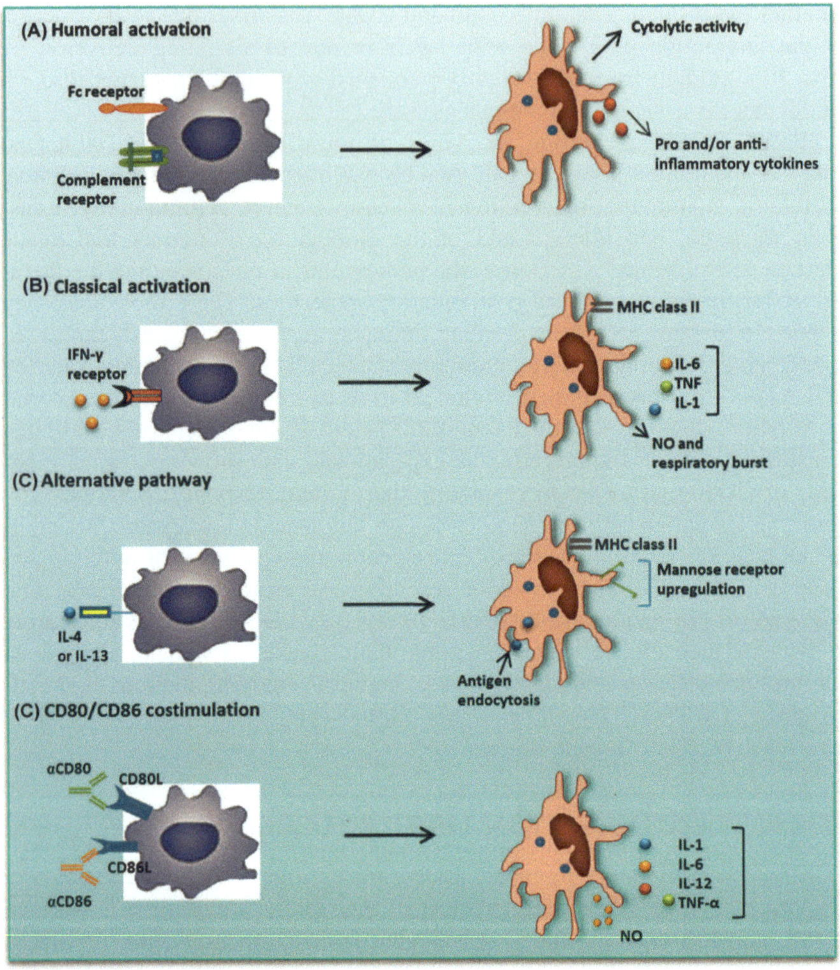

FIGURE 2.6 **Reverse costimulation activation pathways of macrophages.** Macrophages are activated by pathways of innate and acquired immunity. Innate activation of macrophages occurs by microbial stimuli that are recognized TLRs, CD14 (LPS receptor), and a range of nonopsonic receptors. (A) Humoral activation is mediated by some Fc and complement receptors. (B) Classical activation is mediated by the priming stimulus of IFN-γ, followed by a microbial trigger. (C) Alternate activation is mediated by IL-4 and IL-13 acting through a common receptor chain IL-4Rα. (D) Costimulatory activation of macrophages occurs by delivery of signals through CD80 and CD86 molecules. This whole figure depicts that in addition to well-known innate, humoral, classical, and alternate activation, macrophages can also be activated by delivery of signals through CD80 and CD86 molecules.

allow cytolysis of target cells by CTLs *ex vivo*. In contrast, CD80-transfected tumor cells become susceptible to lysis by CTLs *ex vivo*. Although priming of antitumor CTLs can also take place in absence of CD80, the effector T cells are not produced without the expression of CD80 on tumor cells.[75]

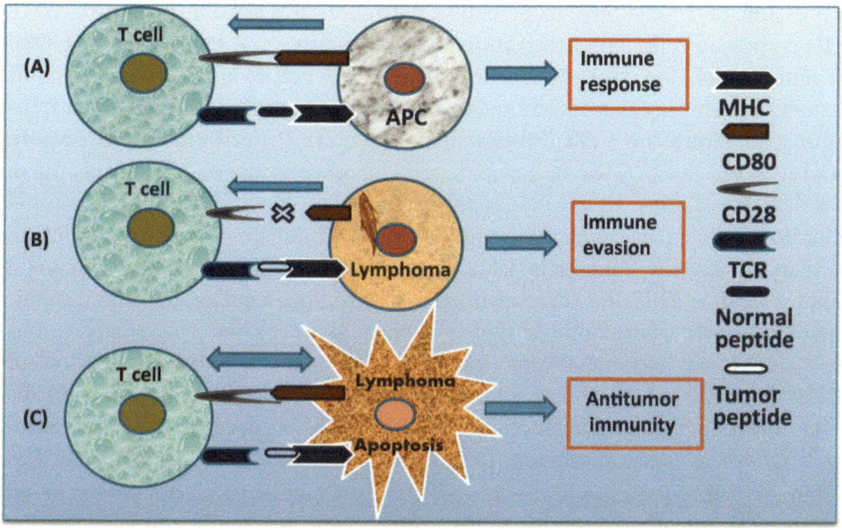

FIGURE 2.7 Reverse costimulation through CD80 in modulating the activity of tumor cells. When a normal cell presents MHC–peptide molecule complex to T cells, the delivery of CD80 costimulatory signal generates an effective immune response (A). Efficient presentation of peptide in association with MHC but in absence of costimulation induces immunological ignorance in T cells and immune evasion in cancer cells (B). Presentation of tumor-peptide–MHC complex and expression of CD80 costimulatory molecule on tumor cells leads to its apoptosis and elicitation of antitumor immunity by the activation of T cells and reverse costimulation (↔) through the CD80 molecule (C).

Interestingly, CD80 has also been known to enhance the memory response in CTLs.[76] This suggests that CD80 expression on tumor is important for antitumor CTL effector function. Expression of CD80 on tumor cells confers direct presentation capacity to prime naive CTLs *in vivo*.[77] Transfection of tumor cells with CD80 will help in generating long-lasting immunity. Therefore, this approach may lead to the development of a successful vaccine against cancer.

CD80 expression is needed for the sustained predominance of CD8+ T cells within a tumor (Figure 2.7C). Transfection of CD80 cDNA into human erythroleukemia DR+ cells induces the allogeneic response of purified T cells from both the cord blood and the peripheral blood of adult donors, demonstrating that CD80 expression could lead to accessory cell-independent activation of naive T cells. Furthermore, in the P815 tumor system, CD86 was substituted for CD80; interestingly, no specific CTL activity was observed. Even though in the tumors that express CD86 there is a need for CD80 expression by host APCs for efficient eradication.[78] Thus, it is apparent that transfection of CD80 in tumor cell serves as a cofactor for IL-2 production and in prevention of anergy by TCR ligation.[79] This suggests that expression of CD80 on cancer cells contributes toward the activation of T cells responsible for imparting anticancer immunity. The expression of CD80 on tumor cells also enhances natural killer (NK) cell recognition and lysis of tumors, which plays an important role in tumor immunity.[80] CD80 costimulation can direct the CD8 T cells to produce IL-2, proliferate, and acquire cytolytic activity.[81] This helper-independent generation of CTLs may have practical application in the development of tumor-specific immunotherapy.[82] Therefore, it is clear that downregulation of CD80 costimulatory molecule by various cancer cells acts as an effective immune evasion mechanism (Figure 2.7B). This has been reported in multiple myelomas, carcinomas, leukemias, and transplantable malignancies. Some of the colon carcinomas such as MC38 and melanomas such as B16 also lack the expression of CD80. This is evident from the fact that silencing of CD80 expression results in tumorigenicity and transfection of CD80 leads to decreased tumorigenicity.[83] CD80 expression triggers *in vitro* NK cell-mediated cytotoxicity. The CD80 gene product functions as a triggering signal for NK cell-mediated cytotoxicity and the strength of this response is such that it overrides the inhibitory signals mediated by MHC-I molecules.[4,84] The efficient control of solid allogeneic tumors by NK cells depends on the codelivery of both CD80 and MHC-I on the tumor cells. The codelivery is required for optimal expansion and effector function of NK cells in response to both melanoma and plasmocytoma that express allogeneic MHC-I. The two signals required for T-cell function can also regulate NK cell immunity and reveal an important similarity between the innate NK cell response and the adaptive T-cell response. Furthermore, it has been reported that NK cells and CD8 + T cells can eliminate CD80-expressing tumors that are resistant to IL-12 gene therapy.[85,86] Hence, expression of CD80 on tumor cells may also have an important bearing on NK cell effector function.

REVERSE COSTIMULATION THROUGH CTLA-4

Recent evidences indicate that engagement of CTLA-4 onto B7 molecules expressed on APCs influence immune responses by delivering suppressive signals into DCs.[23] It was shown that both a soluble form and a membrane-anchored form of CTLA-4 on regulatory T cells can activate the immunosuppressive pathway of tryptophan catabolism in DCs. Engagement of CD80/CD86 on murine DCs by CTLA-4–Ig activates STAT1 and downregulates the SOCS-3 pathway and ultimately stimulates DCs to produce IFN-γ, which acts in an autocrine or paracrine fashion to induce IDO, an enzyme that degrades tryptophan to by-products and inhibit T-cell proliferation.[23] Further, IDO production by this way has been shown to play an important role in maintaining maternal–fetal tolerance and suppressing T-cell responses to MHC-mismatched allograft, tumors and self-antigens.[87] The ligation of CTLA-4 on mouse CD4 + CD25 + regulatory T cells can mediate the same IDO-inducing effect *in vitro*.[47] CTLA-4–Ig, a fusion protein containing the extracellular domain of CTLA-4 linked to an IgG1 Fc region, can block the interaction of CD28 with B7-1 and B7-2 and suppress immune responses in multiple preclinical models of autoimmune and inflammatory disease.[88] However, exacerbations of disease are also seen in these preclinical models after treatment with CTLA-4–Ig,[88,89] complicating predictions for therapeutic use. Exacerbations might result from the blockade of B7-1 and B7-2 interactions with the inhibitory CTLA-4 receptor or from the loss of regulatory T-cell function, which is dependent on CD28 signaling.[90,91] The use of CTLA-4–Ig was first reported in patients with psoriasis vulgaris; some efficacy was observed, although statistical limitations of the trial design precluded identification of a robust therapeutic dose.[92] More recently, CTLA-4–Ig has been tested in combination with methotrexate (MTX) in clinical trials of rheumatoid arthritis.[93] In these studies, 2 or 10 mg/kg doses of CTLA-4–Ig were administered to patients on days 1, 15, and 30, and monthly thereafter for a total of 6 months; patients also received approximately 15 mg MTX per week. Evaluation at 6 months showed that a higher percentage of patients receiving 10 mg/kg CTLA-4–Ig/MTX had improved clinical scores compared with those on MTX alone ($P < 0.001$). Further studies will be needed to assess long-term efficacy and safety for CTLA-4–Ig, and to elucidate its mode of action in humans. However, these promising results suggest that manipulation of costimulatory signals can ameliorate inflammatory disease. CTLA-4 is a negative regulator of T-cell activation, and Abs that block CTLA-4 can enhance T-cell responses.[4] In a recent clinical trial, stage IV melanoma patients were treated with antihuman CTLA-4-Ab in combination with a gp100 melanoma-associated antigen peptide vaccine.[94] Some tumor regression was observed, although patient numbers were too small to draw conclusions on efficacy. Several patients developed manifestations of autoimmune responses in their skin, liver, or intestines, which appeared to resolve after discontinuation of Ab therapy. The autoimmune manifestations limited patient accrual but suggested that the anti-CTLA-4 Ab-enhanced immune responses. Similar autoimmune adverse events were seen in a second small clinical trial.[95] Alternative clinical approaches have explored the use of vaccination strategies with tumor cells expressing high levels of B7-1 or B7-2 to enhance tumor immunity, although robust clinical protocols have yet to emerge.[96–98]

B7-DC Reverse Costimulation

B7-DC does not only costimulate T-cell proliferation and IFN-γ production by T cells, but its cross-linking on DC also modulates DC biology. B7-DC cross-linking on DCs enhanced antigen presentation and IL-12p70 production *in vitro*. Furthermore, anti-B7-DC treatment increased the survival of

DCs *in vitro* and the migration of adoptively transferred DCs reaching draining lymph nodes *in vivo*.[21] B7-DC cross-linking has also been shown to restore the antigen-acquiring function of immature DCs and augments APC function of matured DCs.[28] This shows that B7-DC can function as a means for the communication of signals directly to DCs from ligands in the environment. One of the challenges in targeting the CD28/CTLA-4/B7 pathway has been the shared receptor–ligand interactions. Although CTLA-4–Ig can block stimulatory CD28 signals, it might also interfere with inhibitory CTLA-4 signals. Recent data also indicate that CTLA-4–Ig delivers "reverse signals" mediated by B7 ligands directly into the APC.[23,99] Alternative strategies to block B7 ligands using anti-B7 Abs have been promising in preclinical studies, including primate studies in transplantation[100] and many rodent autoimmune and inflammatory disease models.[90] Recent data indicate that B7-1 and B7-2 can signal into DCs, generating tolerogenic or immunogenic signals depending upon whether the B7s are engaged by CTLA-4 or CD28,[38] respectively, further suggesting that blockade using Abs to B7-1 and B7-2 may differ from using CTLA-4–Ig. Strategies to identify blocking Abs to CD28 for clinical use must consider potential immune activation mediated by unintentional cross-linking of CD28; this would also apply to use of blocking Abs to inducible costimulator (ICOS).[38] Although small molecules have been reported that block the interaction of B7-1 with CD28,[101,102] these are of limited potency, and there are no reports of small molecules that block the interactions of both B7-1 and B7-2 with CD28. Thus, new approaches that specifically target CD28 are needed. Additionally, approaches that spare CD28-dependent regulatory T cells would allow preservation of these important cells in inflammatory and autoimmune diseases. These results suggest that bidirectional B7–CTLA-4 interactions may participate in down-regulation of T-cell responses and induction of T-cell tolerance. Therefore, CTLA-4 not only regulates TCR and CD28 signals in T cells but also delivers signals through CD80/CD86 into DCs to induce IDO and the subsequent biological effects. Binding of CD28 to B7 ligands on DCs leads to up-regulation of IL-6 production by DCs and subsequent immunostimulatory effects on T-cell activation.[38] However, binding of CTLA-4 to B7 ligands upregulates IFN-γ, which then upregulates the expression of the enzyme, IDO, resulting in tryptophan catabolism and suppression of T-cell proliferation.[23,87]

Reverse Costimulation Through CD40L/CD40

The CD40–CD40L receptor–ligand interaction plays a central role in regulating the immune responses by activating and modulating DCs, macrophages, and T cells. CD40–CD40L interaction has been shown to induce CD80 and CD86 expression on other APCs, thereby promoting their costimulatory capacity. CD40 ligation with CD40L on DCs promotes the upregulation of the costimulatory molecules such as CD80 and CD86,[103,104] IL-12 secretion and release of chemokines such as IL-8, MIP-1α, and MIP-1β.[105–107] CD40 ligation has also been shown to upregulate the expression of OX40L, another member of the TNF super family on DCs. CD40L–CD40 interactions mediate B-cell proliferation without further costimulus. Central functions of the B cells, such as proliferation, up-regulation of membrane activation markers, isotype switching (in conjunction with different cytokines), regulation of apoptosis, and memory B-cell formation, are all dependent on signals provided through the CD40–CD40L interactions.[108,109] In order for the B cells to enter the cell cycle, produce Ig, and undergo Ig class switching or somatic hypermutation, it is necessary for them to receive the appropriate T-cell help through CD40–CD40L interaction.[110] It has been reported that CD28 ligation stabilizes CD40L mRNA, allowing for more rapid translation and transport of CD40L onto the T-cell surface, and therefore results in increased B-cell responses.[111]

The interrelationship between the CD28/B7 and CD40L/CD40 pathways plays an important role in the ability of B cells to present antigen. Resting B cells express little if any CD80 or CD86, but CD40 ligation induces their expression. B cells activated with anti-CD40 Ab stimulated an allogeneic MLR more efficiently, and this stimulation was blocked by human cytotoxic T-lymphocyte antigen-4–Ig. Further investigations have revealed that CD40 cross-linking by Ab or the interaction of CD40 with its ligand CD40L upregulated CD80 and CD86.[112] Incubation of resting B cells with activated T cells is another potent means of inducing CD80 and CD86. In this system, CD80 upregulation was inhibited by either anti-CD40 or CD40L Abs, consistent with the notion that CD40L/CD40 regulates CD80 expression. However, the CD40L antagonist did not completely inhibit the ability of activated T cells to upregulate CD86. Therefore, other signals mediated by MHC-II engagement or cytokines are also involved in CD86 regulation by activated T cells.

CD40 is an important regulator of macrophage function as it stimulates the production of TNF-α and other factors.[113] In the presence of IFN-γ, CD40 signaling enhances NO production and anti-*Leishmania* and anti-*Toxoplasma gondii* activity of macrophages.[114,115] However, it is not known whether CD40 can replace IFN-γ as the priming signal for induction of macrophage antimicrobial activity. However, it has been recently shown that CD40 signaling induces the antimicrobial activity of macrophages against intracellular pathogen *T. gondii* despite the lack of two central features of classically activated macrophages, that is, priming with IFN-γ and production of reactive nitrogen intermediates. This CD40 signaling primes macrophages in response to TNF-α to acquire antimicrobial activity.

Interaction between the CD40 receptor on APC and its ligand (CD40L) on activated T cells plays a critical role in immunity to intracellular pathogens by upregulating the production of IL-12.[116] CD40- or CD40L-deficient mice have an increased susceptibility to *Leishmania* infection and show an impaired priming of Th1-type cells, correlating with a lack of activation of the macrophage effector functions required for parasite clearance.[114] CD40 stimulation of bacillus calamite guerin-infected DCs not only promotes their ability to secrete IL-12 but increases the release of other inflammatory mediators such as IL-1α, IL-1β, and IL-6.[117] These may potentiate the development of inflammatory responses, which play a critical role in anti-mycobacterial immunity.

REVERSE SIGNALING THROUGH CD137L/CD137

CD137L is expressed in APCs and other myeloid cells (B cells, macrophages, DCs, mast cells, and eosinophils) and nonhematopoietic cells (endothelial cells, fibroblasts, and epithelial cells).[118] Evidence supporting that CD137L signals play an *in vivo* physiological role in inflammation is just being emerged, even though accumulating evidence has demonstrated the existence of CD137L signals at molecular and cellular levels. For example, CD137L signaling mediates cellular functions ranging from cell differentiation, proliferation, and survival to the production of inflammatory mediators in a variety of cells.[119]

It is now becoming clear that CD137L signaling is critical in multiple phases of inflammation. Inflamed vessels express CD137 and CD137L, and CD137L signaling in endothelial cells leads to the production of proinflammatory cytokines and chemokines.[120,121] Further, CD137L signaling may facilitate transendothelial migration of leukocytes through upregulation of cell adhesion molecules on endothelial cells.[120,121] However, CD137L signaling increases the expression of cell adhesion molecules on monocytes and promotes their extravasation. Because endothelial cells express both CD137 and CD137L, CD137–CD137L interactions between endothelial cells and leukocytes may amplify inflammation in such a way that endothelial cells induce sustained production of inflammatory mediators and prime leukocytes before they arrive at inflamed tissue territories. In the tissues, it seems that CD137L signaling in recruited leukocytes, residential cells, and parenchymal cells is also critical in the amplification of inflammation. Macrophages express CD137L on exposure to an inflammatory environment and produce high levels of proinflamatory cytokines and chemokines in response to CD137L signals.[122–124] In collaboration with other inflammatory inducers, CD137L signaling results in the production of inflammatory mediators in macrophages in a synergistic manner,[125] an indication that CD137L signaling is an amplifier of inflammation. It is noteworthy that CD137L can sustain TLR signaling by binding to TLRs without engagement of CD137.[124] Recently, we have identified a novel inflammatory pathway involving CD137L signaling in epithelial cells.[126] In kidney ischemia–reperfusion injury, CD137 expressed on infiltrated NK cells stimulates CD137L in tubular epithelial cells to produce CXCR1 and CXCR2 that are required for recruitment of neutrophils in the kidney. Because the kidney ischemia–reperfusion injury does not occur without NK cells or neutrophils, it is thought that the axis of NK cell tubular epithelial cell neutrophils is the major pathogenic pathway for kidney ischemia–reperfusion injury.[127]

There are few reports on the roles of CD137L signaling in disease context. As mentioned above, CD137L signaling is indispensable for kidney ischemia–reperfusion injury.[126] Considering that CD137L signaling is critical in inflammatory responses, it is predicted that milder inflammatory diseases will occur in the absence of CD137L signals. Indeed, we have demonstrated that blocking of CD137L can inhibit inflammatory responses and prevent mortality in *C. albicans*-induced sepsis (unpublished data). In this model, CD137 signaling enhances the phagocytic activity of neutrophils, whereas CD137L signaling induces massive cytokine production by macrophages following *C. albicans* infection. In this model, agonistic anti-CD137 mAb has dual beneficial effects on *C. albicans*-induced sepsis by promoting fungal clearance by neutrophils and downregulating cytokine production by macrophages.

Emerging evidence suggests that both CD137 and CD137L signals play an important role in the evolution of inflammation. CD137 signaling in lymphoid cells such as NK cells, NK T cells, and T cells promotes inflammation by producing IFN-γ and TNF-α. However, the outcomes of CD137 signaling in regulatory T cells and neutrophils are connected to the suppression of inflammation. CD137 signaling in regulatory T cells and NK cells induces production of immunosuppressive cytokines that directly decrease inflammation (unpublished result). CD137 signaling in neutrophils can facilitate pathogen clearance and thus contributes to rapid resolution of inflammation (unpublished results, Mir and Agrewala). CD137L signaling seems to always have proinflammatory actions.

Role of Reverse Costimulation in Cancer

Clinical studies have demonstrated that administration of anti-CD80 Ab can decrease tumor burden in patients suffering from lymphomas.[43] CD80 is expressed transiently on the surface of activated B cells and other APCs, including DCs, but is constitutively expressed on a variety of NHLs, including follicular lymphomas. Thus, CD80 is an attractive target for lymphoma therapy. Targeting CD80 on NHLs with anti-CD80 Ab can arrest their growth and therefore can serve as a therapeutic intervention for treating cancer. Engaging costimulatory pathways, as well as blocking coinhibitory pathways, has therapeutic potential for treatment of cancer. However, for tumor immunotherapy, there are multiple barriers to the antitumor response, and coinhibitory pathways participate in shielding tumors from immune eradication. The differential expression of coinhibitory molecules (such as B7-H4) on certain cancers provides an opportunity for selective immunotherapeutic intervention. Interference with multiple coinhibitory pathways may be needed for optimal therapeutic benefit. Despite the expression of antigens by tumor cells, spontaneous immune-mediated rejection of cancer seems to be a rare event. TCR engagement by peptide–MHC constitutes the main signal for the activation of naive T cells but is not sufficient to initiate a productive generation and maintenance of effector cells. Full activation of T cells requires additional signals driven by costimulatory molecules present on activated APCs but rarely on tumors. Following the discovery of B7-1 (CD80), several other costimulatory molecules have been shown to contribute to T-cell activation and have relevance for improving antitumor immunity. Moreover, increasing the understanding of coinhibitory receptors has highlighted key additional pathways that can dominantly inhibit antitumor T-cell function. Improving positive costimulation, and interfering with negative regulation, continues to represent an attractive immunotherapeutic approach for the treatment of cancer. The pathways with the highest potential for clinical application and translation to the clinic summarizing clinical trials aimed at boosting positive costimulation and antitumor immunity with agonistic CD40, 4-1BB, or OX40 Abs, and clinical trials that block the coinhibitory receptors CTLA-4 and PD-1. However, challenges are posed by the development of inflammation or autoimmunity following immune intervention.

A significant number of patients relapse or do not respond to rituximab due to intrinsic or acquired resistance. Hence, mAbs targeting other cell surface antigens on B-cell lymphomas are being studied. CD80 serves as an attractive target in the continued development of mAbs against lymphoma. Preclinical studies with galiximab, an anti-CD80 primatized mAb, have been encouraging and have demonstrated antitumor activity against various B-cell lymphoma models, both as a single agent and in combination with rituximab. Data were reviewed from a PubMed literature search from 1975 to 2009 and also included a review of abstracts from published proceedings of annual meetings from the American Society of Hematology and International Conference of Malignant Lymphoma, Lugano.

Galiximab (Biogen Idec, Inc., San Diego, California) is a chimeric, primatized IgG1 mAb consisting of human constant and primate (cynomolgus macaque) variable regions targeting CD80. It binds specifically to CD80, which is transiently expressed on the surface of activated B cells and APCs, including DCs, but is constitutively expressed on a variety of NHLs, including FL. Thus, CD80 serves as an attractive target for the development of antilymphoma therapy. Galiximab is emerging as an interesting and effective therapy for the treatment of patients with NHL, especially in combination with rituximab. Its favorable toxicity profile makes it an attractive alternative to existing agents. This "primatized" Ab is structurally indistinguishable from human Abs and, therefore, is not significantly immunogenic in humans. Although a number of *in vivo* as well as *in vitro* studies point toward possible "unique" mechanisms of action of galiximab, more studies are needed to fully understand this agent's antitumor activity, as well as to establish strategies by which to optimize its efficacy. However, to further assess the therapeutic role of galiximab in the treatment of patients with follicular and other lymphoma subtypes, as monotherapy or in combination with rituximab or systemic chemotherapy, additional studies are under active consideration.

As established by clinical and experimental results, it is quite evident that anti-CD80 Ab treatment is effective against relapsed and refractory follicular lymphoma. Future studies in other CD80-positive hematological malignancies (e.g., diffuse large B-cell NHL, chronic lymphocytic leukemia, Hodgkin's lymphoma, and multiple myeloma) should also be taken under consideration. Thus, anti-CD80 Ab immunotherapy may have a potent role in the treatment of CD80-bearing cancer cells because their binding can modulate the key molecules in the signaling pathway and enhance antitumor response. Considering the importance of CD80 signaling in the regulation of immune responses against cancer, the manipulation of this signaling pathway to increase immunity against cancer represents a potential therapeutic approach. Understanding the mechanisms by which tumor cells escape immune surveillance will help us to establish new and effective approaches to vaccination and immunotherapy. One of the most important immune evasion mechanism employed by tumor cells is the downregulation of the CD80 costimulatory molecule. The success of novel cancer therapies depends on the identification of functional targets that play an essential role in tumor growth and metastasis, survival, and evasion from immunosurveillance. Anti-CD80 therapy can be used to target tumors expressing CD80. The clinical success of anti-CD80 Ab for the treatment of refractory follicular lymphoma has stimulated great interest in the promise of Ab therapeutics for cancer. The qualities of galiximab, such as long half-life and high specificity and safety compared with other cancer therapeutics together with its ability to bind to and modulate key players in signaling pathways that drive malignant transformation and enhance antitumor immune functions, makes it a highly desirable therapeutic agent.

Most tumors do not regress but continue to grow in spite of the presence of spontaneous or antigen-induced immune responses, due to downregulation of costimulatory molecules such as CD80. The existence of systemic immune responses may not by itself be sufficient to deal with the complex nature of tumor–host interactions because factors such as insufficient costimulation to induce T-cell response may further contribute to the lack of effective immunity. It is now well established that T cells are rendered anergic due to the lack of costimulatory molecule(s) expression by tumor cells. Tumor cells are able to induce antigen-specific tolerance or anergy on the basis of MHC-I-restricted antigen presentation without the expression of costimulatory molecules. This unresponsiveness, however, can be reversed when tumor cells are genetically modified to express costimulatory molecules. A plethora of studies suggest that the insertion of genes encoding CD80 into tumors generally increases their immunogenicity and can be used as vaccine. Recently, fusagene vectors have been developed to encode multiple gene products such as CD80 with cytokines or MHC molecules as fusion proteins from a single cistron to increase the immunogenicity of target tumor cells. The vectors generated could be used in immunotherapy for the treatment of multiple myeloma, leukemias, and other cancers, as they have been shown to stimulate allogeneic mixed lymphocyte proliferation and augment increases in CTL and NK cell responses and IFN-γ release. Considering the importance of costimulation in the regulation of immune responses against relapsed cancer, the manipulation of this pathway to increase immunity represents a potential therapeutic approach. Furthermore, signaling either by anti-CD80 Abs or through CD28-bearing T cells regresses the growth, augments the expression of proapoptotic molecules, and induces apoptosis of CD80 + lymphomas. Therefore, immunotherapy utilizing anti-CD80 Abs is a promising future treatment, especially in the case of relapse and refractory lymphomas.

Therapeutic modalities targeting the B7 and CD28 families of ligands and receptors are showing promise in the clinic. The encouraging results in targeting the B7/CD28/CTLA-4 pathway in psoriasis and rheumatoid arthritis underscore the importance of this costimulatory pathway and validate the pathogenic contributions of T cells in the etiology of these diseases. The costimulatory ICOS pathway might also provide therapeutic opportunities, particularly in diseases in which pathogenic Abs contribute to disease progression. Although the negative regulators CTLA-4 and PD-1 are critical for attenuating normal immune responses, agonistic compounds targeting these proteins to "tune down" inflammatory responses have not yet been identified. This is probably a result of the requirement for coengagement of PD-1 or CTLA-4 with the antigen receptor for delivery of inhibitory signals. However, antagonists of these inhibitory receptors might have utility in enhancing immune responses for cancer, infectious diseases, or vaccine development. The CD28 receptor/B7 ligand families are not yet complete, as receptors for the new B7-H3 and B7-H4 ligands have not been identified, and some data support additional receptors for PD-L1 and PD-L2. Many receptors and their ligands belonging to B7 and TNF/TNFR families of molecules through whom reverse costimulation can be delivered for the activation of APCs and the cells expressing them (Figure 2.8). The role of CD28 in the development of regulatory T cells is further explored, and it has been shown that CD28 is not only required for IL-2 production but also for differentiation of regulatory T cells, independently of IL-2 production. Further support for the costimulatory role of B7-H3 has been demonstrated in allograft rejection models. Treatment of B7-H3-deficient mice with cyclosporin A, rapamycin, or anti-CD154 Ab reduced the incidence of rejection of cardiac or allografts compared with treated wild-type mice. It is postulated that B7-H3 contributes to allograft rejection by induction of IFN-γ or by chemokines induced by IFN-γ. Despite the complex roles and interactions within

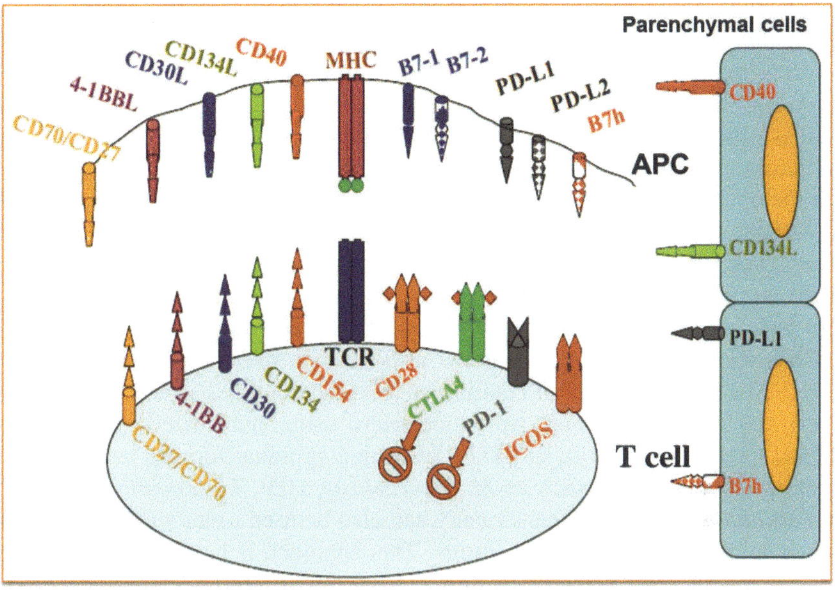

FIGURE 2.8 **Schematic representation of costimulatory molecules through which reverse costimulation can be delivered.** Signal 1 is represented by the TCR interacting with the antigen in the MHC groove. Signals from the CTLA-4 and PD-1 are inhibitory to the T cell. 1BB, CDw137; 1BBL, CDw137 ligand; CTLA-4, cytotoxic T-lymphocyte associated gene-4; ICOS, inducible costimulator; PD, programmed death; TCR, T-cell receptor.

the CD28 and B7 families, we predict that novel approaches targeting these families will yield new therapies for the treatment of inflammation, autoimmunity, transplantation, cancer, and infectious diseases.

Many studies published recently have now established that the CD80 and CD86 costimulatory molecules expressed on the surface of the APCs do not merely have a unidirectional function of stimulating T cells on engagement with CD28 and CD152, but this interaction delivers bidirectional signals affecting the activity of APCs as well. Moreover, based on the kinetics of differential expression, affinity, association and dissociation rates, and structure, indicates that CD80 and CD86 can differentially regulate the cells of immune system. In particular, CD80 delivers similar signals as delivered by CD152 for inhibiting the action of T cells. In contrast, CD86 costimulate APCs in an analogous manner as done by CD28 in activating T cells. Interestingly, the inhibitory role of CD80 on B cells, DCs, neural stem cells, and lymphomas has shown to induce apoptosis by upregulating the expression of proapoptotic molecules and downregulating the expression of antiapoptotic molecules. This inhibitory role of CD80 has been efficiently exploited to treat patients suffering from relapsed and refractory lymphomas. In addition, signaling through CD80 can be explored for inducing tolerance/apoptosis in autoimmune diseases, hypersensitivity reactions, allergies, and transplantation.

Considering the importance of costimulation in the regulation of immune responses against relapsed cancer, the manipulation of this pathway to increase immunity, regresses the growth, augments the expression of proapoptotic molecules, and induces apoptosis of lymphomas represents a potential therapeutic approach. Therapeutic modalities targeting the B7 and CD28 costimulatory families of ligands and receptors are showing promise in the clinic. The encouraging results in targeting the B7/CD28/CTLA-4 pathway in the autoimmune diseases such as psoriasis, multiple sclerosis, and rheumatoid arthritis underscore the importance of this costimulatory pathway and validate the pathogenic contributions of T cells in the etiology of these diseases. This novel strategy of costimulation activation/inhibition can be effectively exploited to develop immunotherapy using humanized Abs against CD80, CD86, and CD40 or CD28 fusogenic proteins for the treatment of intracellular pathogens such as *M. tuberculosis*, HIV, *Leishmania donovani*, and *Trypanosoma cruzi*. This strategy can also be used as an alternative strategy or in combination with the drugs. This approach is based on modulating the immune system of the hosts rather than targeting the pathogen; hence, it significantly diminishes the chance of emergence of drug-resistant strains of pathogens and if applied properly may overcome the rising menace of infectious diseases. To develop alternative or adjunct (with drugs) therapies using costimulatory molecules, an intensive effort has been undertaken in the last decade to understand how intracellular pathogens exploit costimulatory molecules, which are the *tour de force* of the immune system. The potent role of costimulatory molecules is aptly established in the optimum activation of T cells and APCs, the cells that play a cardinal role in curbing the infections. Hence, immunotherapy involving costimulatory molecules can be a breakthrough strategy to treat various diseases, to minimize side effects inflicted by drug therapies, and to restrict the emergence of drug resistance.

To translate this field into the clinic, it is urgent to develop novel methods to target currently appreciated costimulatory pathway and deeply understand pathophysiology of these diseases involving costimulatory molecules. Despite the complex roles and interactions within the CD28 and B7 costimulatory families, we predict that novel approaches targeting these families will yield new therapies for the treatment of inflammation, autoimmunity, transplantation, cancer, and infectious diseases.

REFERENCES

1. Lenschow DJ, Walunas TL, Bluestone JA. CD28/B7 system of T cell co-stimulation. *Annu Rev Immunol* 1996;**14**:233–58.
2. Frauwirth KA, Thompson CB. Activation and inhibition of lymphocytes by co-stimulation. *J Clin Invest* 2002;**109**:295–9.

3. Jenkins MK. The ups and downs of T cell co-stimulation. *Immunity* 1994;**1**:443–6.
4. Chambers CA. The expanding world of co-stimulation: the two-signal model revisited. *Trends Immunol* 2001;**22**:217–23.
5. Turka LA, Linsley PS, Lin H, Brady W, Leiden JM, et al. T-cell activation by the CD28 ligand B7 is required for cardiac allograft rejection in vivo. *Proc Natl Acad Sci USA* 1992; **89**:11102–5.
6. Finck BK, Linsley PS, Wofsy D. Treatment of murine lupus with CTLA4Ig. *Science* 1994;**265**:1225–7.
7. Schweitzer AN, Borriello F, Wong RC, Abbas AK, Sharpe AH. Role of costimulators in T cell differentiation: studies using antigen-presenting cells lacking expression of CD80 or CD86. *J Immunol* 1997;**158**:2713–22.
8. Greenwald RJ, Boussiotis VA, Lorsbach RB, Abbas AK, Sharpe AH. CTLA-4 regulates induction of anergy in vivo. *Immunity* 2000;**14**:145–55.
9. Shahinian A, Pfeffer K, Lee KP, Kundig TM, Kishihara K, Wakeham A, et al. Differential T cell costimulatory requirements in CD28-deficient mice. *Science* 1993;**261**:609–12.
10. Ronchese F, Hausmann B, Hubele S, Lane P. Mice transgenic for a soluble form of murine CTLA-4 show enhanced expansion of antigen-specific CD4 + T cells and defective antibody production in vivo. *J Exp Med* 1994;**179**:809–17.
11. Snapper CM, Paul WE. Interferon-gamma and B cell stimulatory factor-1 reciprocally regulate Ig isotype production. *Science* 1987;**236**:944–7.
12. Ikemizu S, Gilbert RJ, Fennelly JA. Structure and dimerization of a soluble form of B7-1. *Immunity* 2000;**12**:51–60.
13. Bajorath J, Peach RJ, Linsley PS. Immunoglobulin fold characteristics of B7-1 (CD80) and B7-2 (CD86). *Protein Sci* 1994;**3**:2148–50.
14. Heath AW, Chang R, Harada N, Santos-Argumedo L, Gordon J, Hannum C, et al. Antibodies to murine CD40 stimulate normal B lymphocytes but inhibit proliferation of B lymphoma cells. *Cell Immunol* 1993;**152**:468–80.
15. Jeannin P, Delneste Y, Lecoanet-Henchoz S, Gauchat JF, Ellis J, Bonnefoy JY. CD86 (B7-2) on human B cells. A functional role in proliferation and selective differentiation into IgE- and IgG4-producing cells. *J Biol Chem* 1997;**272**:15613–19.
16. Hirokawa M, Kuroki J, Kitabayashi A, Miura AB. Transmembrane signaling through CD80 (B7-1) induces growth arrest and cell spreading of human B lymphocytes accompanied by protein tyrosine phosphorylation. *Immunol Lett* 1996;**50**:95–8.
17. Lumsden JM, Williams JA, Hodes RJ. Differential requirements for expression of CD80/86 and CD40 on B cells for T-dependent antibody responses in vivo. *J Immunol* 2003;**170**:781–7.
18. Podojil JR, Sanders VM. Selective regulation of mature IgG1 transcription by CD86 and beta 2-adrenergic receptor stimulation. *J Immunol* 2003;**170**:5143–51.
19. Suvas S, Singh V, Sahdev S, Vohra H, Agrewala JN. Distinct role of CD80 and CD86 in the regulation of the activation of B cell and B cell lymphoma. *J Biol Chem* 2002;**277**:7766–75.
20. Schmidt CS, Liu J, Zhang T, Song HY, Sandusky G, Mintze K, et al. Enhanced B cell expansion, survival, and humoral responses by targeting death receptor 6. *J Exp Med* 2003; **197**:51–62.
21. Nguyen LT, Radhakrishnan S, Ciric B, Tamada K, Shin T, Pardoll DM, et al. Cross-linking the B7 family molecule B7-DC directly activates immune functions of dendritic cells. *J Exp Med* 2002;**196**:1393–8.
22. Mukherjee S, Maiti PK, Nandi D. Role of CD80, CD86, and CTLA4 on mouse CD4(+) T lymphocytes in enhancing cell-cycle progression and survival after activation with PMA and ionomycin. *J Leukoc Biol* 2002;**72**:921–31.

23. Grohmann U, Orabona C, Fallarino F, Vacca C, Calcinaro F, Falorni A, et al. CTLA-4-Ig regulates tryptophan catabolism in vivo. *Nat Immunol* 2002;**3**(11):1097–101.
24. Yamamoto Y, Gaynor RB. IkappaB kinases: key regulators of the NF-kappaB pathway. *Trends Biochem Sci* 2004;**29**:72–9.
25. Podojil JR, Kin NW, Sanders VM. CD86 and beta2-adrenergic receptor signaling pathways, respectively, increase Oct-2 and OCA-B expression and binding to the 3′-IgH enhancer in B cells. *J Biol Chem* 2004;**279**:23394–404.
26. Podojil JR, Sanders VM. CD86 and beta2-adrenergic receptor stimulation regulate B-cell activity cooperatively. *Trends Immunol* 2005;**26**:180–5.
27. Berberich I, Shu GL, Clark EA. Cross-linking CD40 on B cells rapidly activates nuclear factor-kappa B. *J Immunol* 1994;**153**:4357–66.
28. Radhakrishnan S, Nguyen LT, Ciric B, Ure DR, Zhou B, Tamada K, et al. Naturally occurring human IgM antibody that binds B7-DC and potentiates T cell stimulation by dendritic cells. *J Immunol* 2003;**170**:1830–8.
29. Schjetne KW, Fredriksen AB, Bogen B. Delivery of antigen to CD40 induces protective immune responses against tumors. *J Immunol* 2007;**178**:4169–76.
30. Caux C, Massacrier C, Vanbervliet B, Dubois B, Van Kooten C, et al. Activation of human dendritic cells through CD40 cross-linking. *J Exp Med* 1994;**180**:1263–72.
31. Koch F, Stanzl U, Jennewein P, Janke K, Heufler C, Kampgen E, et al. High level IL-12 production by murine dendritic cells: upregulation via MHC class II and CD40 molecules and downregulation by IL-4 and IL-10. *J Exp Med* 1996;**184**:741–6.
32. Cella M, Scheidegger D, Palmer-Lehmann K, Lane P, Lanzavecchia A, et al. Ligation of CD40 on dendritic cells triggers production of high levels of interleukin-12 and enhances T cell stimulatory capacity: T-T help via APC activation. *J Exp Med* 1996;**184**:747–52.
33. Croft M. Control of Immunity by the TNFR-related molecule OX40 (CD134). *Annu Rev Immunol* 2010;**28**:57–78.
34. Logue EC, Sha WC. CD28-B7 bidirectional signaling: a two-way street to activation. *Nat Immunol* 2004;**5**(11):1103–6.
35. Meyer zum Bueschenfelde CO, Unternaehrer J, Mellman I, Bottomly K. Regulated recruitment of MHC class II and costimulatory molecules to lipid rafts in dendritic cells. *J Immunol* 2004;**173**(10):6119–24.
36. Kovacs B, Parry RV, Ma Z, Fan E, Shivers DK, Freiberg BA. Ligation of CD28 by its natural ligand CD86 in the absence of TCR stimulation induces lipid raft polarization in human CD4 T cells. *J Immunol* 2005;**175**:7848–54.
37. Hiltbold EM, Poloso NJ, Roche PA. MHC class II-peptide complexes and APC lipid rafts accumulate at the immunological synapse. *J Immunol* 2003;**170**:1329–38.
38. Orabona C, Grohmann U, Belladonna ML, Fallarino F, Vacca C, Bianchi R, et al. CD28 induces immuno-stimulatory signals in dendritic cells via CD80 and CD86. *Nat Immunol* 2004;**5**:1134–42.
39. Shin T, Kennedy G, Gorski K, Tsuchiya H, Koseki H, Azuma M, et al. Cooperative B7-1/2 (CD80/CD86) and B7-DC co-stimulation of CD4+ T cells independent of the PD-1 receptor. *J Exp Med* 2003;**198**:31–8.
40. Imitola J, Comabella M, Chandraker AK, Dangond F, Sayegh MH, Snyder EY, et al. Neural stem/progenitor cells express costimulatory molecules that are differentially regulated by inflammatory and apoptotic stimuli. *Am J Pathol* 2004;**164**:1615–25.
41. Kohm AP, Mozaffarian A, Sanders VM. B cell receptor and beta 2-adrenergic receptor-induced regulation of B7-2 (CD86) expression in B cells. *J Immunol* 2002;**168**:6314–22.

42. Kin NW, Sanders VM. CD86 stimulation on a B cell activates the phosphatidyl inositol 3-kinase/Akt and phospholipase C gamma 2/protein kinase C alpha beta signaling pathways. *J Immunol* 2006;**176**:6727–35.
43. Leonard JP, Friedberg JW, Younes A, Fisher D, Gordon LI, Moore J, et al. A phase I/II study of galiximab (an anti-CD80 monoclonal antibody) in combination with rituximab for relapsed or refractory, follicular lymphoma. *Ann Oncol* 2007;**18**(7):1216–23.
44. Greene JL, Leytze GM, Emswiler J, Peach R, Bajorath J, Cosand W, et al. Covalent dimerization of CD28/CTLA-4 and oligomerization of CD80/CD86 regulate T cell costimulatory interactions. *J Biol Chem* 1996;**271**:26762–71.
45. Barragan M, Campas C, Bellosillo B, Gil J. Protein kinases in the regulation of apoptosis in B-cell chronic lymphocytic leukemia. *Leuk Lymphoma* 2003;**44**:1865–70.
46. Lee HH, Dadgostar H, Cheng Q, Shu J, Cheng G. NF-kappa mediated upregulation of Bcl-xL and Bfl-1/A1 is required for CD40 survival signaling in B lymphocytes. *Proc Natl Acad Sci USA* 1999;**96**:9136–41.
47. Fallarino F, Grohmann U, Hwang KW, Orabona C, Vacca C, Bianchi R, et al. Modulation of tryptophan catabolism by regulatory T cells. *Nat Immunol* 2003;**4**(12):1206–12.
48. Van der Merwe PA, Davis SJ. Molecular interactions mediating T cell antigen recognition. *Annu Rev Immunol* 2003;**21**:659–84.
49. Collins AV, Brodie DW, Gilbert RJ, Iaboni A, Manso-Sancho R, Walse B, et al. The interaction properties of costimulatory molecules revisited. *Immunity* 2002;**17**(2):201–10.
50. Zhang X, Schwartz JC, Almo SC, Nathenson SG. Crystal structure of the receptor-binding domain of human B7-2: insights into organization and signaling. *Proc Natl Acad Sci USA* 2003;**100**(5):2586–91.
51. Schwartz JC, Zhang X, Fedorov AA, Nathenson SG, Almo SC. Structural basis for co-stimulation by the human CTLA-4/B7-2 complex. *Nature* 2001;**410**(6828):604–8.
52. Stamper CC, Zhang Y, Tobin JF, Erbe DV, Ikemizu S, Davis SJ, et al. Crystal structure of the B7-1/CTLA-4 complex that inhibits human immune responses. *Nature* 2001;**410**(6828):608–11.
53. Pentcheva-Hoang T, Egen JG, Wojnoonski K, Allison JP. B7-1 and B7-2 selectively recruit CTLA-4 and CD28 to the immunological synapse. *Immunity* 2004;**21**(3):401–13.
54. Sharpe AH, Freeman GJ. The B7-CD28 superfamily. *Nat Rev Immunol* 2002;**2**(2):116–26.
55. Hariharan K, Anderson D, Leigh B. Therapeutic activity of IDEC-114 (anti-CD80) and rituximab (Rituxan) in B-cell lymphoma. *Blood* 2001;**98**:608a. [Abstract 2549].
56. Taylor MW, Feng GS. Relationship between interferon-gamma, indolamine 2,3-dioxygenase, and tryptophan catabolism. *FASEB J* 1991;**5**:2516–22.
57. Hassanain HH, Chon SY, Gupta SL. Differential regulation of human indolamine 2,3-dioxygenase gene expression by interferons-gamma and -alpha. Analysis of the regulatory region of the gene and identification of an interferon-gamma-inducible DNA-binding factor. *J Biol Chem* 1993;**268**:5077–84.
58. Mir MA, Albaradeh R, Agrewala JN. Innate effector immune response elicitation against tuberculosis through anti-B7-1 (CD80) and anti-B7-2 (CD86) signaling in macrophages. *IJBPAS* 2013;**2**(5):1024–43.
59. Sayama S, Nagamatsu T, Schust DJ, Itaoka N, Ichikawa M, Kawana K, et al. Human decidual macrophages suppress IFN-γ production by T cells through costimulatory B7-H1: PD-1 signaling in early pregnancy. *J Reprod Immunol* 2013;**100**(2):109–17.
60. Yu Y, He Y, Yang TT, Jiang H, Xiang YJ, Fang LB, et al. Elevated plasma levels and monocyte-associated expression of CD137 ligand in patients with acute atherothrombotic stroke. *Eur Rev Med Pharmacol Sci* 2014;**18**(10):1525–32.

61. Racke MM, Mosior M, Kovacevic S, Chang CH, Glasebrook AL, Roehm NW, et al. Activation of caspase-3 alone is insufficient for apoptotic morphological changes in human neuroblastoma cells. *J Neurochem* 2002;**80**:1039–48.
62. Ruiz-Ruiz C, Munoz-Pinedo C, Lopez-Rivas A. Interferon-gamma treatment elevates caspase-8 expression and sensitizes human breast tumor cells to a death receptor-induced mitochondria-operated apoptotic program. *Cancer Res* 2000;**60**:5673–80.
63. Lenschow DJ, Ho SC, Sattar H, Rhee L, Gray G, Nabavi N, et al. Differential effects of anti-B7-1 and anti-B7-2 monoclonal antibody treatment on the development of diabetes in the non-obese diabetic mouse. *J Exp Med* 1995;**181**:1145–55.
64. Liang B, Kashgarian MJ, Sharpe AH, Mamula MJ. Autoantibody responses and pathology regulated by B7-1 and B7-2 co-stimulation in MRL/lpr lupus. *J Immunol* 2000;**165**: 3436–43.
65. Liang B, Gee RJ, Kashgarian MJ, Sharpe AH, Mamula MJ. B7 co-stimulation in the development of lupus: autoimmunity arises either in the absence of B7.1/B7.2 or in the presence of anti-B7.1/B7.2 blocking antibodies. *J Immunol* 1999;**163**:2322–9.
66. Zhu XY, Zhou YH, Wang MY, Jin LP, Yuan MM, Li DJ. Blockade of CD86 signaling facilitates a Th2 bias at the maternal-fetal interface and expands peripheral CD4+ CD25+ regulatory T cells to rescue abortion-prone fetuses. *Biol Reprod* 2005;**72**:338–45.
67. Kuchroo VK, Das MP, Brown JA, Ranger AM, Zamvil SS, Sobel RA, et al. B7-1 and B7-2 costimulatory molecules activate differentially the Th1/Th2 developmental pathways: application to autoimmune disease therapy. *Cell* 1995;**80**:707–18.
68. Baskar S, Glimcher L, Nabavi N, Jones RT, Ostrand-Rosenberg S. Major histocompatibility complex class II + B7-1+ tumor cells are potent vaccines for stimulating tumor rejection in tumor-bearing mice. *J Exp Med* 1995;**181**:619–29.
69. Gao JX, Zhang H, Bai XF, Wen J, Zheng X, Liu J, et al. Perinatal blockade of B7-1 and B7-2 inhibits clonal deletion of highly pathogenic autoreactive T cells. *J Exp Med* 2002;**195**:959–71.
70. Abrams JR, Kelley SL, Hayes E, Kikuchi T, Brown MJ, Kang S, et al. Blockade of T lymphocyte co-stimulation with cytotoxic T lymphocyte-associated antigen 4-immunoglobulin (CTLA4Ig) reverses the cellular pathology of psoriatic plaques, including the activation of keratinocytes, dendritic cells, and endothelial cells. *J Exp Med* 2000;**192**:681–94.
71. Sayegh MH, Turka LA. The role of T-cell costimulatory activation pathways in transplant rejection. *N Engl J Med* 1998;**338**:1813–21.
72. Hausen B, Klupp J, Christians U, Higgins JP, Baumgartner RE, Hook LE, et al. Coadministration of either cyclosporine or steroids with humanized monoclonal antibodies against CD80 and CD86 successfully prolong allograft survival after life supporting renal transplantation in cynomologous monkeys. *Transplantation* 2001;**72**:1128–37.
73. Zheng P, Sarma S, Guo Y, Liu Y. Two mechanisms for tumor evasion of preexisting cytotoxic T-cell responses: lessons from recurrent tumors. *Cancer Res* 1999;**59**:3461–7.
74. Matulonis UA, Dosiou C, Lamont C, Freeman GJ, Mauch P, Nadler LM, et al. Role of B7-1 in mediating an immune response to myeloid leukemia cells. *Blood* 1995;**85**:2507–15.
75. Wu TC, Huang AY, Jaffee EM, Levitsky HI, Pardoll DM. A reassessment of the role of B7-1 expression in tumor rejection. *J Exp Med* 1995;**182**:1415–21.
76. Matsumoto K, Anasetti C. The role of T cell costimulation by CD80 in the initiation and maintenance of the immune response to human leukemia. *Leuk Lymphoma* 1999;**35**:427–35.
77. Huang AY, Bruce AT, Pardoll DM, Levitsky HI. Does B7-1 expression confer antigen-presenting cell capacity to tumors in vivo?. *J Exp Med* 1996;**183**:769–76.

78. La Motte RN, Sharpe AH, Bluestone JA, Mokyr MB. Importance of B7-1-expressing host antigen-presenting cells for the eradication of B7-2 transfected P815 tumor cells. *J Immunol* 1998;**161**(12):6552–8.
79. Reiser H, Freeman GJ, Razi-Wolf Z, Gimmi CD, Benacerraf B, Nadler LM. Murine B7 antigen provides an efficient costimulatory signal for activation of murine T lymphocytes via the T-cell receptor/CD3 complex. *Proc Natl Acad Sci USA* 1992;**89**:271–5.
80. Kelly JM, Darcy PK, Markby JL, Godfrey DI, Takeda K, Yagita H, et al. Induction of tumor-specific T cell memory by NK cell-mediated tumor rejection. *Nat Immunol* 2002;**3** (1):83–90.
81. Harding FA, Allison JP. CD28-B7 interactions allow the induction of CD8 + cytotoxic T lymphocytes in the absence of exogenous help. *J Exp Med* 1993;**177**:1791–6.
82. Townsend SE, Allison JP. Tumor rejection after direct costimulation of CD8 + T cells by B7-transfected melanoma cells. *Science* 1993;**259**:368–70.
83. Tirapu I, Huarte E, Guiducci C, Arina A, Zaratiegui M, Murillo O, et al. Low surface expression of B7-1 CD80 is an immunoescape mechanism of colon carcinoma. *Cancer Res* 2006;**66**:2442–50.
84. Chambers BJ, Salcedo M, Ljunggren HG. Triggering of natural killer cells by the costimulatory molecule CD80 B7-1. *Immunity* 1996;**5**:311–17.
85. Heise CP, Shi F, Albertini MR, Mahvi DM. B7.1 expression eliminates tumor resistance to IL-12 gene therapy. *Cancer Gene Ther* 2001;**8**:118–27.
86. Chen L, Ashe S, Brady WA, Hellström I, Hellström KE, Ledbetter JA, et al. Costimulation of antitumor immunity by the B7 counterreceptor for the T lymphocyte molecules CD28 and CTLA-4. *Cell* 1992;**71**:1093–102.
87. Munn DH, Sharma MD, Hou D, Baban B, Lee JR, Antonia SJ, et al. Expression of indoleamine 2,3-dioxygenase by plasmacytoid dendritic cells in tumor-draining lymph nodes. *J Clin Invest* 2004;**114**(2):280–90.
88. Girvin AM1, Dal Canto MC, Rhee L, Salomon B, Sharpe A, Bluestone JA, et al. A critical role for B7/CD28 costimulation in experimental autoimmune encephalomyelitis: a comparative study using costimulatory molecule-deficient mice and monoclonal antibody blockade. *J Immunol* 2000;**164**(1):136–43.
89. Racke MK, Scott DE, Quigley L, Gray GS, Abe R, June CH, et al. Distinct roles for B7-1 (CD-80) and B7-2 (CD-86) in the initiation of experimental allergic encephalomyelitis. *J Clin Invest* 1995;**96**(5):2195–203.
90. Salomon B, Lenschow DJ, Rhee L, Ashourian N, Singh B, Sharpe A, et al. B7/CD28 costimulation is essential for the homeostasis of the CD4 + CD25 + immunoregulatory T cells that control autoimmune diabetes. *Immunity* 2000;**12**(4):431–40.
91. Tang Q, Henriksen KJ, Boden EK, Tooley AJ, Ye J, Subudhi SK, et al. Cutting edge: CD28 controls peripheral homeostasis of CD4+CD25+ regulatory T cells. *J Immunol* 2003;**171**(7):3348–52.
92. Abrams JR, Lebwohl MG, Guzzo CA, Jegasothy BV, Goldfarb MT, et al. CTLA4Ig-mediated blockade of T-cell costimulation in patients with psoriasis vulgaris. *J Clin Invest* 1999;**103**(9):1243–52.
93. Kremer JM, Westhovens R, Leon M, Di Giorgio E, Alten R, Steinfeld S, et al. Treatment of rheumatoid arthritis by selective inhibition of T-cell activation with fusion protein CTLA4Ig. *N Engl J Med* 2003;**349**(20):1907–15.
94. Phan GQ, Yang JC, Sherry RM, Hwu P, Topalian SL, Schwartzentruber DJ, et al. Cancer regression and autoimmunity induced by cytotoxic T lymphocyte-associated antigen 4 blockade in patients with metastatic melanoma. *Proc Natl Acad Sci USA* 2003;**100**(14):8372–7.

95. Sanderson K, Scotland R, Lee P, Liu D, Groshen S, Snively J, et al. Autoimmunity in a phase I trial of a fully human anti-cytotoxic T-lymphocyte antigen-4 monoclonal antibody with multiple melanoma peptides and Montanide ISA 51 for patients with resected stages III and IV melanoma. *J Clin Oncol* 2005;**23**(4):741–50.
96. Dols A, Smith II JW, Meijer SL, Fox BA, Hu HM, et al. Vaccination of women with metastatic breast cancer, using a costimulatory gene (CD80)-modified, HLA-A2-matched, allogeneic, breast cancer cell line: clinical and immunological results. *Hum Gene Ther* 2003;**14**(11):1117–23.
97. Antonia SJ, Seigne J, Diaz J, Muro-Cacho C, Extermann M, Farmelo MJ, et al. Phase I trial of a B7-1 (CD80) gene modified autologous tumor cell vaccine in combination with systemic interleukin-2 in patients with metastatic renal cell carcinoma. *J Urol* 2002;**167**(5):1995–2000.
98. Raez LE, Cassileth PA, Schlesselman JJ, Sridhar K, Padmanabhan S, Fisher EZ, et al. Allogeneic vaccination with a B7.1 HLA-A gene-modified adenocarcinoma cell line in patients with advanced non-small-cell lung cancer. *J Clin Oncol* 2004;**22**(14):2800–7.
99. Boasso A, Herbeuval JP, Hardy AW, Winkler C, Shearer GM. Regulation of indoleamine 2,3-dioxygenase and tryptophanyl-tRNA-synthetase by CTLA-4-Fc in human CD4+ T cells. *Blood* 2005;**105**(4):1574–81.
100. Bîrsan T, Hausen B, Higgins JP, Hubble RW, Klupp J, Stalder M, et al. Treatment with humanized monoclonal antibodies against CD80 and CD86 combined with sirolimus prolongs renal allograft survival in cynomolgus monkeys. *Transplantation* 2003;**75**(12):2106–13.
101. Huxley P1, Sutton DH, Debnam P, Matthews IR, Brewer JE, et al. High-affinity small molecule inhibitors of T cell costimulation: compounds for immunotherapy. *Chem Biol* 2004;**11**(12):1651–8.
102. Green NJ, Xiang J, Chen J, Chen L, Davies AM, Erbe D, et al. Structure-activity studies of a series of dipyrazolo[3,4-b:3′,4′-d]pyridin-3-ones binding to the immune regulatory protein B7.1. *Bioorg Med Chem* 2003;**11**(13):2991–3013.
103. Hancock WW, Sayegh MH, Zheng XG, Peach R, Linsley PS, Turka LA. Costimulatory function and expression of CD40 ligand, CD80, and CD86 in vascularized murine cardiac allograft rejection. *Proc Natl Acad Sci USA* 1996;**93**:13967–72.
104. Elgueta R, Benson MJ, de Vries VC, Wasiuk A, Guo Y, Noelle RJ. Molecular mechanism and function of CD40/CD40L engagement in the immune system. *Immunol Rev* 2009;**229**:152–72.
105. Croft M, So T, Duan W, Soroosh P. The significance of OX40 and OX40L to T-cell biology and immune disease. *Immunol Rev* 2009;**229**:173–91.
106. Wang C, Lin GHY, McPherson AJ, Watts TH. Immune regulation by 4-1BB and 4-1BBL: complexities and challenges. *Immunol Rev* 2009;**229**:192–215.
107. Nolte MA, van Olffen RW, Van Gisbergen KPJM, van Lier RAW. Timing and tuning of CD27-CD70 interactions: the impact of signal strength in setting the balance between adaptive responses and immunopathology. *Immunol Rev* 2009;**229**:216–31.
108. Wang Y, Zhu M, Miller M, Fu YX. Immunoregulation by tumor necrosis factor superfamily member LIGHT. *Immunol Rev* 2009;**229**:232–43.
109. Cai G, Freeman GJ. The CD160, BTLA, LIGHT/HVEM pathway: a bidirectional switch regulating T-cell activation. *Immunol Rev* 2009;**229**:244–58.
110. Kwon BS, Weissman SM. cDNA sequences of two inducible T-cell genes. *Proc Natl Acad Sci USA* 1989;**86**(6):1963–7.
111. Pollok KE, Kim YJ, Zhou Z, Hurtado J, Kim KK, Pickard RT, et al. Inducible T cell antigen 4-1BB. Analysis of expression and function. *J Immunol* 1993;**150**(3):771–81.

112. Schwarz H, Valbracht J, Tuckwell J, von Kempis J, Lotz M. ILA, the human 4-1BB homologue, is inducible in lymphoid and other cell lineages. *Blood* 1995;**85**(4):1043–52.
113. Goodwin RG, Din WS, Davis-Smith T, Anderson DM, Gimpel SD, Sato TA, et al. Molecular cloning of a ligand for the inducible T cell gene 4-1BB: a member of an emerging family of cytokines with homology to tumor necrosis factor. *Eur J Immunol* 1993;**23**(10):2631–41.
114. Kamanaka M, Yu P, Yasui T, Yoshida K, Kawabe T, Horii T, et al. Protective role of CD40 in *Leishmania major* infection at two distinct phases of cell-mediated immunity. *Immunity* 1996;**4**(3):275–81.
115. Reichmann G, Walker W, Villegas EN, Craig L, Cai G, Alexander J, et al. The CD40/CD40 ligand interaction is required for resistance to toxoplasmic encephalitis. *Infect Immun.* 2000;**68**(3):1312–18.
116. Grewal IS, Borrow P, Pamer EG, Oldstone MB, Flavell RA. The CD40-CD154 system in anti-infective host defense. *Curr Opin Immunol* 1997;**9**(4):491–7.
117. Demangel C, Palendira U, Feng CG, Heath AW, Bean AG, Britton WJ. Stimulation of dendritic cells via CD40 enhances immune responses to *Mycobacterium tuberculosis* infection. *Infect Immun* 2001;**69**(4):2456–61.
118. Kim J, Kim W, Kim HJ, Park S, Kim HA, Jung D, et al. Superscript CD25+CD4+Foxp3+ regulatory T cells primed by anti-CD137 mAbs inhibit graft-versus-host disease. *Biol Blood Marrow Transplant* 2012;**18**:44–54.
119. Shao Z, Schwarz H. CD137 ligand, a member of the tumor necrosis factor family, regulates immune responses via reverse signal transduction. *J Leukoc Biol* 2011;**89**:21–9.
120. Olofsson PS, Söderström LA, Wågsäter D, Sheikine Y, Ocaya P, et al. CD137 is expressed in human atherosclerosis and promotes development of plaque inflammation in hypercholesterolemic mice. *Circulation* 2008;**117**:1292–301.
121. Jeon HJ, Choi JH, Jung IH, Park JG, Lee MR, Lee MN, et al. CD137 (4-1BB) deficiency reduces atherosclerosis in hyperlipidemic mice. *Circulation* 2010;**121**:1124–33.
122. Ho WT, Pang WL, Chong SM, Castella A, Al-Salam S, Tan TE, et al. Expression of CD137 on Hodgkin and Reed-Sternberg cells inhibits T-cell activation by eliminating CD137 ligand expression. *Cancer Res* 2013;**73**(2):652–61.
123. Kim DK, Lee SC, Lee HW. CD137 ligand-mediated reverse signals increase cell viability and cytokine expression in murine myeloid cells: involvement of mTOR/p70S6 kinase and Akt. *Eur J Immunol* 2009;**39**:2617–28.
124. Kang YJ, Kim SO, Shimada S, Otsuka M, Seit-Nebi A, Kwon BS, et al. Cell surface 4-1BBL mediates sequential signaling pathways “downstream” of TLR and is required for sustained TNF production in macrophages. *Nat Immunol* 2007;**8**:601–9.
125. Kim JD, Lee EA, Quang NN, Cho HR, Kwon B. Recombinant TAT-CD137 ligand cytoplasmic domain fusion protein induces the production of IL-6 and TNF-α in peritoneal macrophages. *Immune Netw* 2011;**11**:216–22.
126. Kim HJ, Lee JS, Kim JD, Cha HJ, Kim A, Lee SK, et al. Reverse signaling through the costimulatory ligand CD137L in epithelial cells is essential for natural killer cell-mediated acute tissue inflammation. *Proc Natl Acad Sci USA* 2012;**109**:E13–22.
127. Park SJ, Kim HJ, Lee JS, Cho HR, Kwon B. Reverse signaling through the co-stimulatory ligand, CD137L, as a critical mediator of sterile inflammation. *Mol Cells* 2012;**33**:533–7.

Chapter 3

Costimulation Immunotherapy in Infectious Diseases

INTRODUCTION

The immune system is a sophisticated and complex weapon that has evolved to destroy invading pathogens. Multicellular organisms possess very sophisticated defense mechanisms that are designed to effectively counter the continual microbial insult of the environment within the vertebrate host. However, successful microbial pathogens have in turn evolved complex and efficient methods to overcome innate and adaptive immune mechanisms, which can result in disease or chronic infections. Although the various virulence strategies used by viral and bacterial pathogens are numerous, there are several general mechanisms that are used to subvert and exploit immune systems that are shared between these diverse microbial pathogens. The success of each pathogen is directly dependent on its ability to mount an effective anti-immune response within the infected host, which can ultimately result in acute disease, chronic infection, or pathogen clearance.[1] The three biggest global infectious disease threats to humans are human immunodeficiency virus (HIV), tuberculosis, and malaria, each killing one to two million people worldwide each year. Each of these three causative agents (which represent a virus, a bacterium, and a parasite) have developed highly effective mechanisms to subvert the human immune system, which explains why developing vaccines and controlling these pathogens have been so difficult. Successful pathogens have evolved a range of anti-immune strategies to overcome both innate and acquired immunity (Table 3.1), which play critical roles in their abilities to cause disease. Although at first glance the immunomodulatory mechanisms used by viruses and bacteria might appear quite different, there are a surprising number of similarities and shared mechanistic concepts. Both types of pathogens have to overcome the same host immune mechanisms, and it is illustrative to see how they have developed parallel strategies to neutralize host immunity. Moreover, viral and bacterial diseases are often linked, exploiting weaknesses in host defenses that are caused by another pathogen.[2–5]

Developing Costimulatory Molecules for Immunotherapy of Diseases.
DOI: http://dx.doi.org/10.1016/B978-0-12-802585-7.00003-0

TABLE 3.1 Various Strategies Used by Pathogens (Bacteria and Viruses) to Evade Effective Immune Responses of the Host

Strategy Used by Pathogens	Examples from Bacteria	Examples from Viruses
Subvert or kill immune cells/phagocytes	– Superantigens – Avoid phagolysosomal fusion – Block inflammatory pathways by injecting effectors – Replicate within and overrun immune cells	– Infect and kill immune cells (DCs, APCs, lymphocytes, macrophage, etc.) – Inhibit CTL/NK cell killing pathways – Alter immune cell signaling, effector functions, or differentiation – Express superantigens
Block acquired immunity	– IgA proteases – Block antigen presentation	– Downregulate MHC-I or -II – Block antigen presentation/proteosome – Prevent induction of immune response genes
Inhibit complement	– Proteases to degrade complement – Produce capsules and long chain LPS to avoid complement deposition and MAC attack	– Soluble inhibitors of complement cascade – Viral Fc receptors
Inhibit cytokines/interferon/chemokines	– Block inflammatory pathways – Activate alternate pathways – Secrete proteases to degrade	– Inhibit ligand gene expression – Ligand/receptor signaling inhibitors – Block secondary antiviral gene induction – Interfere with effector proteins
Modulate apoptosis/autophagy	– Inhibit apoptosis – Activate death signaling pathways – Alter apoptotic signaling pathways	– Inhibit or accelerate cell death – Block death signaling pathways – Scavenge free radicals – Downregulate death receptors or ligands – Inactivate death sensor pathways

Interfere with TLRs	– Alter TLR ligands to decrease recognition – Bind to TLR to dampen inflammation – Inject effectors to inhibit downstream inflammation signaling	– Block or hijack TLR signaling – Prevent TLR recognition
Block antimicrobial small molecules	– Secrete proteases to degrade – Alter cell surface to avoid peptide insertion – Use pumps to transport peptide – Directly sense small molecules to trigger defense mechanism	– Prevent inducible nitric oxide synthase (iNOS) induction – Inhibit antiviral RNA silencing
Block intrinsic cellular pathways	– Alter ubiquitin pathway – Alter transcriptional programs	– Inhibit RNA editing – Regulate ubiquitin/ISGylation pathways
Secreted modulators or toxins	– Many toxins – Proteases	– Ligand mimics (virokines) – Receptor mimics (viroceptors)
Modulators on the pathogen surface	– Lipid A of LPS – Carbohydrates such as capsules – Outer membrane proteins – Adhesins and invasins	– Complement inhibitors – Coagulation regulators – Immune receptors – Adhesion molecules
Hide from immune surveillance	– Avoid phagolysosomal fusion – Inhibit phagocytosis	– Latency – Infect immunoprivileged tissues
Antigenic hypervariability	– Vary many surface structures – Pili, outer membrane proteins, LPS – Strain to strain variation	– Express error-prone replicase – Escape from antibody recognition – "Outrun" T-cell recognition

For intracellular bacteria, entry into host cells represents the central requirement for survival in, as well as elimination by, the host. Host-cell-directed uptake, called "phagocytosis," is a feature of the so-called professional phagocytes that comprise polymorphonuclear granulocytes and mononuclear phagocytes. Entry induced by the pathogen and termed invasion allows entry into nonphagocytic cells (nonprofessional phagocytes). Contact between host cells and pathogens proceeds either directly via receptor–ligand interactions or indirectly via deposition on the surface of the pathogen of host molecules for which physiologic receptors exist on the target cell. Depending on the cellular target, the final outcome of host cell entry varies markedly. Nonprofessional phagocytes are nonphagocytic, and hence entry depends on expression of surface receptors that can be misused for invasion. Benefits of having a well-performing immune system are clearly shown by the pathologies associated with congenital and/or acquired immunodeficiency. The protective function of the immune system resides in the capacity of immune cells to discriminate between self- and nonself-antigens. Major histocompatibility complex (MHC) molecules expressed on the surface of all nucleated cells (class I), and "professional" antigen-presenting cells (APCs) (class II) are an essential tool for the recognition of nonself-antigens.[6,7] The vertebrate immune system is highly evolved to combat and eliminate pathogens (Figure 3.1), however, some pathogens can successfully subvert the host immune system to establish their intracellular survival via strategies like immunosuppression, molecular mimicry, disguise or sequestration of antigens, circumvention of complements and cytokines cascade, blockade of antigen presentation, escape from apoptosis and autophagy, and modulation of costimulatory signals.[1] It is well known that development of immune response, especially in case of naive T cells needs at least two distinct signals for full activation to proliferate and differentiate.[8] The first signal is provided by the specific antigen (MHC–peptide complex) recognition by the T-cell receptor (TCR) and the second signal is provided by the costimulatory molecules.[9] This requirement for second signal explains why adaptive immune responses are stimulated by microbes but not by most self-antigens, which are not normally recognized by the innate immune system and therefore do not elicit adaptive immune responses. The second signal, which is not delivered via the TCR and is not antigen specific, has been termed as costimulatory signal because, while essential, it does not by itself induce any response in T cells. However, when a T cell has its receptor ligated and receives a costimulatory signal, the T cell will proliferate and differentiate into an effector cell. Moreover, T cells that bind antigen but do not receive a costimulatory signal are thought to die or to become anergic,[10] a state in which the cell cannot be activated even if it receives both of the signals required to activate a T cell. Thus, an encounter with antigen can lead to two quite distinct outcomes: proliferation and differentiation into effector cells, or inactivation or death, which outcome occurs is determined by the appropriate delivery of costimulatory signals (Figure 3.2). With the continuous discovery of new

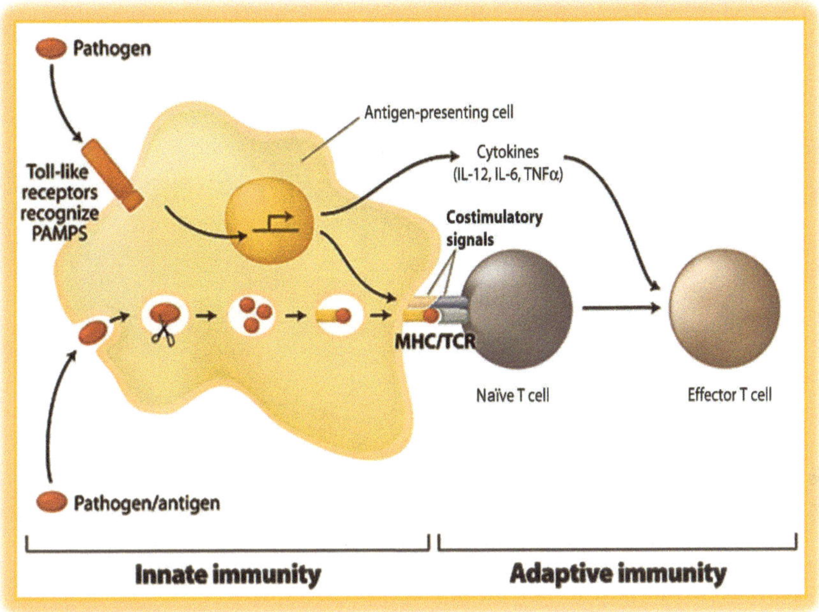

FIGURE 3.1 **Processing of pathogens (antigens) by vertebrate immune system to generate immune response against pathogens.** Pathogens have PAMPS on their surface that are recognized by PRRs on host cells which phagocytose the pathogen. After chopping down the pathogen in the phagosome–lysosome system, they present the antigens to T cells in context with their own MHC molecules to be recognized by naive T cells specific for that antigen so the T cell can mount an effective immune response.

costimulatory molecules on APCs and their receptors on T cells, the story is very much an evolving one. But to date, B7-1 (CD80) and B7-2 (CD86) remain the best-defined costimulatory molecules on APCs[11] which provide the second signals for activation of naive T cells.[12,13] For the first time Suvas et al. from our lab gave a concept of bidirectional costimulation and demonstrated that costimulation through CD80 and CD86 not only influence the activation of T cells but by bidirectional costimulation they can also affect the activity of B cells.[14] Since then many studies have shown the significance of CD80 and CD86 in influencing the activity of B cells, stem cells, and dendritic cells (DCs) but nothing is known about the role of these molecules in the case of macrophages. For instance, it is not known how these molecules regulate the activation of macrophages, which are the important cells of the immune system and the host for a plethora of intracellular pathogens,[6,15] especially the causative agent of tuberculosis. So what is needed is an integrated picture of how signals delivered through major costimulatory molecules CD80 and CD86 expressed on the surface of macrophages regulate the type of immune response generated during infection. Hence the main aim of the present study is to

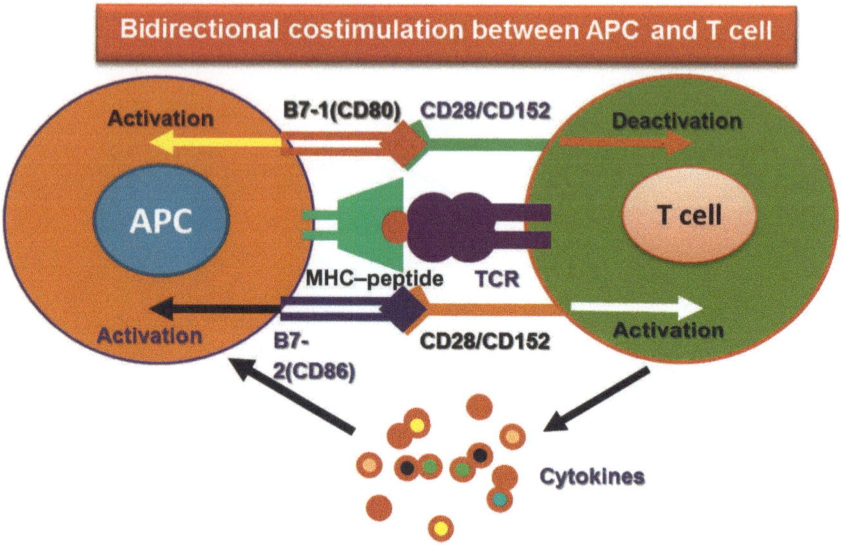

FIGURE 3.2 **Innate and adaptive arms of immune responses against pathogens.** Pathogens have PAMPS on their surface which are recognized by PRRs on professional APCs like DCs which then move to lymph nodes where they interact with the naive or memory T cell generating the humoral or cell-mediated immune response against the pathogen. Without the involvement of costimulatory signals the naive T cells will not be activated as the costimulatory signals are important for their activation.

monitor whether bidirectional costimulation can affect the performance of macrophages. Further, we will investigate whether costimulatory signals can be selectively delivered to activate and inhibit the function of macrophages. Further, we will investigate whether the delivery of costimulatory signals can curb the growth of intracellular pathogens. The use of agents that block or activate costimulatory pathways will undoubtedly require a better understanding of how the diverse biologic activities of these pathways are orchestrated. Also we will seek to find the better biomarkers to predict outcomes of the manipulation of T-cell and APC costimulation in humans and to find preclinical studies with established predictive value. Signaling through CD80 and CD86 can be explored for inducing tolerance/apoptosis in autoimmune diseases, hypersensitivity reactions, allergies, transplantation, and in killing the intracellular pathogens.

Some of the most dreadful pathogens of humans such as *Mycobacterium tuberculosis* (*Mtb*), HIV, and *Leishmania donovani* cause chronic infections and remain a serious global threat to humanity[16] and a challenge to scientific community to find a solution for their control. These three organisms are representatives of successful pathogens from the class of bacteria, virus, and parasites. Innovative strategies have been developed by these pathogens to evade immune responses such as subversion of phagocytosis, antigenic shift and drift, induction of immune regulatory pathways, interference with antigen processing/presentation, and more often the manipulation of the costimulatory molecules. Exploitation of the behavior of costimulation pathways provides evolutionary incentive to the pathogens and thereby abates the functioning of immune system. Impairment by pathogens in the signaling events delivered by costimulatory molecules may be responsible for defective T-cell responses; consequently organisms grow unhindered in the host cells. These molecules expressed on the surface of various cells play a decisive role in the initiation and sustenance of immunity. These pathogens have devised various convergent devices that pathogens employ to tune and tame the immune system using costimulatory molecules. Studying host–pathogen interaction in context with costimulatory signals may unveil the molecular mechanism that will help in understanding the survival/death of the pathogens. Hence, the very same pathways can potentially be exploited to develop immunotherapeutic strategies to eliminate intracellular pathogens.

The organisms mentioned above are representatives of successful pathogens from the class of bacteria, virus, and parasites. It appears that these pathogens adopt a common evolutionarily convergent mechanism to evade host immune reaction. In this chapter we will discuss the mechanisms by which pathogens suppress host immunity by modulating the expression of costimulatory molecules. Table 3.2 shows the modulation of costimulatory molecules by intracellular pathogens. We therefore, in this chapter, suggest avenues of therapeutic intervention by exploiting costimulatory pathways for treating infections caused by pathogens.

Costimulation Biology Modulation by Pathogens

Costimulatory molecules of CD80/CD28, tumor necrosis factor (TNF)/TNFR, and T-cell immunoglobulin mucin (TIM) superfamilies have revealed a plethora of the possible ligand–receptor interactions that has elaborated the understanding of regulatory mechanisms of the immune responses mediated by APCs and T cells. For example, a positive regulator like CD40L (on T cells) when associated with CD40 (on APCs), not only activates T cells but also results in the activation of DCs; a process that is popularly called "T-cell licensing."[17,18] Similarly, ligation of CD28 with CD80 and CD86 is known to induce the secretion of interleukin-6 (IL-6) and interferon-γ (IFN-γ) by DCs and activation, proliferation, and differentiation of B cells.[19,20] It is reported that 4-1BBL expressed on DCs, binds to 4-1BB on T cells, to bolster DCs help to T cells.[21] Many reports have highlighted the inhibitory roles of cytotoxic T lymphocyte-associated antigen (CTLA-4; CD152) and programmed death (PD)-1 (expressed on T cells) with ligands CD80/CD86 and PDL-1/PDL-2 (on APCs), respectively.[22,23] It clearly suggests that costimulation not only amplifies the magnitude of the activation of T cells and APCs, but fine tunes the immune response as well, thereby controlling the hyper activation.

TABLE 3.2 Modulation of Costimulatory Molecules by Various Intracellular Pathogens such as Protozoa, Bacteria, and Viruses

Intracellular Pathogen Type	Name of the Intracellular Pathogen	Costimulatory Molecule Upregulated/Downregulated	Loss of Function
Viruses	HIV	PD-1↑, PDL-1↑, CTLA-4↑, CD80↓, CD86↓, CD33↓, CD40L↓, 4-1BB↓, OX40↓	Blocks IL-2 but augments IL-10 secretion, induces exhaustion of T cells, defective CTLs, respectively, and hampers antigen uptake ability of APCs
	HBV	PDL-1↑, PD-1↑	Induces IL-10 secretion, enhances apoptosis and anergy in T cells
	HCV	CD83↓, CD86↓	Reduces stimulatory capacity of DCs
	Measles	CD40↓, CD80↓, CD86↓, CD25↓, CD83↓, CD69↓	Abnormal DCs differentiation improper CD8 T-cell proliferation
	Herpes simplex virus	ICAM-1↓	Blocks APCs T-cell communication
Protozoa	*L. donovani*	CD80↓	Inefficient T-cell response
	T. gondii	CD80↓	Inhibits T-cell stimulatory activity
Bacteria	*Mtb*	CD80↓, CD86↓, CD40↓, PDL-1/PDL-2↑, PD-1↑	Hampers effective T-cell activation; induces anergy or apoptosis in T cells, paralyzes IL-2 and chemokines secretion, and inhibits NK cell function
	M. leprae	CD80↓, CD28↓	Blockade of IL-12 secretion, defective T-cell response
	S. typhimurium	ICAM-1↓	Impedes antigen uptake ability of APCs
	B. anthracis	CD40↓, CD80↓, CD86↓	Impairment of antigen-specific B- and T-cell immunity, suppresses the function of DCs
	H. pylori	PDL-1↑, CTLA-4↑	Exhaustion of DCs, obstructs cytokines secretion, induces anergy in T cells
	B. bronchiseptica	CD40↓	Hampers maturation of DCs
	B. pertussis	CD40↓, ICAM↓	Promotes differentiation of Tregs

Note: Symbol (↑) means upregulation or enhancement in the expression while symbol (↓) means downregulation or suppression of expression.

T-cell interaction with APC involving TCR and costimulatory molecules activates a plethora of downstream signaling molecules, leading to the induction of the expression of CD40L, PD-1, and CD28.[24]

Intracellular pathogens utilize an array of mechanisms to manipulate costimulatory molecules. Upon infection, pathogens trigger IL-10 secretion by inhibiting p38 mitogen-activated protein kinases (MAPKs) and promoting ERK phosphorylation.[25] IL-10 blocks the degradation of IκB-α which inhibits the NF-κB activation eventually inhibiting the expression of costimulatory molecules.[26] Interference in Toll-Like Receptor (TLRs) signaling by the intracellular pathogens is considered to be a foremost event in the suppression of costimulatory molecules. Mannosylated lipoarabinomannan (ManLAM) of *Mtb* binds to DC-SIGN and compromises the lipopolysaccharide (LPS)-induced activation of DCs by interfering in the TLRs' signaling.[27] Binding of *Mtb* early secreted antigenic target protein 6 (ESAT-6) to TLR-2 activates AKT and prevents interaction between the MyD88 and IRAK4, consequently abrogating NF-κB activation that suppresses CD80 expression.[28] Similarly, HIV upregulates PDL-1 on DCs and monocytes by attenuating the signaling of TLR-7 and TLR-8.[29] In addition, HIV-mediated PI3K activation upregulates PDL-1 on APCs and thus suppresses the activation of HIV-specific CD8+ T cells.[30] Rapid endocytosis of costimulatory molecules upon infection is suggested as one of the mechanisms to interrupt the function of APCs. For instance, Nef protein of HIV modulates the actin-dependent trafficking mechanism to remove CD80/CD86 from the monocytes surface, making them inefficient to activate T cells.[31]

TCR signaling is central for the optimum expression of costimulatory molecules and effector function of T cells. Therefore, it may serve as an important target for pathogens to paralyze T-cell activity.[32] *Mtb* glycolipids interfere with TCR signaling and block the activation of CD4+ T cells.[32] HIV gp120 interacts with CD4 (a coreceptor for TCR) that inhibits intracellular signal transduction through TCR, leading to decreased hydrolysis of polyphosphoinositide (PI), Ca^{2+} influx, activation of protein kinase C (PKC), and eventually failure of nulear factor of activated T cells (NFAT) translocation. These events culminate in the inhibition of CD40L expression. Decline of CD40L on T cells abrogates the bidirectional signaling and reduces the exhibition of CD80 on APCs.[33] In contrast, Nef activates NFAT and stimulates IL-2 release to overcome the exogenous requirement of IL-2 to promote T-cell proliferation, consequently disseminating the infection.[34] However, Nef retards CD28 and CD4 expression, thereby making T cells incapable of promoting cell-mediated immunity (CMI).[35] Corroborative with these observations, Nef-mutated HIV is unable to cause persistent infection. Similarly, core protein of HCV inhibits TCR signaling and upregulates PD-1.[36] The above-mentioned mechanisms imply that pathogens can effectively utilize various costimulatory pathways to subvert immune response to persist in the host.

MODULATION OF COSTIMULATORY MOLECULES BY VIRUSES

The vertebrate immune system has evolved complex antiviral innate and adaptive immune mechanisms like production of IFNs which limit the viral replication by the host cells. Other wonderful examples involve the natural killer (NK) cell-mediated lysis and apoptosis of the infected cells[37,38] to counter viral infestation. Adaptive antiviral immunity relies greatly on the lysis of infected cells by cytotoxic CD8+ T cells and neutralizing antibodies secreted by B cells. HIV is a retrovirus that is responsible for 1.9 million deaths annually. It predominantly infects CD4+ T helper (Th) cells. Further, it invades DCs, monocytes, and macrophages expressing CD4 and one of its coreceptors CCR5 or CXCR4. HIV can also bind to DC-SIGN and mannose receptors.[39,40] However, the virus preferentially replicates in the activated HIV-specific CD4+ T cells. Indeed, excessive loss of CD4+ T cells is the hallmark of HIV infection.

Like many other intracellular pathogens, HIV efficiently exploits the costimulatory molecules to override the immune responses. Its infection is associated with decreased expression of CD40L on CD4+ T cells.[41] Upon activation, CD4+ T cells from individuals with progressive disease show very little upregulation of CD40L, which corroborates with their inability to help APCs and failure to induce IL-12 in DCs.[42] Further, CD40–CD40L interaction has been demonstrated to be important in engendering a robust HIV-specific CD8+ T-cell response. Furthermore, HIV interferes in the CD40 signaling pathway in B cells and hinders T cell help, thereby impairing the secretion of immunoglobulin G (IgG) and IgA antibodies.[43] AIDS patients suffer from a defective humoral immunity (HI), which may be due to loss of T-cell function or B-cell intrinsic defects.[44] HIV upregulates Fas and FasL (members of TNF superfamily) on CD8+ T cells and APCs, respectively, which leads to the apoptosis of the interacting CD8+ T cells.[45,46] Thus, in HIV infections, the hunter becomes the hunted! During viral infections, continual expression of CD80/CD86 on DCs is decisive to maintain the effector function of CD8+ T cells.[47] Intriguingly, HIV downregulates the expression of CD80/CD86 and their ligand CD28 on infected APCs and T cells, respectively. The expression of costimulatory molecules such as 4-1BBL, CD70, OX40, and OX40L is affected during HIV-1 infection.[48] Measles, herpes, and hepatitis C viruses (HCVs) retard the expression of CD80, CD86, CD25, CD83, and CD40 that leads to poor CD8+ T-cell priming.[49,50] In addition, herpes virus suppresses intracellular cell adhesion molecule (ICAM)-1 on APCs, thereby obstructing immunological synapse with T cells.[51]

Chronic viral infections are associated with loss of function in T cells, a phenomenon popularly known as T-cell exhaustion. Exhausted T cells highly express PD-1 and have poor effector function.[52] PD-1 expression on HIV-specific T cells is associated with T-cell exhaustion and disease progression.[53] PD-1 is known to make CD8+ T cells more susceptible to Fas-mediated lysis.[54] Signaling through PD-1 can suppress IL-2 secretion by CD8+ T cells. IL-2 is known to rescue T cells from anergy and boost the memory response.[55] In addition, upregulation of PDL-1 on APCs during HIV or hepatitis B virus (HBV) infection supports the survival of pathogens[56] (Table 3.2). In essence, viruses can exploit costimulatory molecules in restraining the function of both T cells and APCs.

MODULATION OF COSTIMULATORY MOLECULES BY BACTERIA

The bacterial intracellular pathogens like *Salmonella typhi* (*S. typhi*), *Helicobacter pylori* (*H. pylori*), *Mtb*, *Mycobacteria avium*, *M. leprae*, etc., infect both DCs and macrophages. These APCs have pathogen recognition receptors (PRRs) on their surface which recognize bacterial components known as pathogen-associated molecular patterns (PAMPs) thus triggering innate immunity that initiates antimicrobial defense mechanisms involving autophagy, apoptosis, release of antimicrobial compounds like IFN-γ and TNF-α, etc.[57] It is followed by activation of adaptive immunity which is highly specific and has immunological memory. The adaptive immune response involves the clonal selection of B cells and T cells that confer HI and CMI to pathogens, respectively (Figure 3.3). Pathogen-specific Th1 cells release cytokines, especially IFN-γ and TNF-α, which plays an imperative role in activating infected macrophages and restraining the microbial growth.[58] Moreover the interaction of costimulatory molecule ligand receptor between CD80/CD86 with CD28 is essential for preventing apoptosis and anergy in T cells. Further, interaction of CD40/CD40L costimulatory receptor ligand results in efficient IL-12 production together with an upregulation of costimulatory molecules, in addition to enhanced antigen presentation by APCs thereby leading to an enhanced T-cell response.[18,59] Hence, interference in the downmodulation of any of these pathways by the pathogens would be detrimental to the host. *Mtb* is one of the most successful pathogens in the history of mankind.

There are numerous reports indicating the role of mycobacteria in downregulating the expression of CD80, CD86, and CD40 on APCs.[60] An elegant study demonstrated that the expression of costimulatory molecules and MHC are downregulated in macrophages infected with fluorescent reporter bacteria.[61] A recent study showed, albeit for BCG, that MHC-II, CD80, CD86, and CD40 are downtuned during chronic phase of infection. In such studies, it is important to delineate the expression of these molecules on infected versus noninfected cells, as by-stander inflammation could interfere in the interpretation of results. Defect caused by bacterial infections in APCs in the CD80/CD86 (downregulation) and CTLA-4 (upregulation) signaling pathway in APC and T cells is known to induce anergy/apoptosis of interacting T cells, and to paralyze the release of IL-2, which may compromise the generation of T-cell memory.[62,63] Impediment in CD28 signaling interferes in IFN-γ production

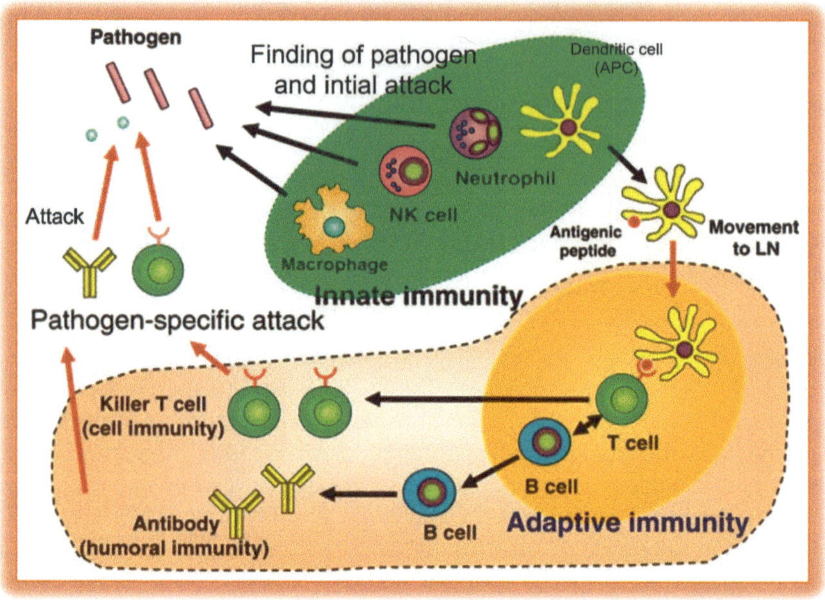

FIGURE 3.3 **CD80 and CD86 deliver bidirectional signaling for the activation of T cell and APC.** Cognate association between T cell and APC lead to interaction between MHC–peptide with TCR, and CD80/86 with CD28/CD152. This steers toward the activation and differentiation of T cell. Activated T cell secretes cytokines that ultimately help in the activation and differentiation of APC. The arrows shown in the diagram depict that there occur as well an alternative pathway of bidirectional signaling through costimulatory molecules CD80/CD86 and CD28/CD152 that activates both T cell and APC.

and hence promotes the survival of pathogens. *M. leprae* has been shown to obstruct the CD28/B7 signaling pathway for rendering antigen-specific T cell unresponsive in lepromatous leprosy patients. Protective CMI is always associated with the release of chemokines and migration of immune cells to the site of infection. *Mtb* impairs the secretion of chemokines by interfering with the CD28-CD80/CD86 signaling pathway thereby obstructing the surveillance of immune cells and enhancing the propagation of the bacterium.[64,65] Recently, the importance of CD80/CD86 in controlling mycobacterial infection has been demonstrated in CD80/CD86 double knockout mice.[66] The down-modulation of CD80/CD86 in chronic phase of the infection suggests that mycobacteria may actively exploit this pathway to anergize the T cells. It has been shown that the most abundant cell wall lipid trehalose 6,6′-dimycolate of *Mtb* and MTSA-10 inhibit the expression of costimulatory molecules on the surface of the macrophages.[67,68] Similarly, CD40–CD40L interaction is very important in mediating efficient protection against mycobacteria.[69] Indeed, it has been shown *in vitro* and in lepromatous patients that CD40 is downregulated by

M. leprae.[70] There is indirect evidence indicating the involvement of *Mtb* manipulating CD40/CD40L expression. In humans, CD40L expression on Th1 cells of tuberculosis patients has been correlated with the intensity of IFN-γ secretion. However, CD40 but not CD40L knockout mice are susceptible to *Mtb* infection. It is reported that the heat shock protein 70 (HSP70) of *Mtb* acts as an alternate ligand for CD40. Corroboratively, overexpression of HSP70 interferes with long-time persistence of *Mtb* and allows its clearance.[71] Interestingly, in chronic mycobacterial infections, CD40 is suppressed on infected cells.[61,72] Therefore, it is intriguing to speculate that in the chronic phase of infection, mycobacteria may hamper CD40 expression or manipulate CD40L signaling through binding with HSP70 instead of CD40L in order to evade host defense mechanisms.

The expression of PD-1 and its ligands PDL-1/PDL-2 is upregulated by the mycobacteria.[73] Blockade of PD-1 interaction with PDL-1/PDL-2 enhances immune response. Several studies have shown that T cells and NK cells from tuberculosis patients have increased PD-1 expression.[74,75] These observations suggest that mycobacteria may exploit PD-1 and PDL-1/PDL-2 pathways to dampen the host immune responses. In contrast, some studies have suggested that these pathways may be involved in controlling exuberant T-cell responses in tuberculosis and hence may be beneficial for both the host and the pathogen.[76,77] *Mtb* retards the development and maturation of monocyte-derived DCs to limit the immune response.[78] These immature DCs have a tolerogenic effect *in vivo* that can result in the generation of regulatory T cells (Tregs). Tregs can restrain the proliferation of naive and memory T cells, thereby suppressing preexisting T-cell immunity.[79,80]

Not only mycobacterial species but many other bacterial pathogens can exploit CD80/CD86-CD28/CTLA-4 pathways for their persistence (modulation of costimulatory pathways; Table 3.2). *S. typhi* is known to suppress ICAM-1 and as a consequence reduces the antigen uptake by APCs and inadequate T-cell response.[81,82] *Yersinia pseudotuberculosis* decreases CD86 expression on B cells and impedes the function of both B and T cells.[83] *H. pylori* causes chronic infection in the gut resulting in peptic ulcers. Further, it is known to induce the expression of CTLA-4, resulting in the anergy of T cells and poor clearance of the bacteria.[84] *H. pylori* diminishes the expression of CD40L on T cells and therefore employs CD40/CD40L pathway for its survival. Furthermore, it upregulates PDL-1 expression on gastric epithelial cells and inhibits the activation of T cells recruited to gastric mucosa.[85] In addition, it has been reported that PDL-1 upregulation not only blocks T-cell proliferation and IL-2 secretion, but also promotes the development of Tregs.[86] *Bordetella pertussis* and *B. bronchiseptica* decrease the manifestation of CD40 and ICAM-1 on DCs, and subsequently, render DCs tolerogenic and promote chiefly Tregs but not Th1 cells.[87] Hence, costimulatory molecules could serve as attractive targets for bacteria to modulate in order to prolong their own survival.

MODULATION OF COSTIMULATORY MOLECULES BY PROTOZOAN PARASITES

T cells play a significant role in controlling the protozoa-inflicted diseases like malaria, visceral leishmaniasis, and trypanosomiasis. Humoral responses play a less important role. However, complement-mediated killing or opsonization is responsible for control of pathogen during the intermittent extracellular phase of its replication cycle within the vertebrate host.[88] Parasites like *Leishmania donovani, L. chagasi, Toxoplasma gondii (T. gondii), T. cruzi,* and *Plasmodium falciparum* can manipulate the costimulatory molecules for evading immune system. *L. donovani* and *L. chagasi* infect macrophages and are reported to downregulate both CD80 and ICAM-1[89] Such APCs fail to optimally activate T cells. *T. gondii* and *T. cruzi*, selectively dampen the exhibition of CD80 and CD28, respectively to impair the function of T cells.[89] CD40 deficient mice succumb to plasmodium infection. *Plasmodium* interferes in the signaling mechanism of CD40 in DCs.[90] This signifies that this pathway is detrimental in providing sterilizing immunity to parasites, as it activates APCs and protective Th1 responses. CD40-CD40L signaling is crucial for Th1 immunity against *L. major*, because CD40L/CD40 knockout mice sparsely secrete IL-12, favoring Th2-biased response. Interestingly, *L. major* can differentially modulate the expression of CD40 and thus anergizes T cells and promotes Tregs population.[91] In nutshell, parasites can efficiently enable the immune system by dampening the expression of costimulatory molecules.

COSTIMULATORY MOLECULES IN THERAPEUTIC VACCINATION

In order to develop successful vaccines against chronic viral diseases it is widely thought that a cell-mediated immune response is required to eliminate or control intracellular viruses. For a protective immune response it is important to induce long-term immunological memory. The initial activation of T cells requires both an antigen-specific signal, involving the recognition of a peptide–MHC complex by the TCR as well as additional costimulatory signals. Only when the T cell recognizes both the antigen and a costimulatory signal on the DCs is an immune response initiated. The idea of a therapeutic vaccine is that the natural immune response, although present, may be suboptimal. By providing antigens and costimulatory molecules together, one may be able to provide a strong enough response to eliminate, or at least better contain, the virus.

Coinhibitory pathways also have become therapeutic targets for combating chronic viral infections. Blockade of the PD-1/PD-L pathway identified the key role of inhibitory receptors in mediating T-cell exhaustion. Exhausted CD8+ T cells express multiple inhibitory receptors, including PD-1, lymphocyte-activation gene 3 (Lag-3), CD160, 2B4 (CD244), and CTLA-4. The coexpression of multiple inhibitory receptors has been associated with greater T-cell exhaustion and more severe infection. Co-blockade of PD-1 and LAG-3 synergistically improved T-cell responses and reduced viral load, demonstrating that distinct inhibitory pathways can uniquely regulate T-cell exhaustion. Further studies are needed to define the unique and overlapping functions of coinhibitory pathways in exhausted T cells and to test the therapeutic benefits of targeting multiple coinhibitory pathways during chronic viral infection. Recent technological advances in structural biology provide new opportunities for understanding the structural and chemical features of costimulatory receptors and ligands, and their mechanisms of costimulation. The crystal structures of costimulatory receptors and ligands in the Ig, TNF, and TIM families, illustrate how structural understanding can provide important mechanistic insights through defining chemical and physical features that underlie receptor/ligand specificity, affinity, and oligomeric state. These approaches also may guide the development of improved therapeutic agents and reveal new therapeutic strategies for targeting costimulatory pathways.[92]

We have recently shown that signals delivered through costimulatory molecules:

i) not only are responsible for optimum activation of T cells but through bidirectional signaling can also influence macrophages;
ii) can modulate the secretion of proinflammatory molecules;
iii) can regress the growth of intracellular pathogens like *M. tuberculosis*, *M. microti*, *etc.*;
iv) this novel strategy can be effectively exploited to develop immunotherapy either using humanized antibodies against CD80, CD86 and CD40 or CD28 fusogenic proteins for the treatment of intracellular pathogens like *M. tuberculosis*, *HIV*, *L. donovani*, *T. cruzi*, etc.;
v) since this approach is based on modulating the immune system of the hosts rather than targeting the pathogen; hence it significantly diminishes chance of emergence of drug resistant strains of bacteria. It may be concluded from the results that macrophages are not only activated and kills intracellular pathogens by cytokines secreted by T cells but also through bidirectional costimulation through signals delivered by costimulatory molecules.[92a,92b,92c]

Latest reports suggest that 4-1BBL can provide a costimulatory signal to the human CD28-T cells, leading to cytokine production, cell survival and the upregulation of molecules associated with cellular cytotoxicity.[93] Memory CD8+ T cells specific for chronic viral pathogens (HCV, HIV, cytomegalovirus, Epstein–Barr virus) are found among the CD28-T cell population in human blood.[94,95] The proportion of T cells lacking CD28 is increased in people with chronic viral infections or other persistent conditions such as multiple myeloma. The observation that 4-1BBL can stimulate CD28-T cells makes it an attractive candidate for boosting immunity in chronic viral infection, where the lack of CD28 on the memory cells will make this population of cells insensitive to B7 stimulation. As will be discussed below, stimulatory anti-4-1BB antibodies have been tested *in vivo* in mouse models. Provision of anti-4-1BB can systemically increase both anticancer and antiviral immunity.[96]

Further work has shown that the systemic administration of stimulatory anti-4-1BB antibodies can correct the defect in CD28−/− mice when a single dose is provided during the primary influenza infection. This results in full restoration of the memory T-cell response, suggesting that for CD8+ T cells, CD28 is only required for initial T-cell activation and not for recall responses. Conversely, a single dose of anti-4-1BB antibody corrects the defect in the CD8+ T cell recall response in 4-1BBL−/− mice only when added at the time of viral challenge, arguing that the 4-1BB costimulatory signal is more important during recall responses (unpublished data from Mir and Agrewala et al.) Why the immune system switches from CD28 to 4-1BB as a costimulatory molecule during primary versus secondary responses is not clear. Interestingly, administration of anti-4-1BB (100 μg) during viral challenge results in a two fold increase in the recall response to influenza virus, even in wild-type mice. The physiological levels of 4-1BBL in mice appear to be very low, as the ligands are difficult to detect except after extensive stimulation of the cells *in vitro*.[97] This is consistent with the finding that the provision of extra 4-1BBL or stimulatory anti-4-1BB antibodies is immune stimulatory even in immunocompetent mice.[98] These findings suggest that 4-1BBL, rather than B7, may be the better choice of immune stimulatory agents to use in an immunotherapeutic regimen for antiviral immunity.

THERAPEUTIC VACCINATION USING COSTIMULATORY MOLECULES IN HIV

With chronic viral diseases such as HIV there may well have been a vigorous initial immune response to the pathogen, but the combination of viral escape variants and viral interference with the immune system results in the establishment of a chronic infection. One model for applying a therapeutic vaccine to the problem of HIV is to first use antiviral therapy to reduce viral load as much as possible. This would be followed by the interruption of antiviral therapy and provision of HIV antigens together with costimulatory molecules, in the hope that the enhanced immune response could eradicate the residual virus and prevent further erosion of the immune system. A key issue becomes how to deliver the antigen and costimulatory molecules. As has been demonstrated in mouse models of cancer or acute viral infection, systemic administration of stimulatory antibodies against receptors involved in immune triggering is one possible approach. However, the need to produce large amounts of protein product for therapy could be prohibitively expensive. On the other hand, the recent success of a recombinant protein therapy for arthritis (soluble TNFR) suggests that such approaches might be feasible.[99] An alternative approach that may be cheaper to administer would be to use recombinant replication-defective viruses containing both viral epitopes and the genes encoding costimulatory molecules as a therapeutic vaccine. Replication-defective adenoviruses, modified canary pox, and other viral vectors are being developed for immunotherapy.[100,101] Recombinant replication-defective adenoviruses are particularly attractive as there are two regions of their genome that can readily accommodate foreign DNA so that one could independently incorporate both antigens and costimulatory molecules. Furthermore, multiple serotypes of a virus should allow for more than one immunization.

Another approach being considered for HIV therapy is known as adoptive immunotherapy. In this approach, patient lymphocytes are obtained by leukophoresis and stimulated *in vitro* before reinfusion into the same patient. In a recent example, Levine and colleagues used anti-CD3 (a component of the TCR) and anti-CD28 coated beads to stimulate HIV patient T cells in a nonspecific way. The T cells were then infused back into the patients and their CD4+ T cell counts were found to improve, at least temporarily.[102] The advantage of this approach is that the stimulatory agents are not delivered systemically, which reduces toxicity concerns. This approach, using antigen-specific activation together with costimulatory molecules, such as 4-1BBL, could be used to generate useful T cells for reinfusion into patients. This approach could also use a replication-defective viral delivery vector containing HIV epitopes and costimulatory molecules delivered to the patient's APCs *ex vivo*. These would be used to activate the patients' T cells, and the activated T cells are subsequently reinfused, again avoiding systemic delivery of the virus. Although great strides have been made over the last few years in our understanding of T-cell activation and responses during infection, many challenges remain in the development of therapeutic vaccines for chronic viral infections. These advances suggest that we will see a number of new therapeutic vaccine approaches developed over the next few years.

B7 COSTIMULATORY MOLECULES IN INFECTIOUS DISEASES

Because microbial products can affect the expression of costimulatory molecules, these molecules participate in the pathogenesis of infectious diseases. They also participate in the pathogenesis of autoimmune diseases, the rejection of grafted organs, and graft-versus-host disease, and antagonists of these molecules can prevent or ameliorate these conditions. Although B7 molecules are important in the pathogenesis of graft rejection, graft-versus-host disease, infections, and autoimmune diseases; in addition, they participate in immunity against tumors,[103] but here we will focus on the role of B7 molecules in infectious diseases. The B7:CD28 costimulatory pathway participates in the pathogenesis of several bacterial, parasitic, and viral diseases.

Certain bacteria or their products can increase the expression of B7. One of these bacterial products, LPS, increases the expression of B7-1 and B7-2 by APCs.[103,104] The incubation of macrophages with heat-killed *Listeria monocytogenes* also causes increased production of B7.[105] A series of proteins isolated from pathogenic strains of neisseria, *Neisseria meningitidis* and *N. gonorrhoeae*, upregulate the expression of B7-2, which may explain the adjuvant effect of these neisserial proteins in antibody production.[106] In contrast, *Mtb* deficient expression of costimulatory molecules and the intracellular protozoan *L. donovani* inhibit the expression of B7-1 molecules after they infect macrophages *in vitro*.[107] The toxic shock syndrome and food poisoning are serious side effects of the immune system's defense against extracellular bacteria. These complications are caused by a class of microbial products, called superantigens, that can activate all T cells that express a particular family of T-cell antigen-receptor genes. The immune response to certain bacterial superantigens, such as the staphylococcal enterotoxins and the related toxic shock syndrome toxin, also depends on costimulation by B7-1 and B7-2.[108] Only a few studies have addressed the role of the B7:CD28 pathway in viral infections. After infection with the HIV, the expression of CD28 is reduced in both CD4 and CD8 T cells.[109,110] It is not known whether stimulation of the remaining CD28 molecules promotes or inhibits[111] viral infection. In mice carrying a targeted mutation in the CD28 gene, the response of helper T cells to infection with vesicular-stomatitis virus is diminished, but cytotoxic T-cell responses to infection with lymphocytic-choriomeningitis virus are normal.[112]

These findings suggest that the B7:CD28 pathway plays a more important part in viral infections in which viral clearance depends on antibody responses. Infection with the HBV may be one of these, but this issue has not yet been examined. Infection with *Leishmania major* perhaps best exemplifies the consequences of the dominance of a particular subgroup of helper T cells on the immune response. Strains of mice that use type-1 helper T cells to respond to *L. major* produce large amounts of IFN-γ, and thus resist the parasite. By contrast, strains of mice that use type-2 helper T cells, and consequently produce IL-4 and IL-10, succumb to the organism. CTLA-4−Ig, if administered early after infection, reduces the production of IL-4 and halts the progression of disease in susceptible BALB/c mice but has no effect in the genetically resistant C57BL/6 strain of mice. These different effects in susceptible and resistant mice indicate that the priming of type-2 helper T cells is more dependent on the B7:CD28 pathway than is the priming of type-1 cells,[113] and provides evidence for the interpretation of analogous results in mice deficient in CD28. Infection with the trematode helminth *Schistosoma mansoni* may be an instance in which the levels of B7 expression on APCs correlate with, if they do not dictate, the severity of disease. *S. mansoni* antigens sensitize type-1 and type-2 helper T cells to form large granulomas in the liver around eggs of the parasite. However, the response of the type-1 helper T cells and the intensity of granulomatous inflammation spontaneously subside after the acute stage of the infection. There is substantial expression of B7-2 in cells of granulomas during the acute schistosomal disease; it rapidly diminishes thereafter.[114] It is likely that the downregulation of B7 expression and of the granulomatous reaction are precipitated by IL-10 given that macrophages from egg granulomas secrete IL-10 and induce unresponsiveness in type-1 helper T cells.[115] Neutralization of IL-10 by specific antibodies increases the expression of B7-2 by these macrophages and thus restores costimulatory activity.[116] A similar process has been observed in humans infected with *S. haematobium.* Taken together, these findings suggest that the inhibition of B7 expression may permit therapeutic control of schistosomal egg granulomas. In fact, injection of IL-10 at a time when its endogenous expression is low or absent results in decreased formation of granulomas and decreased cytokine production by type-1 helper T cells.[117] The observation that, as compared with type-2 effector CD4 T cells, type-1 effectors depend more on costimulation and are more susceptible to anergy has implications for chronic infections in which immune defenses depend on type-1 helper T cells. Very recently we have shown that macrophages can be activated not only through classical and alternate pathways but also by costimulation. Upon costimulation macrophages produce nitric oxide and proinflammatory cytokines and also upregulate the cell surface molecules thereby showing a state of activation. These costimulated macrophages effectively inhibit the growth of *Mtb* see Figure 3.4. In tuberculosis, leprosy, schistosomiasis, filariasis, and leishmaniasis, the waning of the B7:CD28 costimulatory pathway may change the clinical form of the disease by depressing CMI and inducing T-cell anergy. To what extent this downregulation of T-cell immunity is caused by the organisms themselves or mediated by cytokines is not known.

COSTIMULATORY MOLECULES IN ALLERGIES AND ASTHMA

The prevalence of allergy is increasing worldwide, especially in Western countries.[118,119] This trend may be due to increased hygiene which prevents early exposure to microorganisms in infancy and increases the risk of developing an allergic disease in the future.[120] Air pollution may also favor the development of allergies.[121] Among allergic diseases, asthma is of particular concern as it can evolve into a life-threatening chronic pulmonary disease. It is now recognized that inhalation of aeroallergens by sensitized patients initiates a massive Th2 cell response resulting in the production of IL-4, IL-5, and IL-13 by CD4+ T cells.[122] This triggers the development of typical signs of bronchial asthma including airway hyperresponsiveness, bronchoconstriction, mucus secretion, and airway remodeling. The recruitment, differentiation, and activation of Th2 cells play a cardinal role in the development of allergic disease. This Th2 polarization is mainly controlled by APCs that provide signals capable of supporting the differentiation of naive T cells into Th2 cells. Initially,

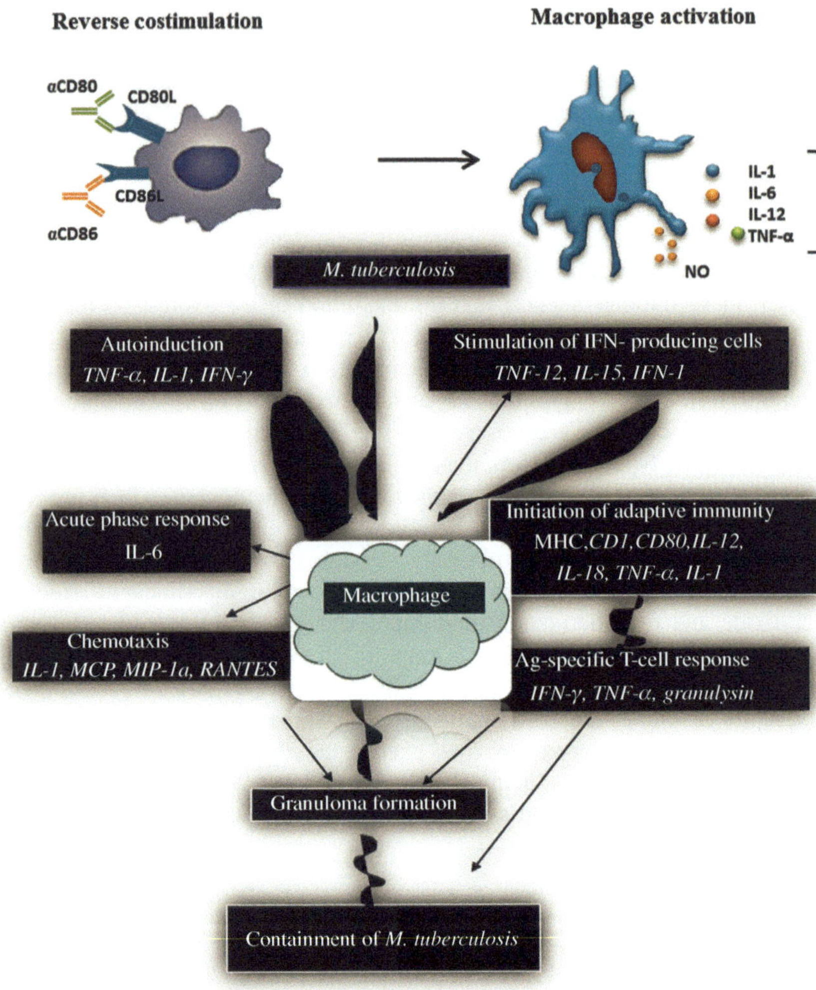

FIGURE 3.4 **Activation of macrophages through costimulation to enhance the production of cytokines and nitric oxide.** Macrophages are activated through reverse costimulation through anti-CD80 and anti-CD86 to enhance the production of cytokines and nitric oxide, both of which play an important role in protection against pathogens (*Mtb*).

Lafferty et al.[123] suggested that T lymphocytes require two coordinate signals to be fully activated. The first signal confers specificity to the immune response and plays an important role in the recognition of the MHC class–peptide complex at the surface of APCs by T lymphocytes. However, this primary signal is not sufficient to completely activate these T cells. To become fully effective, a second, nonspecific costimulatory signal is often required by T cells. These signals are provided by interactions between APCs and T cells through surface molecules expressed on T lymphocytes. APCs express costimulatory molecules such as CD80 (B7-1) and CD86 (B7-2) which belong to the B7 family. They provide modulation of T-cell function by ligation to their receptors, CD28 or CTLA-4. Engagement of CD28 or CTLA-4 has been observed to have opposite effects. CD28 promotes T-cell activation and survival while CTLA-4 inhibits T-cell responses and regulates peripheral T-cell tolerance.[124] This demonstration provides clear evidence that costimulatory molecules are involved in the fine-tuning of the T-cell response by mediating both stimulatory as well as inhibitory signals. In many recent studies, numerous new costimulatory molecules have been described leading to the recognition that costimulation pathways are more complex than the classical two-signal model. In general, costimulatory molecules are divided into two main families: molecules from the B7:CD28 family, such as CTLA-4 or PD-L1, and from the tumor necrosis factor receptor (TNFR) superfamily such as OX40 or CD27.[125] All these costimulatory molecules have particular effects on T-cell activation, function, and survival and are implicated in nearly all inflammatory diseases. Studies to better characterize the specific role of these molecules in allergy and asthma are still ongoing. In this chapter, we summarize current knowledge concerning the role of costimulatory molecules in allergy and analyze the potential functions of the emerging new subsets of costimulatory molecules recently described.

Involvement of the B7:CD28 Family Molecules in the Regulation of Allergic Diseases

The first costimulatory molecules described were the ligands of CD28: CD80 (B7-1) and CD86 (B7-2). The CD28 costimulation pathway is an important factor for the promotion of an effective antigen-specific immune response. However, CD28-deficient mice are still able to develop allergic airway inflammation showing that CD28 cannot be solely responsible for the development of an allergic response.[126] The expression of CD28 ligands (CD80 and CD86) has been extensively studied in clinical samples from asthmatic patients. Hofer et al.[127a] reported that B lymphocytes from asthmatic patients exposed to allergens express higher levels of surface CD86, but not CD80, compared with those from asthmatic patients not exposed to allergen or with those from healthy individuals (Table 3.3). Another study demonstrated that CD80 and, to a lesser extent, CD86 were upregulated at the surface of alveolar macrophages from allergic patients compared with those from pulmonary sarcoidosis, extrinsic allergic alveolitis patients, or from normal subjects.[127b] In contrast, Burastero et al.[128] observed that in allergic individuals, CD80, but not CD86, is highly expressed by alveolar macrophages. CD86 can also be expressed in a soluble form, where the transmembrane domain is deleted. This form is mostly produced by circulating monocytes and, like membrane-bound CD86, crosslinks CD28 or

TABLE 3.3 Important Roles Played by Various Costimulatory Molecules in Allergic Diseases and Asthma

Costimulatory Molecule Family	APC	Effector Cell	Functions and Characteristics
B7 Family	CD80	CTLA-4	Contributes to the suppressive activity of allergen-specific regulatory cells during sensitization
	CD86		Polymorphism in Ctla-4 promoter and gene favors allergic diseases
		CD28	CD80 and CD86 expression is upregulated on the surface of various cells of allergic patients. Soluble CD86 is increased in the sera of allergic patients
	ICOS-L	ICOS	Regulates Th2-effector cell function and their infiltration in the lungs, production of Th2 cytokine, promotes B-cell differentiation and IgE production
			Expression on iNKT cells contributes to airway hyperreactivity
			Contributes to the differentiation of regulatory cells in pulmonary lymph nodes
	PD-L1	PD-1	Drives the differentiation of Foxp3+ CD4+ T cells
			Downregulates contact hypersensitivity reaction
	PD-L2	PD-1	Regulates asthma by an IFN-γ-dependent mechanism
			Downregulates airway hyperreactivity, prevents eosinophil infiltration in the lungs, and prevents IgE production
	B7-H3	Receptor unknown	Promotes Th2 differentiation, eosinophil infiltration, and development of airway hyperreactivity
			Decreases the severity of allergic conjunctivitis

TNFR Family	OX40L	OX40L	Promotes the development of Th2 cells
			Prevents differentiation of Treg cells
			Abrogates mast cell degranulation
	CD30-L	CD30	CD30 is expressed by Langerhans cells, CD4+ and T cells of atopic patients
			Soluble CD30 is increased in the sera of allergic patients
	4-1BB-L	4-1BB	Promotes airway hyperreactivity, eosinophil infiltration, and IgE production
			Upregulates Th2 cell proliferation and mast cell cytokine production
	Fas	FasL	Delays resolution of airway hyperresponsiveness
			Promotes eosinophil apoptosis in the lungs
	CD27	CD70	Increases production of IgE by B cells
	CD40	CD40L	Contributes to isotype class switching toward IgE
			Enhances development of airway inflammation
			Increases production of Th2 cytokine and decreases number of Treg cells
Others	CD2	CD58	Promotes differentiation of Th2 cells and the production of IgE
			Expressed on monocytes of allergic patients

CTLA-4 and activates T lymphocytes.[129] In patients with acute asthma, the level of soluble CD86 has been shown to be increased relative to that in patients with stable asthma or in healthy individuals. Monocytes from allergic patients produce more soluble CD86 compared with those of healthy individuals.[130] It was also observed that the level of soluble CD86 is correlated with the severity of the airway hyperreactivity (AHR). These results are consistent with studies which show that the concentrations of soluble CD80 and soluble CD86 are elevated in asthmatic patients. Interestingly, the administration of a glucocorticoid (e.g., prednisolone), used to reduce airway inflammation in allergic patients, reduces the level of circulating CD86.[131] Recently, Ritprajak et al.[132] demonstrated that the topical administration of a silencer RNA specific to the CD86 gene reduced local inflammation in a mouse model of atopic dermatitis by decreasing the recruitment of DCs into the skin, production of antigen-specific IL-4, and induction of serum IgE and IgG1. It has also been reported that pulmonary tolerogenic DCs stimulated by allergen exposure express high levels of both CD80 and CD86.[133,134] Taken together, these studies suggest that overexpression of CD80 and/or CD86 is correlated with the development of allergic disease and asthma. Within the B7 family, CD28 and inducible costimulator (ICOS) are most homologous with respect to structure and function. Both are type I transmembrane receptors expressed as homodimers, with an extracellular (Ig)V-like domain, a hallmark of receptors of the B7-related family. ICOS expression is induced *in vitro* within 24–48 h of activation on all Th-primed cells.[135] ICOS has been shown to regulate the production of Th2 cytokines[136] and plays a critical role in lung mucosal inflammatory responses.[137] Further, this costimulatory molecule has been suggested not only to intensify some of the functions of CD28 during an already established immune response but also to induce additional T-effector cell functions.[138] Recent studies suggest that ICOS-mediated costimulation may regulate Th2-effector cell function without affecting Th2 differentiation. Another study showed that transfer of ICOS-enriched T cells followed by allergen airway challenge-induced infiltration of recipient T and B cells as well as local production of allergen-specific IgE by intrapulmonary plasma cells.[139] In contrast, transfer of the ICOS-depleted T-cell fraction resulted in the recruitment of significantly lower numbers of B cells with no local IgE production. These data indicate that expression of ICOS defines a subset of T-effector cells that are required for B-cell infiltration and local IgE production in lung tissue. According to Tesciuba et al.,[138] ICOS stimulation increases the migration of lymphocytes into draining lymph nodes by augmenting the expression of attractant chemokines CCL21 and CXCL13. In other reports, the increased production of IL-5, which is a main factor for the differentiation, maturation, and recruitment of eosinophils, is attributed to ICOS+ cells. ICOS+ T cells also promote the differentiation of B cells and IgE-producing plasma cells through the enhanced production of IL-4 and IL-10. ICOS-deficient mice are unable to induce high IgE responses which demonstrates their role in the induction of IgE production. Some studies also suggest that intermediate ICOS expression is associated with high production of Th2 cytokines, whereas high levels of ICOS predominantly translate into high IL-10 production. Surprisingly, ICOS/ICOS-L interaction not only promotes the development of Th2-driven inflammation but also mediates mucosal tolerance, as studies have indicated that pulmonary DCs in the bronchial lymph nodes of mice exposed to respiratory allergen induced the costimulation of Tregs via the ICOS/ICOS-L pathway.[133,134,140,141] These Treg cells produce IL-10, show inhibitory activity and, when adoptively transferred into sensitized mice, have the ability to inhibit the development of AHR. These reports suggest that both the development and inhibitory function of Treg cells depend upon the presence of IL-10 and ICOS/ICOS-L interaction.

CTLA-4 has been described to be an important regulator of T-cell activation. CTLA-4 is constitutively and exclusively expressed by T lymphocytes in both mice and humans.[124] CTLA-4 expression confers to T-lymphocyte regulatory functions. Indeed, the contribution of CTLA-4 in the regulation of the immune system is demonstrated by the development of multiple organ autoimmune pathologies and lymphoproliferative disease in CTLA-4-deficient mice. Blockade of CTLA-4 activity abolishes the suppressive function of CD4+ CD25+ T cells.[142] In a mouse model of inflammatory bowel disease, the effect of transfer of a population of CD4+ CD45RB low Treg cells in decreasing intestinal inflammation is abrogated by the co-administration of a blocking anti-CTLA-4 antibody. These studies suggest that the engagement of CTLA-4 at the surface of Treg cells by its ligands CD80 or CD86 contributes to the regulation of suppressive functions of Treg cells. Polymorphism in CTLA-4 gene is also considered a risk factor for allergy and asthma. Howard et al.[143a] characterized four single nucleotide polymorphisms which were related to allergic and asthma phenotypes. They demonstrated that these specific polymorphisms alone or in combinations are correlated with an elevated IgE titer or bronchial hyperresponsiveness in patients with asthma. Interestingly, in the same study, no correlation between allergic phenotype and single nucleotide polymorphisms for CD28 was observed. These findings confirm that CTLA-4 is indeed involved in the course of allergic diseases. Interestingly, CTLA-4 seems to play a more important role in the sensitization phase than in established allergy.

REGULATION OF THE IMMUNE RESPONSES TO PATHOGENS THROUGH COSTIMULATORY MOLECULES

Immune response to pathogens is regulated by stimulatory and inhibitory costimulatory signals. Positive costimulation is critical for the development of T-cell immune responses against foreign pathogens, while negative regulation is critical for the termination of immune responses, for peripheral tolerance and to avoid inflammation-induced tissue damage.[143b–145] Up to now four different families of costimulatory and coinhibitory molecules have been identified which are able to modulate TCR signaling in APC–T-cell interaction. These families include (1) B7-CD28 family including CD28, cytotoxic T-lymphocyte antigen-4 (CTLA-4, CD152), PD-1 (CD279), inducible costimulatory molecule (ICOS, CD278), and B- and T-lymphocyte attenuator (BTLA, CD272); (2) TNFR superfamily including CD27; (3) CD2/signaling lymphocyte activation molecule (SLAM) family including SLAM (CD150), 2B4 (CD244), and CD48; and (4) Ig family including TIM-3, CD160, and Lag-3 (Figure 3.5).

In the presence of a pathogen, a specific and effective immune response must be induced and naive T cells undergo activation upon encounter with their specific antigens.[146,147] This leads to antigen-specific T-cell proliferation,[148,149] cytokines production, and induction of T-cell differentiation toward an effector phenotype[150] combined to survival signals.[151,152] After clearance or control of the pathogen, the immune response must be terminated in order to avoid tissue damage and chronic inflammation.[152,153] Two main mechanisms are involved in the contraction of the effector phase of immune responses, that is, either the inhibition of T-cell expansion[154] or the elimination of activated cells by apoptosis.[155] The latter is referred to as activation-induced cell death (AICD).[155,156] Direct inhibition of T-cell proliferation is induced via signals through coinhibitory molecules such as CTLA-4 or PD-1, while 2B4 and SLAM are considered to be critical in the regulation of AICD.[157] The role of coinhibitory molecules in regulating the immune system is also evidenced by severe autoimmune and lymphoproliferative diseases resulting from the lack or aberrant expression of these molecules.[158]

Expression of Coinhibitory Molecules on Effector T Cells

T cells play an important role in the defense against infectious agents. Upon recognition of their cognate antigen, naive T cells get activated and differentiate into effector cells.[159] This activation results in both phenotypic and functional changes that will determine the fate of effector T cells and the efficacy of the immune response.[150] Several studies have aimed to better define the profile of effector cells associated with the efficient control of infectious agents.[160] Viganò et al.[161a] has recently performed and observed a comprehensive investigation of the expression of PD-1, 2B4, CD160, CTLA-4, TIM-3, Lag-3, and SLAM on CD4 and CD8 T-cell subsets identified according to their differentiation state (i.e., naive, memory, effector/memory). These analyses showed that whereas virtually none of the coinhibitory molecules tested was present on naive cells, they were present on memory T cells but at low levels, and more importantly, that effector/memory T cells expressed a significantly higher density of coinhibitory molecules simultaneously.

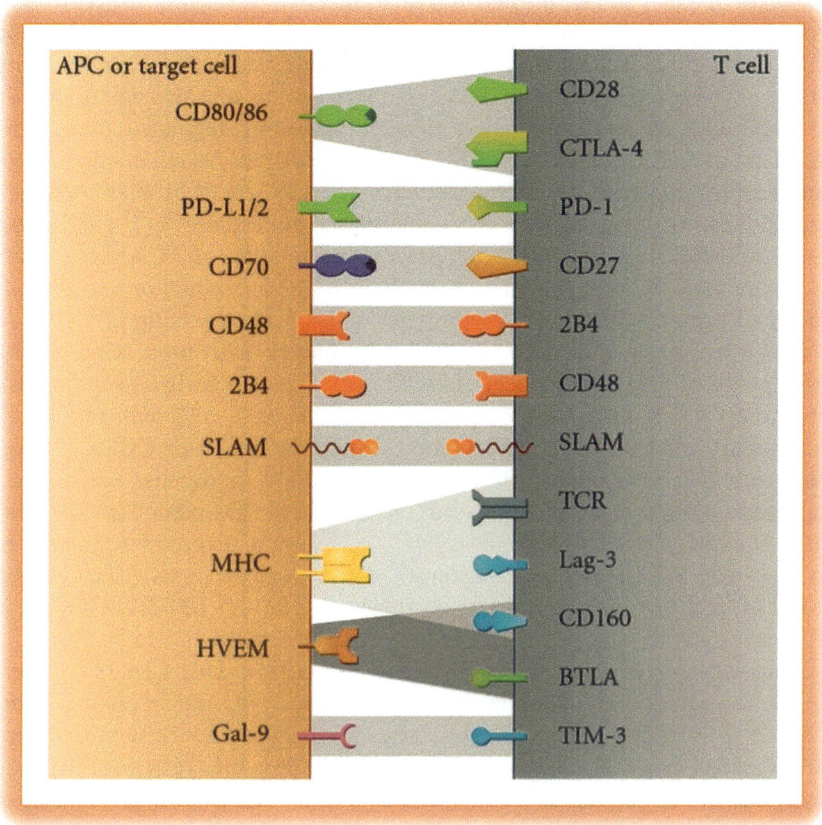

FIGURE 3.5 **Regulatory molecules and their ligands. Schematic overview of the different costimulatory and coinhibitory molecules expressed by T cells (right panel) and association with their respective ligands expressed by APCs or target cells (left panel).** Coinhibitory molecules are color coded according to their relevant families. The four families of regulatory molecules include (1) B7-CD28 family including CD28, cytotoxic T-lymphocyte antigen-4 (CTLA-4; CD152), programmed death-1 (PD-1; CD279), inducible costimulatory molecule (ICOS; CD278), and B- and T-lymphocyte attenuator (BTLA; CD272); (2) TNF-receptor superfamily including CD27 (3) CD2/signaling lymphocyte activation molecule (SLAM) family including SLAM (CD150), 2B4 (CD244), and CD48; and (4) Ig family including T-cell immunoglobulin mucin-3 (TIM-3), CD160, and lymphocyte-activation gene 3 (Lag-3).

ROLE OF COINHIBITORY MOLECULES IN THE CONTRACTION OF THE EFFECTOR PHASE OF IMMUNE RESPONSES

The immune system is able to mount strong and efficient immune responses against pathogens without damaging organs. This is notably achieved by the induction of the contraction and termination of the immune response after control or elimination of the infectious agent. During the contraction, the majority of effector T cells die, while remaining cells survive as memory cells.[152,153] The contraction of the immune response and the determination of T-cell fate depend on many transcription factors regulated during the course of the immune response.[161b] These factors can be either induced or repressed by different signaling pathways provided, with different strength and kinetics, by costimulatory and coinhibitory molecules.[162,163] One of the best-established mechanisms involved in the regulation of TCR signaling is the interaction between costimulatory (CD28) and coinhibitory (CTLA-4) molecules with CD80 or CD86 expressed by DCs. Crosslinking of CD28 on T cells synergizes with TCR signaling to induce activation. Conversely, crosslinking of CTLA-4 induces an inhibitory signal, which prevents T-cell activation.[154,164] CTLA-4 is upregulated on activated T cells and, as a structural homologous to CD28 with higher affinity for CD80 or CD86, it competes with CD28 to inhibit TCR signaling.[154] PD-1 is another well-known regulatory molecule. It is expressed on activated CD4 and CD8 T cells, NKT, B cells, and activated monocytes,[124,143b] and its expression is induced by TCR- and BCR-mediated signaling[165] The two PD-1 ligands (i.e., PD-L1 and PD-L2) differ in their expression pattern.[166] PD-L1 (B7-H1, CD274) is expressed by a broad array of cells (e.g., vascular endothelial cells, epithelial cells, muscles cells, hepatocytes) whereas PD-L2 (B7-DC, CD273) expression is restricted to hematopoietic cell types (i.e., DC, macrophages, mast cells).[167] PD-1/PD-Ls pathway regulates the balance between stimulatory and inhibitory signals needed for effective immune responses against pathogens.[168–171] Engagement of PD-1 by PD-L1 leads to the inhibition of CD28-mediated costimulation and thus of TCR-mediated lymphocyte proliferation and cytokines secretion. The relative levels of expression of inhibitory (PD-Ls) and stimulatory (CD80/CD86) ligands by APCs can determine the extent of T-cell activation while PD-L1 expression on nonlymphoid tissues may determine the extent of effector immune responses at sites of inflammation.[168] Also member of the B7-CD28 family, BTLA, is an inhibitory receptor able to recruit phosphatases to dampen TCR signaling[172] through the interaction with herpes virus entry mediator (HVEM) expressed on naive T and B cells. HVEM-BTLA signaling was shown to limit T-cell activity *in vivo* and to negatively regulate homeostatic expansion of CD4 and CD8 T cells.[173] Finally, HVEM can also interact with CD160, resulting in an inhibitory signaling dampening T-cell activation.[174]

Functional Exhaustion and Loss of Effector Functions

During chronic viral infections such as HIV and HCV, several inhibitory molecules are overexpressed on virus-specific CD4 and CD8 T cells, and this is associated with a state of functional deficiency also called functional exhaustion. Exhaustion is characterized by the progressive loss of T-cell functionality, leading ultimately to the deletion of exhausted T cells. The loss of the distinct T-cell functions occurs sequentially.[52] IL-2 production and T-cell proliferation potential are lost first. TNF-α production and cytotoxic capacity disappear later followed, ultimately, by the loss of IFN-γ production. Finally, deeply exhausted T cells are deleted via apoptosis.[175]

The current hypothesis is that functional exhaustion occurs as a consequence of the attempt of the immune system to limit the magnitude of effector T-cell responses in order to safeguard against autoimmune responses and inflammatory damages. Nonetheless, this mechanism of protection may compromise effective immunity against persistent infectious agents and tumors.[176]

More recently, the severity of lymphocytic choriomeningitis virus (LCMV) infection was associated to the number and the intensity of coinhibitory receptors expressed by virus-specific CD8 T cells.[177] Among these molecules, TIM-3, Lag-3, 2B4, CTLA-4, CD160, BTLA, KLRG1, CD305, and CD200R have been further investigated in the context of several human chronic virus infections and established tumors. In particular, the coexpression of TIM-3 and PD-1 was observed on both CD4 and CD8 T cells from patients with HIV[178] or HCV[179–181] chronic infections and correlated with T-cell exhaustion and disease progression. In addition, TIM-3- and PD-1-expressing CD8 T cells represented a major population within tumor-infiltrating lymphocytes in several murine models of cancer and in the blood of patients with advanced melanoma.[182,183] In all cases, TIM-3/PD-1-expressing cells represented the most impaired population of CD8 T cells. Of note, the blockade of both molecules could restore CD8 T-cell effector functions (proliferation potential and cytotoxic capacity) of antigen-specific CD8 T cells and was associated with the control of tumor growth.[178–182]

CTLA-4 is another coinhibitory receptor upregulated in the context of chronic infections and tumors.[183] It has been shown that CTLA-4 was overexpressed on CD4, but not CD8, T cells of simian immunodeficiency virus (SIV)-infected macaques,[184] and HIV-infected patients.[185,186] Furthermore, the combination of CTLA-4 blockade and 4-1BB (CD137) activation enhanced tumor rejection by increasing T-cell infiltration, proliferation capacity, and cytokines production.[187] Of interest, BTLA was reported to be persistently expressed by melanoma-specific CD8 T cells, thus inhibiting their antitumor function.[188] On the other hand, BTLA expression on CD4 and CD8 T cells decreased during HIV infection and this was associated with CD4 T-cell differentiation and activation.[189,190] Enhancing BTLA pathway may therefore represent an alternative therapeutic strategy to overcome immune activation during chronic HIV infection.

Lag-3 is an activation-induced cell-surface molecule, whose overexpression during chronic virus infection is also commonly associated with T-cell exhaustion and functional impairment. Blocking of Lag-3 alone failed in rescuing

T-cell function or in decreasing plasma viremia during chronic LCMV infection, while blockade of both PD-1 and Lag-3 synergistically improved T-cell responses and decreased viral loads *in vivo*.[177] Elevated levels of Lag-3 and CTLA-4 were found in PD1+ CD4 T cells from HIV-infected patients[191] and in tumor-derived NY-ESO-1-specific CD8 T cells.[124] Functionality of these T-cell subsets was more impaired than in Lag-3 − PD-1− or single Lag-3+ subsets.[192]

SLAM family members are immunomodulatory receptors with a role in the regulation of costimulation, T-cell cytokines production, and cytotoxic activity. 2B4, which is a key molecule from this family, is involved in CD8 T- and NK-cell cytotoxicity. However, the proportion of 2B4+ CD8 T cells in HIV-infected patients correlated with immune activation of memory T cells and was increased in patients with progressive disease.[193] In addition, IFN-γ secretion and cytotoxic activity of 2B4+ CD8 T cells were significantly lower following stimulation with HIV as compared to influenza-derived antigens, respectively.[194] Furthermore, during infectious mononucleosis, the expression of SLAM and 2B4 on CD8 T cells correlated with severity of symptoms and viral loads.[195]

The coexpression of molecules such as 2B4 and CD160, which have been related to potent cytolytic functions, was associated with exhaustion and regulation of virus-specific CD8 and CD4 T cells in the context of chronic virus infections.[196] A recent study showed a high frequency of CD8 T cells coexpressing PD-1, 2B4, CD160, KLRG1, LAG-3, and CTLA-4 in HCV infection. The coexpression of these molecules was associated with low levels of CD127 expression and correlated with impaired proliferation capacity.[196]

The expression of another set of inhibitory molecules (i.e., PD-1, CTLA-4, CD305, and CD200R) has been investigated on CD4 T cells from HCV-infected patients. PD-1 and CTLA-4 were upregulated by HCV-specific CD4 T cells from patients with chronic infection, while CD305 and CD200R were upregulated in patients with cleared infection. Of note, the blockade of PD-Ls increased the expansion of CD4 T cells.[197]

In the context of HIV infection, the presence of HIV-specific CD8 T cells coexpressing CD160, 2B4, and PD-1 but not Lag-3 was reported. The simultaneous expression of these molecules correlated with the level of virus replication and decreased cytokines production. The proliferative capacity was restored by blocking both PD-1/PD-L1 and 2B4/CD48 interactions.[198] Along the same line, another group showed that more than 30% of HIV-specific CD4 T cells expressed simultaneously PD-1, CTLA-4, and TIM-3, whereas less than 2% of simian immunodeficiency virus (CMV)- or varicella-zoster virus-specific CD4 T cells coexpressed all three receptors. The coexpression of these molecules on HIV-specific CD4 T cells was more strongly correlated with the viral load compared with the expression of each receptor individually.

Potential Therapeutic Applications of Costimulatory Molecules in Infections

The well-established immunosuppressive properties of coinhibitory molecules and the potential to revert exhausted or inactivated T-cell responses following selective blocking of their function made these markers interesting targets for therapeutic intervention in patients with persistent viral infections or cancer. To date, clinical and preclinical data are available for anti-CTLA-4 and anti-PD-1 blocking agents.[199–202] Initial human clinical trials assessing the effects of a blocking anti-CTLA-4 antibody demonstrated not only a reduction in tumor mass and clinical benefit in a minority of treated subjects but also an increase in systemic inflammation.[203,204] Improvement in safety of these antibodies resulted in the recent approval by the U.S. Food and Drug Administration of a human monoclonal antibody against CTLA-4 (Ipilimumab, MDX-010, Yervoy) for the treatment of metastatic melanoma. In both early and late phase trials, Ipilimumab has demonstrated consistent activity against melanoma. However, serious (grade 3–5) immune-related adverse events occurred in 10–15% of patients. Thus, while providing a clear survival benefit, Ipilimumab administration requires careful patient monitoring combined to, sometimes, treatment with immune-suppressive therapy.[199,200] In contrast, anti-CTLA-4 blockade failed to show benefit in terms of plasma viral load or survival in acutely or chronically SIV-infected macaques.[205,206] Since CTLA-4 is preferentially upregulated on CD4 T cells and not on CD8 T cells,[185] it might be possible that the blockade of anti-CTLA-4 induced an expansion and activation of CD4 T cells thus providing additional targets to HIV without significant improvement of CD8 T-cell functions.

Preclinical data showed how prevention of *in vivo* interactions between PD-1 and PD-L1 enhanced T-cell responses via the restoration of their ability to undergo proliferation, secrete cytokines, and lyse-infected cells and ultimately induce substantial reduction in viral loads. Of note, blockade of the PD-1/PD-L1 inhibitory pathway *in vivo* demonstrated a beneficial effect on CD8 T cells in mice that were lacking CD4 T-cell help.[166] This study identified a potentially effective immunotherapeutic strategy for chronic viral infections. This has then been further explored in nonhuman primates in a recent study evaluating the safety and immunomodulatory potential of an anti-PD-1 blocking antibody in SIV-infected macaques. The treatment was well tolerated and led to a rapid increase in virus-specific CD8 T-cell responses with improved functional quality, both in peripheral and in gut associated lymphoid tissue (GALT). PD-1 blockade also resulted in the expansion of virus-specific CD4 T cells, memory B cells, and higher titers of virus-specific antibodies. In contrast, one additional study showed an increase in CD4 T-cell activation and viral replication in mucosal sites.[206] Furthermore, a humanized anti-PD-1 monoclonal antibody (ONO-4538) is currently being tested in a Phase 1 study in patients with recurrent or treatment-refractory cancer. Preliminary data support the safety, tolerability, and pharmacokinetic profile of a single dose of the drug. In addition, preliminary evidences of antitumor activity were observed.[201,202]

There is currently a strong interest in the potential for clinical interventions targeting immunoregulatory networks to enhance immunity against cancer cells and persistent viruses or to boost the efficacy of preventive and therapeutic vaccines. The studies discussed previously have yielded promising results but have also highlighted important safety issues. This strongly indicates the importance to better understand mechanisms of immune regulation in order to exploit them for potential therapeutic applications.

SUMMARY

Coinhibitory molecules are involved in maintaining the balance between the capacity to generate effector T cells able to control pathogens and the preservation of tolerance. During the development of immune responses, key coinhibitory molecules are upregulated with different kinetics and play a role in regulating the development and the fate of effector and memory T-cell responses. In most cases, pathogens replication is controlled by the immune system leading to the contraction of effector T cells. Many different coinhibitory molecules, that is, PD-1, CTLA-4, BTLA, SLAM, and 2B4, play a role during this phase. The remaining memory T cells express some coinhibitory molecules, which depend on the type and biology of the pathogens, and also on the level of differentiation. However, a hallmark of memory T cells is the lack of simultaneous expression of multiple coinhibitory molecules. Conversely, when pathogens replication is not controlled, continuous stimulation of T cells, due to antigen persistence, prevents the full contraction and leads to functional exhaustion of effector T cells. In contrast to memory T cells (see previous paragraph), a hallmark of exhausted effector cells is the simultaneous expression of several coinhibitory molecules. The simultaneous expression of these coinhibitory molecules is associated with their functional anergy, also called exhaustion. However, several findings both *in vitro* and *in vivo* suggest that this anergic state can be reverted by blocking the interactions between coinhibitory molecules and their ligands. For this reason, coinhibitory molecules are now targets of preclinical and clinical studies aimed to identify new therapeutic strategies in the context of chronic infections and tumors. To date, only two coinhibitory molecules have been investigated in clinical trials, that is, PD-1 and CTLA-4, but recent evidences have underlined the importance of targeting multiple pathways in order to improve functional restoration. It is very likely that in the close future many additional targets will be assessed in preclinical and clinical studies. In addition, while most studies focused their attention on the reversion of functional exhaustion, additional parallel strategies may be envisioned, such as the prevention of exhaustion in the context of therapeutic immunization.

Moreover, preventing/reverting exhaustion as a therapy for chronic conditions might be difficult to achieve notably for safety issues. On the one hand, the prevention/reversion of exhaustion counteracts a physiological mechanism that is probably settled in order to avoid tissue damages and autoimmunity. On the other hand, restoration of functionality might not be sufficient since it will restore the functions of cells that failed to control the infection or to eliminate the pathogens. Therefore, it seems wise to plan to combine the functional restoration of T cells to other immunotherapeutic interventions.

Induction of the expression of costimulatory molecules on exposure to various inflammatory cytokines (IL-6, IL-12, TNF-α, IFN-c) or PAMPs/damage-associated molecular patterns (DAMPs) is regulated by transcription factors such as NF-κB, IRF-3, AP-1, and NFAT.[86,87] Activation of these transcription factors is tightly regulated by various kinases or phosphatases that include MAPKs, TNF-receptor-associated factor proteins (TRAF), IL-1 receptor-associated kinase 4 (IRAK4), phosphoinositide 3-kinase (PI3K), and Janus-kinase. For example, triggering of TLR-4 with LPSs elicits pathways dependent on myeloid differentiation primary response gene 88 (MyD88) and TIR-domain-containing adapter-inducing interferon-b (TRIF). Both the molecules inducc downstream signaling to activate MAPKs, NF-κB, and IRF family proteins, which are responsible for the enhanced expression of CD40 and CD86. Further, T-cell interaction with APC involving TCR and costimulatory molecules activates a plethora of downstream signaling molecules, which leads to the induction of the expression of CD40L, PD-1, and CD28. Intracellular pathogens utilize an array of mechanisms to manipulate costimulatory molecules. Upon infection, pathogens trigger IL-10 secretion by inhibiting p38MAP kinases and promoting ERK phosphorylation. IL-10 blocks the degradation of IkB-α that inhibits the NF-κB activation eventually inhibiting the expression of costimulatory molecules. Interference in TLRs signaling by the intracellular pathogens is considered to be a foremost event in the suppression of costimulatory molecules. ManLAM of *Mtb* binds to DC-SIGN and compromises the LPS-induced activation of DCs by interfering in the TLRs' signaling. Binding of *Mtb* ESAT-6 to TLR-2 activates AKT and prevents interaction between the MyD88 and IRAK4, consequently abrogating NF-κB activation that suppresses CD80 expression. Similarly, HIV upregulates PDL-1 on DCs and monocytes by attenuating the signaling of TLR-7 and TLR-8. In addition, HIV-mediated PI3K activation upregulates PDL-1 on APCs and thus suppresses the activation of HIV-specific CD8+ T cells. Rapid endocytosis of costimulatory molecules upon infection is suggested as one of the mechanisms to interrupt the function of APCs. For instance, Nef protein of HIV modulates the actin-dependent trafficking mechanism to remove CD80/CD86 from the monocytes surface, making them inefficient to activate T cells. TCR signaling is central for the optimum expression of costimulatory molecules and effector function of T cells. Therefore, it may serve as an important target for pathogens to paralyze T-cell activity. *Mtb* glycolipids interfere with TCR signaling and block the activation of CD4+ T cells. HIV gp120 interacts with CD4 (a coreceptor for TCR) that inhibits intracellular signal transduction through TCR, which leads to decreased hydrolysis of PI, Ca^{2+} influx, activation of PKC, and eventually failure of NFAT translocation. These events culminate in the inhibition of CD40L expression. Decline of CD40L on T cells abrogates the bidirectional signaling and reduces the exhibition of CD80 on APCs. In contrast, Nef activates NFAT and stimulates IL-2 release to overcome the exogenous requirement of IL-2 to promote T-cell proliferation, consequently disseminating the infection. However, Nef retards CD28 and CD4 expression, thereby making T cells incapable of promoting CMI. Corroborative with these observations, Nef-mutated HIV is unable to cause persistent infection. Similarly, core protein of HCV inhibits TCR signaling and upregulates PD-1. The above-mentioned mechanisms imply that pathogens can effectively utilize various costimulatory pathways to subvert immune response to persist in the host. The noncompliance with the relatively high dose and extended therapeutic regime reduces the effectiveness of current drugs, which leads to global emergence of MDR/XDR/TDR pathogenic strains. Interestingly, costimulatory molecules have been suggested for therapeutic intervention to treat lymphoma patients. To develop alternative or adjunct (with drugs) therapies, an intensive effort has been undertaken in the last decade to understand how intracellular pathogens exploit costimulatory molecules, which are the tour de force of the immune system. The potent role of costimulatory molecules is aptly established in the optimum activation of T cells and APCs; the cells that play a cardinal role in curbing the infections. Hence, immunotherapy involving costimulatory molecules can be a breakthrough strategy to treat various diseases, minimizing side effects inflicted by drug therapies and in restricting the emergence of drug resistance.

The prevalence of allergic diseases has increased rapidly in recent years. It is well established that the deleterious allergic response is initiated by T-cell recognition of MHC class II–peptide complexes at the surface of APCs. While this first signal gives antigen specificity to the adaptive immune response, a second nonspecific costimulatory signal is required by T cells to become fully activated. This signal is provided by interactions between APCs and T cells through molecules borne at the surfaces of the two cell types. Depending on the type of molecules involved, this secondary signal can promote the development of an inflammatory allergic reaction or may favor immune regulation. Several molecules of the B7 family (CD80, CD86, PD-1, ICOS, CTLA-4) and TNFR family (OX40, CD30, 4-1BB, Fas, CD27, CD40) play an important role in delivering costimulatory signals in early and late phases of allergic response. Therefore, costimulatory molecules involved in the promotion or prevention of allergic immune responses are potential targets for the development of novel therapeutic approaches. Families of costimulatory molecules are involved in the regulation of most inflammatory diseases by finely controlling the intensity of the immune response. Costimulatory molecules are implicated in the development and control of allergic inflammation characterized by the establishment of an acute Th2 polarization. Elucidation of the role of costimulation pathways in the development of new subsets of Th cells has just begun, and most of the mechanisms underlying the regulation of atopic diseases by costimulatory molecules are unknown and require further investigation. With an increased understanding of these immunological mechanisms, new therapeutic strategies in the treatment of allergic airway diseases can be created by analyzing the role of costimulatory molecules that are critically involved in the induction and maintenance of allergen-induced airway diseases. Taken together, recent studies have begun to provide insight into the role of costimulatory molecules and give us new clues to design more efficient therapies to fight the increasing public health problem that allergies represent.

Some of the most successful pathogens of humans, such as *Mtb*, HIV, and *L. donovani* not only establish chronic infections but also remain a grave global threat. These pathogens have developed innovative strategies to evade immune responses such as antigenic shift and drift, interference with antigen processing/presentation, subversion of phagocytosis, induction of immune regulatory pathways, and manipulation of the costimulatory molecules. Costimulatory molecules expressed on the surface of various cells play a decisive role in the initiation and sustenance of immunity. Exploitation of the "code of conduct" of costimulation pathways provides evolutionary incentive to the pathogens and thereby abates the functioning of the immune system. Here we review how *Mtb*, HIV, *Leishmania* sp., and other pathogens manipulate costimulatory molecules to establish chronic infection. Impairment by pathogens in the signaling events delivered by costimulatory molecules may be responsible for defective T-cell responses; consequently organisms grow unhindered in the host cells. This review summarizes the convergent devices that pathogens employ to tune and tame the immune system using costimulatory molecules. Studying host–pathogen interaction in context with costimulatory signals may unveil the molecular mechanism that will help in understanding the survival/death of the pathogens. We emphasize that the very same pathways can potentially be exploited to develop immunotherapeutic strategies to eliminate intracellular pathogens.

REFERENCES

1. Finlay BB, McFadden G. Anti-immunology: evasion of the host immune system by bacterial and viral pathogens. *Cell* 2006;**124**(4):767–82.

2. Fauci AS. The global challenge of infectious diseases: the evolving role of the National Institutes of Health in basic and clinical research. *Nat Immunol* 2005;**6**:743–7.
3. Morens DM, Folkers GK, Fauci AS. The challenge of emerging and re-emerging infectious diseases. *Nature* 2004;**430**:242–9.
4. Hilleman MR. Strategies and mechanisms for host and pathogen survival in acute and persistent viral infections. *Proc Natl Acad Sci USA* 2004;**101**(Suppl. 2):14560–6.
5. Coombes BK, Valdez Y, Finlay BB. Evasive maneuvers by secreted bacterial proteins to avoid innate immune responses. *Curr Biol* 2004;**14**:R856–67.
6. Kaufmann SHE, Sher A, Ahmed AM. *Immunology of infectious diseases*. Washington, DC: ASM Press; 2002.
7. Hornef MW, Wick MJ, Rhen M, Normark S. Bacterial strategies for overcoming host innate and adaptive immune responses. *Nat Immunol* 2002;**3**:1033–40.
8. Jenkins MK. The ups and downs of T cell costimulation. *Immunity* 1994;**1**:443–6.
9. Janeway Jr CA, Bottomly K. Signals and signs for lymphocyte responses. *Cell* 1994;**76**: 275–85.
10. Jenkins MK, Pardoll DM, Mizuguchi J, Chused TM, Schwartz RH. Molecular events in the induction of a nonresponsive state in interleukin 2-producing helper T-lymphocyte clones. *Proc Natl Acad Sci USA* 1987;**84**:5409–13.
11. Lenschow DJ, Sperling AI, Cooke MP, Freeman G, Rhee L. Differential up-regulation of the B7-1 and B7-2 costimulatory molecules after Ig receptor engagement by antigen. *J Immunol* 1994;**153**:1990–7.
12. Harding FA, McArthur JG, Gross JA, Raulet DH, Allison JP. CD28-mediated signalling co-stimulates murine T cells and prevents induction of anergy in T-cell clones. *Nature* 1992; **356**:607–9.
13. Linsley PS, Peach R, Gladstone P, Bajorath J. Extending the B7 (CD80) gene family. *Protein Sci* 1994;**3**:1341–3.
14. Suvas S, Singh V, Sahdev S, Vohra H, Agrewala JN. Distinct role of CD80 and CD86 in the regulation of the activation of B cell and B cell lymphoma. *J Biol Chem* 2002;**277**: 7766–75.
15. Kaufmann S. Protection against tuberculosis: cytokines, T cells, and macrophages. *Ann Rheum Dis* 2002;**61**(Suppl. 2):ii54–8.
16. Khan N, Gowthaman U, Pahari S, Agrewala JN. Manipulation of costimulatory molecules by intracellular pathogens: Veni, Vidi, Vici!! *PLoS Pathog* 2012;**8**(6):e1002676.
17. Cella M, Sallusto F, Lanzavecchia A. Origin, maturation and antigen presenting function of dendritic cells. *Curr Opin Immunol* 1997;**9**:10–16.
18. Cella M, Scheidegger D, Palmer-Lehmann K, Lane P, Lanzavecchia A, Alber G. Ligation of CD40 on dendritic cells triggers production of high levels of interleukin-12 and enhances T cell stimulatory capacity: T-T help via APC activation. *J Exp Med* 1996;**184**: 747–52.
19. Orabona C, Grohmann U, Belladonna ML, Fallarino F, Vacca C, Bianchi R, et al. CD28 induces immuno-stimulatory signals in dendritic cells via CD80 and CD86. *Nat Immunol* 2004;**5**:1134–42.
20. Banchereau J, Bazan F, Blanchard D, Briere F, Galizzi JP, et al. The CD40 antigen and its ligand. *Annu Rev Immunol* 1994;**12**:881–922.
21. De Keersmaecker B, Heirman C, Corthals J, Empsen C, van Grunsven LA, et al. The combination of 4-1BBL and CD40L strongly enhances the capacity of dendritic cells to stimulate HIV-specific T cell responses. *J Leukoc Biol* 2011;**89**:989–99.

22. Walunas TL, Lenschow DJ, Bakker CY, Linsley PS, Freeman GJ, et al. CTLA-4 can function as a negative regulator of T cell activation. *Immunity* 1994;**1**:405–13.
23. Keir ME, Butte MJ, Freeman GJ, Sharpe AH. PD-1 and its ligands in tolerance and immunity. *Annu Rev Immunol* 2008;**26**:677–704.
24. Lenschow DJ, Walunas TL, Bluestone JA. CD28/B7 system of T cell costimulation. *Annu Rev Immunol* 1996;**14**:233–58.
25. Rub A, Dey R, Jadhav M, Kamat R, Chakkaramakkil S, et al. Cholesterol depletion associated with *Leishmania major* infection alters macrophage CD40 signalosome composition and effector function. *Nat Immunol* 2009;**10**:273–80.
26. Ding L, Linsley PS, Huang LY, Germain RN, Shevach EM. IL-10 inhibits macrophage costimulatory activity by selectively inhibiting the up-regulation of B7 expression. *J Immunol* 1993;**151**:1224–34.
27. Geijtenbeek TB, Van Vliet SJ, Koppel EA, Sanchez-Hernandez M, Vandenbroucke-Grauls CM, et al. Mycobacteria target DC-SIGN to suppress dendritic cell function. *J Exp Med* 2003;**197**:7–17.
28. Pathak SK, Basu S, Basu KK, Banerjee A, Pathak S, et al. Direct extracellular interaction between the early secreted antigen ESAT-6 of *Mycobacterium tuberculosis* and TLR2 inhibits TLR signaling in macrophages. *Nat Immunol* 2007;**8**:610–18.
29. Meier A, Bagchi A, Sidhu HK, Alter G, Suscovich TJ, et al. Upregulation of PD-L1 on monocytes and dendritic cells by HIV-1 derived TLR ligands. *AIDS* 2008;**22**:655–8.
30. Muthumani K, Shedlock DJ, Choo DK, Fagone P, Kawalekar OU, et al. HIV-mediated phosphatidylinositol 3-kinase/serine-threonine kinase activation in APCs leads to programmed death-1 ligand upregulation and suppression of HIV-specific CD8 T cells. *J Immunol* 2010;**187**:2932–43.
31. Chaudhry A, Das SR, Jameel S, George A, Bal V, et al. A two-pronged mechanism for HIV-1 Nef-mediated endocytosis of immune costimulatory molecules CD80 and CD86. *Cell Host Microbe* 2007;**1**:37–49.
32. Swigut T, Shohdy N, Skowronski J. Mechanism for down-regulation of CD28 by Nef. *EMBO J* 2001;**20**:1593–604.
33. Chirmule N, McCloskey TW, Hu R, Kalyanaraman VS, Pahwa S. HIV gp120 inhibits T cell activation by interfering with expression of costimulatory molecules CD40 ligand and CD80 (B71). *J Immunol* 1995;**155**:917–24.
34. Manninen A, Renkema GH, Saksela K. Synergistic activation of NFAT by HIV-1 nef and the Ras/MAPK pathway. *J Biol Chem* 2000;**275**:16513–17.
35. Yao ZQ, King E, Prayther D, Yin D, Moorman J. T cell dysfunction by hepatitis C virus core protein involves PD-1/PDL-1 signaling. *Viral Immunol* 2007;**20**:276–87.
36. Leonard JP, Friedberg JW, Younes A, Fisher D, Gordon LI, et al. A phase I/II study of galiximab (an anti-CD80 monoclonal antibody) in combination with rituximab for relapsed or refractory, follicular lymphoma. *Ann Oncol* 2007;**18**:1216–23.
37. Everett H, McFadden G. Apoptosis: an innate immune response to virus infection. *Trends Microbiol* 1999;**7**:160–5.
38. Price DA, Klenerman P, Booth BL, Phillips RE, Sewell AK. Cytotoxic T lymphocytes, chemokines and antiviral immunity. *Immunol Today* 1999;**20**:212–16.
39. Davis CB, Dikic I, Unutmaz D, Hill CM, Arthos J, et al. Signal transduction due to HIV-1 envelope interactions with chemokine receptors CXCR4 or CCR5. *J Exp Med* 1997;**186**:1793–8.
40. Geijtenbeek TB, van Kooyk Y. DC-SIGN: a novel HIV receptor on DCs that mediates HIV-1 transmission. *Curr Top Microbiol Immunol* 2003;**276**:31–54.

41. Kornbluth RS. An expanding role for CD40L and other tumor necrosis factor superfamily ligands in HIV infection. *J Hematother Stem Cell Res* 2002;**11**:787–801.
42. Smed-Sorensen A, Lore K, Walther-Jallow L, Andersson J, Spetz AL. HIV-1-infected dendritic cells up-regulate cell surface markers but fail to produce IL-12 p70 in response to CD40 ligand stimulation. *Blood* 2004;**104**:2810–17.
43. Kornbluth RS. The emerging role of CD40 ligand in HIV infection. *J Leukoc Biol* 2000; **68**:373–82.
44. De Milito A, Nilsson A, Titanji K, Thorstensson R, Reizenstein E, et al. Mechanisms of hypergammaglobulinemia and impaired antigen-specific humoral immunity in HIV-1 infection. *Blood* 2004;**103**:2180–6.
45. Boudet F, Lecoeur H, Gougeon ML. Apoptosis associated with ex vivo down-regulation of Bcl-2 and up-regulation of Fas in potential cytotoxic CD8+ T lymphocytes during HIV infection. *J Immunol* 1996;**156**:2282–93.
46. Gehri R, Hahn S, Rothen M, Steuerwald M, Nuesch R, et al. The Fas receptor in HIV infection: expression on peripheral blood lymphocytes and role in the depletion of T cells. *AIDS* 1996;**10**:9–16.
47. Dolfi DV, Duttagupta PA, Boesteanu AC, Mueller YM, Oliai CH, et al. Dendritic cells and CD28 costimulation are required to sustain virus-specific CD8+ T cell responses during the effector phase in vivo. *J Immunol* 2011;**186**:4599–608.
48. De Keersmaecker B, Thielemans K, Aerts JL. Fighting with the enemy's weapons? The role of costimulatory molecules in HIV. *Curr Mol Med* 2011;**11**:172–96.
49. Servet-Delprat C, Vidalain PO, Bausinger H, Manie S, Le Deist F, et al. Measles virus induces abnormal differentiation of CD40 ligand-activated human dendritic cells. *J Immunol* 2000;**164**:1753–60.
50. Auffermann-Gretzinger S, Keeffe EB, Levy S. Impaired dendritic cell maturation in patients with chronic, but not resolved, hepatitis C virus infection. *Blood* 2001;**97**: 3171–6.
51. Coscoy L, Ganem D. A viral protein that selectively downregulates ICAM-1 and B7-2 and modulates T cell costimulation. *J Clin Invest* 2001;**107**:1599–606.
52. Wherry EJ. T cell exhaustion. *Nat Immunol* 2011;**12**:492–9.
53. Day CL, Kaufmann DE, Kiepiela P, Brown JA, Moodley ES, et al. PD-1 expression on HIV-specific T cells is associated with T-cell exhaustion and disease progression. *Nature* 2006;**443**:350–4.
54. Petrovas C, Casazza JP, Brenchley JM, Price DA, Gostick E, et al. PD-1 is a regulator of virus-specific CD8+ T cell survival in HIV infection. *J Exp Med* 2006;**203**: 2281–92.
55. Chikuma S, Terawaki S, Hayashi T, Nabeshima R, Yoshida T, et al. PD-1-mediated suppression of IL-2 production induces CD8+ T cell anergy in vivo. *J Immunol* 2009;**182**: 6682–9.
56. Chen L, Zhang Z, Chen W, Zhang Z, Li Y, et al. B7-H1 up-regulation on myeloid dendritic cells significantly suppresses T cell immune function in patients with chronic hepatitis B. *J Immunol* 2007;**178**:6634–41.
57. Krutzik SR, Sieling PA, Modlin RL. The role of Toll-like receptors in host defense against microbial infection. *Curr Opin Immunol* 2001;**13**:104–8.
58. Cooper AM. Cell-mediated immune responses in tuberculosis. *Annu Rev Immunol* 2009; **27**:393–422.
59. Grewal IS, Flavell RA. The role of CD40 ligand in costimulation and T-cell activation. *Immunol Rev* 1996;**153**:85–106.

60. Bonato VL, Medeiros AI, Lima VM, Dias AR, Faccioliti LH, et al. Downmodulation of CD18 and CD86 on macrophages and VLA-4 on lymphocytes in experimental tuberculosis. *Scand J Immunol* 2001;**54**:564–73.
61. Schreiber HA, Hulseberg PD, Lee J, Prechl J, Barta P, et al. Dendritic cells in chronic mycobacterial granulomas restrict local anti-bacterial T cell response in a murine model. *PLoS One* 2010;**5**:e11453.
62. Fuse S, Zhang W, Usherwood EJ. Control of memory CD8+ T cell differentiation by CD80/CD86-CD28 costimulation and restoration by IL-2 during the recall response. *J Immunol* 2008;**180**:1148–57.
63. Saha B, Das G, Vohra H, Ganguly NK, Mishra GC. Macrophage-T cell interaction in experimental mycobacterial infection. Selective regulation of co-stimulatory molecules on Mycobacterium-infected macrophages and its implication in the suppression of cell-mediated immune response. *Eur J Immunol* 1994;**24**:2618–24.
64. Herold KC, Lu J, Rulifson I, Vezys V, Taub D, et al. Regulation of C-C chemokine production by murine T cells by CD28/B7 costimulation. *J Immunol* 1997;**159**:4150–3.
65. Arias MA, Jaramillo G, Lopez YP, Mejia N, Mejia C, et al. *Mycobacterium tuberculosis* antigens specifically modulate CCR2 and MCP-1/CCL2 on lymphoid cells from human pulmonary hilar lymph nodes. *J Immunol* 2007;**179**:8381–91.
66. Bhatt K, Uzelac A, Mathur S, McBride A, Potian J, et al. B7 costimulation is critical for host control of chronic *Mycobacterium tuberculosis* infection. *J Immunol* 2009;**182**:3793–817.
67. Kan-Sutton C, Jagannath C, Hunter Jr. RL. Trehalose 6,6′-dimycolate on the surface of *Mycobacterium tuberculosis* modulates surface marker expression for antigen presentation and costimulation in murine macrophages. *Microbes Infect* 2009;**11**:40–8.
68. Singh B, Singh G, Trajkovic V, Sharma P. Intracellular expression of *Mycobacterium tuberculosis*-specific 10-kDa antigen down-regulates macrophage B7.1 expression and nitric oxide release. *Clin Exp Immunol* 2003;**134**:70–7.
69. Grewal IS, Borrow P, Pamer EG, Oldstone MB, Flavell RA. The CD40-CD154 system in anti-infective host defense. *Curr Opin Immunol* 1997;**9**:491–7.
70. Murray RA, Siddiqui MR, Mendillo M, Krahenbuhl J, Kaplan G. *Mycobacterium leprae* inhibits dendritic cell activation and maturation. *J Immunol* 2007;**178**:338–44.
71. Stewart GR, Snewin VA, Walzl G, Hussell T, Tormay P, et al. Overexpression of heat-shock proteins reduces survival of *Mycobacterium tuberculosis* in the chronic phase of infection. *Nat Med* 2001;**7**:732–7.
72. Co DO, Hogan LH, Kim SI, Sandor M. Mycobacterial granulomas: keys to a long-lasting host-pathogen relationship. *Clin Immunol* 2004;**113**:130–6.
73. Sakai S, Kawamura I, Okazaki T, Tsuchiya K, Uchiyama R, et al. PD-1-PD-L1 pathway impairs T(h)1 immune response in the late stage of infection with *Mycobacterium bovis* bacillus Calmette-Guerin. *Int Immunol* 2010;**22**:915–25.
74. Jurado JO, Alvarez IB, Pasquinelli V, Martinez GJ, Quiroga MF, et al. Programmed death (PD)-1:PD-ligand 1/PD-ligand 2 pathway inhibits T cell effector functions during human tuberculosis. *J Immunol* 2008;**181**:116–25.
75. Alvarez IB, Pasquinelli V, Jurado JO, Abbate E, Musella RM, et al. Role played by the programmed death-1-programmed death ligand pathway during innate immunity against *Mycobacterium tuberculosis*. *J Infect Dis* 2010;**202**:524–32.
76. Lazar-Molnar E, Chen B, Sweeney KA, Wang EJ, Liu W, et al. Programmed death-1 (PD-1)-deficient mice are extraordinarily sensitive to tuberculosis. *Proc Natl Acad Sci USA* 2010;**107**:13402–7.

77. Barber DL, Mayer-Barber KD, Feng CG, Sharpe AH, Sher A. CD4 T cells promote rather than control tuberculosis in the absence of PD-1-mediated inhibition. *J Immunol* 2010;**186**:1598–607.
78. Hanekom WA, Mendillo M, Manca C, Haslett PA, Siddiqui MR, et al. *Mycobacterium tuberculosis* inhibits maturation of human monocyte-derived dendritic cells in vitro. *J Infect Dis* 2003;**188**:257–66.
79. Shortman K, Heath WR. Immunity or tolerance? That is the question for dendritic cells. *Nat Immunol* 2001;**2**:988–9.
80. Levings MK, Sangregorio R, Roncarolo MG. Human cd25(+)cd4(+) T regulatory cells suppress naive and memory T cell proliferation and can be expanded in vitro without loss of function. *J Exp Med* 2001;**193**:1295–302.
81. Pryjma J, Baran J, Ernst M, Woloszyn M, Flad HD. Altered antigen-presenting capacity of human monocytes after phagocytosis of bacteria. *Infect Immun* 1994;**62**:1961–7.
82. Wyant TL, Tanner MK, Sztein MB. Potent immunoregulatory effects of *Salmonella typhi* flagella on antigenic stimulation of human peripheral blood mononuclear cells. *Infect Immun* 1999;**67**:1338–46.
83. Yao T, Mecsas J, Healy JI, Falkow S, Chien Y. Suppression of T and B lymphocyte activation by a *Yersinia pseudotuberculosis* virulence factor, yopH. *J Exp Med* 1999;**190**:1343–50.
84. Anderson KM, Czinn SJ, Redline RW, Blanchard TG. Induction of CTLA-4-mediated anergy contributes to persistent colonization in the murine model of gastric *Helicobacter pylori* infection. *J Immunol* 2006;**176**:5306–13.
85. Das S, Suarez G, Beswick EJ, Sierra JC, Graham DY, et al. Expression of B7-H1 on gastric epithelial cells: its potential role in regulating T cells during *Helicobacter pylori* infection. *J Immunol* 2006;**176**:3000–9.
86. Beswick EJ, Pinchuk IV, Das S, Powell DW, Reyes VE. Expression of the programmed death ligand 1, B7-H1, on gastric epithelial cells after *Helicobacter pylori* exposure promotes development of CD4+ CD25+ FoxP3+ regulatory T cells. *Infect Immun* 2007;**75**:4334–41.
87. Skinner JA, Reissinger A, Shen H, Yuk MH. Bordetella type III secretion and adenylate cyclase toxin synergize to drive dendritic cells into a semimature state. *J Immunol* 2004;**173**:1934–40.
88. Hall BF, Joiner KA. Strategies of obligate intracellular parasites for evading host defences. *Immunol Today* 1991;**12**:A22–7.
89. Kaye PM, Rogers NJ, Curry AJ, Scott JC. Deficient expression of co-stimulatory molecules on *Leishmania*-infected macrophages. *Eur J Immunol* 1994;**24**:2850–4.
90. Mukherjee P, Chauhan VS. *Plasmodium falciparum*-free merozoites and infected RBCs distinctly affect soluble CD40 ligand-mediated maturation of immature monocyte-derived dendritic cells. *J Leukoc Biol* 2008;**84**:244–54.
91. Campbell KA, Ovendale PJ, Kennedy MK, Fanslow WC, Reed SG, et al. CD40 ligand is required for protective cell-mediated immunity to *Leishmania major. Immunity* 1996;**4**:283–9.
92. Chattopadhyay K, Lazar-Molnar E, Yan Q, Rubinstein R, et al. Sequence, structure, function, immunity: structural genomics of costimulation. *Immunol Rev* 2009;**229**(1):356–86.
92a. Mir MA, Albaradie RS, Agrewala JN. Reverse costimulation through anti-B7-1 and anti-B7-2 in the survival of Mycobacterium tuberculosis in antigen presenting cells. *IJBPAS* 2013;**2**(5):1024–43.
92b. Mir MA, Agrewala JN. Influence of CD80 and CD86 costimulation in the modulation of the activation of APCs. *Curr Immunol Rev* 2007;**3**(3):160–9.

92c. Mir MA, Albaradie RS. Tuberculosis time bomb a global emergency: urgent need for alternative vaccines. *Majmaah J Health Sci* 2013;**1**(1):87–93.

93. Watts TH, Bertram EM, Bukczynski J, Wen T. T cell costimulatory molecules in anti-viral immunity: potential role in immunotherapeutic vaccines. *Can J Infect Dis* 2003;**14**(4):221–9.

94. Papagno L, Appay V, Sutton Y, Rostron T, Gillespie GMA, Ogg GS, et al. Comparison between HIV- and CMV-specific T cell responses in long-term HIV infected donors. *Clin Exp Immunol* 2002;**130**(3):509–17.

95. Scott-Algara D, Aboulker JP, Durier C, Badell E, Marcellin F, Prud'homme M. CD4 T cell recovery is slower in patients experiencing viral load rebounds during HAART. *Clin Exp Immunol* 2001;**126**(2):295–303.

96. Shuford WW, Klussman K, Tritchler DD, Loo DT, Jan Chalupny AW, et al. 4-1BB costimulatory signals preferentially induce CD8+ T cell proliferation and lead to the amplification in vivo of cytotoxic T cell responses. *J Exp Med* 1997;**186**(1):47–55.

97. Hernandez-Chacon JA, Li Y, Wu RC, Bernatchez C, Wang Y, et al. Co-stimulation through the CD137/4-1BB pathway protects human melanoma tumor-infiltrating lymphocytes from activation-induced cell death and enhances anti-tumor effector function. *J Immunother* 2011;**34**(3):236–50.

98. Guinn BA, Mohamedali A, Mills KI, Czepulkowski B, Schmitt M, Greiner J. Leukemia associated antigens: their dual role as biomarkers and immunotherapeutic targets for acute myeloid leukemia. *Biomark Insights* 2007;**2**:69–79.

99. Zhu FG, Pisetsky DS. Role of the heat shock protein 90 in immune response stimulation by bacterial DNA and synthetic oligonucleotides. *Infect Immun* 2001;**69**(9):5546–52.

100. Loeh BI, Willson P, Babiuk LA, van Drunen Littel-van den Hurk S. Gene gun-mediated DNA immunization primes development of mucosal immunity against bovine herpesvirus 1 in cattle. *J Virol* 2000;**74**(13):6077–86.

101. Stephenson JR. Understanding dengue pathogenesis: implications for vaccine design. *Bull World Health Organ* 2005;**83**(4):308–14.

102. Riley JL, Levine BL, Craighead L, Francomano T, Kim D, et al. Naïve and memory CD4 T cells differ in their susceptibilities to human immunodeficiency virus type 1 infection following CD28 costimulation: implications for transmission and pathogenesis. *J Virol* 1998;**72**(10):8273–80.

103. Bluestone JA. New perspectives of CD28-B7-mediated T cell costimulation. *Immunity* 1995;**2**:555–9.

104. Razi-Wolf Z, Freeman GJ, et al. Expression and function of the murine B7 antigen, the major costimulatory molecule expressed by peritoneal exudate cells. *Proc Natl Acad Sci USA* 1992;**89**:4210–14.

105. Hathcock KS, Laszlo G, et al. Comparative analysis of B7-1 and B7-2 costimulatory ligands: expression and function. *J Exp Med* 1994;**180**:631–40.

106. Wetzler LW, Ho Y, Reiser H. Neisserial porins induce B lymphocytes to express costimulatory B7-2 molecules and to proliferate. *J Exp Med* 1996;**183**:1151–9.

107. Kaye PM, Rogers NJ, et al. Deficient expression of costimulatory molecules on *Leishmania*-infected macrophages. *Eur J Immunol* 1994;**24**:2850–4.

108. Muraille E, De Smedt T, et al. Activation of murine T cells by bacterial superantigens requires B7-mediated costimulation. *Cell Immunol* 1995;**162**:315–20.

109. Haffar OK, Smithgall MD, et al. Costimulation of T-cell activation and virus production by B7 antigen on activated CD41 T cells from human immunodeficiency virus type 1-infected donors. *Proc Natl Acad Sci USA* 1993;**90**:11094–8.

110. Lewis DE, Tang DS. Anergy and apoptosis in CD81 T cells from HIV-infected persons. *J Immunol* 1994;**153**:412–20.
111. Levine BL, Mosca JD. Antiviral effect and ex vivo CD41 T cell proliferation in HIV-positive patients as a result of CD28 costimulation. *Science* 1996;**272**:1939–43.
112. Shahinian A, Pfeffer K, et al. Differential T cell costimulatory requirements in CD28-deficient mice. *Science* 1993;**261**:609–12.
113. Corry DB, Reiner SL, et al. Differential effects of blockade of CD28-B7 on the development of Th1 or Th2 effector cells in experimental leishmaniasis. *J Immunol* 1994;**153**: 4142–8.
114. Rathore A, Sacristán C, et al. In situ analysis of B7-2 costimulatory, major histocompatibility complex class II, and adhesion molecule expression in schistosomal egg granulomas. *Am J Pathol* 1996;**149**:187–94.
115. Flores-Villanueva PO, Harris TS, et al. Macrophages from schistosomal egg granulomas induce unresponsiveness in specific cloned Th-1 lymphocytes in vitro and down-regulate granulomatous disease in vivo. *J Immunol* 1994;**152**:1847–55.
116. Flores-Villanueva PO. Regulation of T helper cell responses in experimental schistosomiasis by IL-10: effect on expression of B7 and B7-2 costimulatory molecules by macrophages. *J Immunol* 1994;**153**:5190–9.
117. Flores-Villanueva PO, Zheng XX, et al. Recombinant IL-10 and IL-10/Fc treatment down-regulate egg antigen-specific delayed hypersensitivity reactions and egg granuloma formation in schistosomiasis. *J Immunol* 1996;**156**:3315–20.
118. Masoli M, Fabian D, et al. The global burden of asthma: executive summary of the GINA dissemination committee report. *Allergy* 2004;**59**:469–78.
119. Bousquet J, Khaltaev N. *Global surveillance: Prevention and control of chronic respiratory diseases*. Geneva, Switzerland: World Health Organization; 2007. pp. 15–20.
120. Tse K, Horner AA. Allergen tolerance versus the allergic march: the hygiene hypothesis revisited. *Curr Allergy Asthma Rep* 2008;**8**:475–83.
121. Kim H, Jin HS, Lee SY, Kim J, Kim B, Park S, et al. The effect of rush immunotherapy with house dust mite in the production of IL-5 and IFN-γ from the peripheral blood T cells of asthmatic children. *J Korean Med Sci* 2009;**24**(3):392–7.
122. Meiler F, Zimmermann M, et al. T cell subsets in the pathogenesis of human asthma. *Curr Allergy Asthma Rep* 2006;**6**:91–6.
123. Lafferty KJ, Cunningham AJ. A new analysis of allogeneic interactions. *Aust J Exp Biol Med Sci* 1975;**53**:27–42.
124. Greenwald RJ, Freeman GJ, Sharpe AH. The B7 family revisited. *Annu Rev Immunol* 2005;**23**:515–48.
125. Croft M. Co-stimulatory members of the TNFR family: keys to effective T cell immunity? *Nat Rev Immunol* 2003;**3**:609–20.
126. Burr JS, Kimzey SL, et al. CD28 and CTLA4 coordinately regulate airway inflammatory cell recruitment and T helper cell differentiation after inhaled allergen. *Am J Respir Cell Mol Biol* 2001;**24**:563–8.
127a. Hofer MF, Jirapongsananuruk O, Trumble AE, Leung DY. Upregulation of B7.2, but not B7.1, on B cells from patients with allergic asthma. *J Allergy Clin Immunol* 1998;**101**: 96–102.
127b. Agea E, Forenza N, et al. Expression of B7 co-stimulatory molecules and CD1a antigen by alveolar macrophages in allergic bronchial asthma. *Clin Exp Allergy* 1998;**28**:1359–67.
128. Burastero SE, Magnani Z, et al. Increased expression of the CD80 accessory molecule by alveolar macrophages in asthmatic subjects and its functional involvement in allergen

presentation to autologous Th2 lymphocytes. *J Allergy Clin Immunol* 1999;**103**: 1136–42.
129. Jeannin P, Magistrelli G, et al. Soluble CD86 is a costimulatory molecule for human T lymphocytes. *Immunity* 2000;**13**:303–12.
130. Shi HZ, Xie ZF, et al. Soluble CD86 protein in serum samples of patients with asthma. *Thorax* 2004;**59**:870–5.
131. Deng JM, Shi HZ, et al. Effects of allergen inhalation and oral glucocorticoid on concentrations of serum-soluble CD86 in allergic asthmatics. *Clin Immunol* 2005;**115**:178–83.
132. Ritprajak P, Hashiguchi M, Azuma M. Topical application of cream-emulsified CD86 siRNA ameliorates allergic skin disease by targeting cutaneous dendritic cells. *Mol Ther* 2008;**16**:1323–30.
133. Akbari O, DeKruyff RH, Umetsu DT. Pulmonary dendritic cells producing IL-10 mediate tolerance induced by respiratory exposure to antigen. *Nat Immunol* 2001;**2**:725–31.
134. Lombardi V, Singh AK, Akbari O. The role of costimulatory molecules in allergic disease and asthma. *Int Arch Allergy Immunol* 2010;**151**(3):179–89.
135. Hutloff A, Dittrich AM, et al. ICOS is an inducible T cell costimulator structurally and functionally related to CD28. *Nature* 1999;**397**:263–6.
136. McAdam AJ, Chang TT, et al. Mouse inducible costimulatory molecule (ICOS) expression is enhanced by CD28 costimulation and regulates differentiation of CD4+ T cells. *J Immunol* 2000;**165**:5035–40.
137. Gonzalo JA, Tian J, et al. ICOS is critical for T helper cell-mediated lung mucosal inflammatory responses. *Nat Immunol* 2001;**2**:597–604.
138. Tesciuba AG, Subudhi S, et al. Inducible costimulator regulates Th2-mediated inflammation, but not Th2 differentiation, in a model of allergic airway disease. *J Immunol* 2001; **167**:1996–2003.
139. Beier KC, Hutloff A, et al. Inducible costimulator positive T cells are required for allergen-induced local B-cell infiltration and antigen-specific IgE production in lung tissue. *J Allergy Clin Immunol* 2004;**114**:775–82.
140. Akbari O, Stock P, et al. ICOS/ICOSL interaction is required for CD4+ invariant NKT cell function and homeostatic survival. *J Immunol* 2008;**180**:5448–56.
141. Akbari O, Freeman GJ, et al. Antigen-specific regulatory T cells develop via the ICOS-ICOS-ligand pathway and inhibit allergen induced airway hyperreactivity. *Nat Med* 2002;**8**:1024–32.
142. Takahashi T, Tagami T, et al. Immunologic self-tolerance maintained by CD25(+)CD4(+) regulatory T cells constitutively expressing cytotoxic T lymphocyte-associated antigen 4. *J Exp Med* 2000;**192**:303–10.
143a. Howard TD, Postma DS, Hawkins GA, Koppelman GH, Zheng SL, Wysong AK, et al. Fine mapping of an IgE-controlling gene on chromosome 2q: analysis of CTLA4 and CD28. *J Allergy Clin Immunol* 2002;**110**:743–51.
143b. Chen L. Co-inhibitory molecules of the B7-CD28 family in the control of T-cell immunity. *Nat Rev Immunol* 2004;**4**(5):336–47.
144. Goodnow CC, Sprent J, Fazekas de St Groth B, Vinuesa CG. Cellular and genetic mechanisms of self tolerance and autoimmunity. *Nature* 2005;**435**(7042):590–7.
145. Bour-Jordan H, Esensten JH, Martinez-Llordella M, et al. Intrinsic and extrinsic control of peripheral T-cell tolerance by costimulatory molecules of the CD28/B7 family. *Immunol Rev* 2011;**241**(1):180–205.
146. Goeken NE. Differential stimulatory requirements and regulation of naive and primed human lymphocytes. *Hum Immunol* 1984;**10**(4):251–63.

147. Inaba K, Metlay JP, Crowley MT, Steinman RM. Dendritic cells pulsed with protein antigens in vitro can prime antigen-specific, MHC-restricted T cells in situ. *J Exp Med* 1990;**172**(2):631–40.
148. Henrickson SE, Mempel TR, Mazo IB, et al. In vivo imaging of T cell priming. *Sci Signaling* 2008;**1**(12). pt 2.
149. Henrickson SE, Mempel TR, Mazo IB, et al. T cell sensing of antigen dose governs interactive behavior with dendritic cells and sets a threshold for T cell activation. *Nat Immunol* 2008;**9**(3):282–91.
150. Kaech SM, Wherry EJ, Ahmed R. Effector and memory T-cell differentiation: implications for vaccine development. *Nat Rev Immunol* 2002;**2**(4):251–62.
151. Kaech SM, Wherry EJ. Heterogeneity and cell-fate decisions in effector and memory $CD8^+$ T cell differentiation during viral infection. *Immunity* 2007;**27**(3):393–405.
152. Mackay CR, Marston WL, Dudler L. Naive and memory T cells show distinct pathways of lymphocyte recirculation. *J Exp Med* 1990;**171**(3):801–17.
153. Badovinac VP, Harty JT. Programming, demarcating, and manipulating $CD8^+$ T-cell memory. *Immunol Rev* 2006;**211**:67–80.
154. Chambers CA, Kuhns MS, Egen JG, Allison JP. CTLA-4-mediated inhibition in regulation of T cell responses: mechanisms and manipulation in tumor immunotherapy. *Annu Rev Immunol* 2001;**19**:565–94.
155. Hildeman DA, Zhu Y, Mitchell TC, Kappler J, Marrack P. Molecular mechanisms of activated T cell death in vivo. *Curr Opin Immunol* 2002;**14**(3):354–9.
156. Arnold R, Brenner D, Becker M, Frey CR, Krammer PH. How T lymphocytes switch between life and death. *Eur J Immunol* 2006;**36**(7):1654–8.
157. Chen G, Tai AK, Lin M, Chang F, Terhorst C, Huber BT. Increased proliferation of CD8+ T cells in SAP-deficient mice is associated with impaired activation-induced cell death. *Eur J Immunol* 2007;**37**(3):663–74.
158. Mueller DL. Mechanisms maintaining peripheral tolerance. *Nat Immunol* 2010;**11**(1): 21–7.
159. Butz EA, Bevan MJ. Massive expansion of antigen-specific $CD8^+$ T cells during an acute virus infection. *Immunity* 1998;**8**(2):167–75.
160. Harari A, Enders FB, Cellerai C, Bart PA, Pantaleo G. Distinct profiles of cytotoxic granules in memory CD8 T cells correlate with function, differentiation stage, and antigen exposure. *J Virol* 2009;**83**(7):2862–71.
161a. Viganò S, Perreau M, Pantaleo G, Harari A. Positive and negative regulation of cellular immune responses in physiologic conditions and diseases. *Clin Dev Immunol* 2012;**2012**. Article ID 485781, 11 pages, 2012.
161b. Hughes PD, Belz GT, Fortner KA, Budd RC, Strasser A, Bouillet P. Apoptosis regulators Fas and Bim cooperate in shutdown of chronic immune responses and prevention of autoimmunity. *Immunity* 2008;**28**(2):197–205.
162. Iezzi G, Karjalainen K, Lanzavecchia A. The duration of antigenic stimulation determines the fate of naive and effector T cells. *Immunity* 1998;**8**(1):89–95.
163. Salomon B, Bluestone JA. Complexities of CD28/B7:CTLA-4 costimulatory pathways in autoimmunity and transplantation. *Annu Rev Immunol* 2001;**19**:225–52.
164. Collins AV, Brodie DA, Gilbert RJC, et al. The interaction properties of costimulatory molecules revisited. *Immunity* 2002;**17**(2):201–10.
165. Nakae S, Suto S, Iikura M, et al. Mast cells enhance T cell activation: importance of mast cell costimulatory molecules and secreted TNF. *J Immunol* 2006;**176**(4):2238–48.

166. Ishida M, Iwai Y, Tanaka Y, et al. Differential expression of PD-L1 and PD-L2, ligands for an inhibitory receptor PD-1, in the cells of lymphohematopoietic tissues. *Immunol Lett* 2002;**84**(1):57–62.
167. Latchman Y, Wood CR, Chernova T, et al. PD-L2 is a second ligand for PD-1 and inhibits T cell activation. *Nat Immunol* 2001;**2**(3):261–8.
168. Freeman GJ, Long AJ, Iwai Y, et al. Engagement of the PD-1 immunoinhibitory receptor by a novel B7 family member leads to negative regulation of lymphocyte activation. *J Exp Med* 2000;**192**(7):1027–34.
169. Okazaki T, Honjo T. The PD-1-PD-L pathway in immunological tolerance. *Trends Immunol* 2006;**27**(4):195–201.
170. Nishimura N, Nose M, Hiai H, Minato N, Honjo T. Development of lupus-like autoimmune diseases by disruption of the PD-1 gene encoding an ITIM motif-carrying immunoreceptor. *Immunity* 1999;**11**(2):141–51.
171. Nishimura H, Okazaki T, Tanaka Y, et al. Autoimmune dilated cardiomyopathy in PD-1 receptor-deficient mice. *Science* 2001;**291**(5502):319–22.
172. Sedy JR, Gavrieli M, Potter KG, et al. B and T lymphocyte attenuator regulates T cell activation through interaction with herpesvirus entry mediator. *Nat Immunol* 2005;**6**(1):90–8.
173. Krieg C, Boyman O, Fu YX, Kaye J. B and T lymphocyte attenuator regulates CD8+ T cell-intrinsic homeostasis and memory cell generation. *Nat Immunol* 2007;**8**(2):162–71.
174. Cai G, Anumanthan A, Brown JA, Greenfield EA, Zhu B, Freeman GJ. CD160 inhibits activation of human CD4+ T cells through interaction with herpesvirus entry mediator. *Nat Immunol* 2008;**9**(2):176–85.
175. Wherry EJ, Blattman JN, Murali-Krishna K, Van Der Most R, Ahmed R. Viral persistence alters CD8 T-cell immunodominance and tissue distribution and results in distinct stages of functional impairment. *J Virol* 2003;**77**(8):4911–27.
176. Sharpe AH, Wherry EJ, Ahmed R, Freeman GJ. The function of programmed cell death 1 and its ligands in regulating autoimmunity and infection. *Nat Immunol* 2007;**8**(3):239–45.
177. Blackburn SD, Shin H, Haining WN, et al. Coregulation of CD8+ T cell exhaustion by multiple inhibitory receptors during chronic viral infection. *Nat Immunol* 2009;**10**(1): 29–37.
178. Jones RB, Ndhlovu CL, Barbour JD, et al. Tim-3 expression defines a novel population of dysfunctional T cells with highly elevated frequencies in progressive HIV-1 infection. *J Exp Med* 2008;**205**(12):2763–79.
179. Golden-Mason L, Palmer BE, Kassam N, et al. Negative immune regulator Tim-3 is overexpressed on T cells in hepatitis C virus infection and its blockade rescues dysfunctional CD4+ and $CD8^+$ T cells. *J Virol* 2009;**83**(18):9122–30.
180. McMahan RH, Golden-Mason L, Nishimura MI, et al. Tim-3 expression on PD-1+ HCV-specific human CTLs is associated with viral persistence, and its blockade restores hepatocyte-directed in vitro cytotoxicity. *J Clin Invest* 2010;**120**(12):4546–57.
181. Vali B, Jones RB, Sakhdari A, et al. HCV-specific T cells in HCV/HIV co-infection show elevated frequencies of dual Tim-3/PD-1 expression that correlate with liver disease progression. *Eur J Immunol* 2010;**40**(9):2493–505.
182. Sakuishi K, Apetoh L, Sullivan JM, Blazar BR, Kuchroo VK, Anderson AC. Targeting Tim-3 and PD-1 pathways to reverse T cell exhaustion and restore anti-tumor immunity. *J Exp Med* 2010;**207**(10):2187–94.
183. Contardi E, Palmisano GL, Tazzari PL, et al. CTLA-4 is constitutively expressed on tumor cells and can trigger apoptosis upon ligand interaction. *Int J Cancer* 2005;**117**(4):538–50.

184. Boasso A, Vaccari M, Hryniewicz A, et al. Regulatory T-cell markers, indoleamine 2,3-dioxygenase, and virus levels in spleen and gut during progressive simian immunodeficiency virus infection. *J Virol* 2007;**81**(21):11593–603.
185. Kaufmann DE, Kavanagh DG, Pereyra F, et al. Upregulation of CTLA-4 by HIV-specific CD4+ T cells correlates with disease progression and defines a reversible immune dysfunction. *Nat Immunol* 2007;**8**(11):1246–54.
186. Kaufmann DE, Walker BD. PD-1 and CTLA-4 inhibitory cosignaling pathways in HIV infection and the potential for therapeutic intervention. *J Immunol* 2009;**182**(10):5891–7.
187. Curran MA, Kim M, Montalvo W, Al-Shamkhani A, Allison JP. Combination CTLA-4 blockade and 4-1BB activation enhances tumor rejection by increasing T-cell infiltration, proliferation, and cytokine production. *PLoS One* 2011;**6**(4):e19499.
188. Derre L, Rivals JP, Jandus C, et al. BTLA mediates inhibition of human tumor-specific $CD8^+$ T cells that can be partially reversed by vaccination. *J Clin Invest* 2010;**120**(1): 157–67.
189. Xu XS, Zhang Z, Gu LL, Wang FS. BTLA characterization and its association with disease progression in patients with chronic HIV-1 infection. *Chin J Cell Mol Immunol* 2009;**25**:1158–60.
190. Zhang Z, Xu X, Lv J, et al. B and T lymphocyte attenuator down-regulation by HIV-1 depends on type I interferon and contributes to T-cell hyperactivation. *J Infect Dis* 2011; **203**(11):1668–78.
191. Antonelli LRV, Mahnke Y, Hodge JN, et al. Elevated frequencies of highly activated $CD4^+$ T cells in HIV+ patients developing immune reconstitution inflammatory syndrome. *Blood* 2010;**116**(19):3818–27.
192. Matsuzaki J, Gnjatic S, Mhawech-Fauceglia P, et al. Tumor-infiltrating NY-ESO-1-specific CD8+ T cells are negatively regulated by LAG-3 and PD-1 in human ovarian cancer. *Proc Natl Acad Sci USA* 2010;**107**(17):7875–80.
193. Peritt D, Sesok-Pizzini DA, Schretzenmair R, et al. C1.7 antigen expression on CD8+ T cells is activation dependent: increased proportion of C1.7+CD8+ T cells in HIV-1-infected patients with progressing disease. *J Immunol* 1999;**162**(12):7563–8.
194. Aldy KN, Horton NC, Mathew PA, Mathew SO. 2B4+ CD8+ T cells play an inhibitory role against constrained HIV epitopes. *Biochem Biophys Res Commun* 2011;**405**(3):503–7.
195. Williams H, Macsween K, McAulay K, et al. Analysis of immune activation and clinical events in acute infectious mononucleosis. *J Infect Dis* 2004;**190**(1):63–71.
196. Bengsch B, Seigel B, Ruhl M, et al. Coexpression of PD-1, 2B4, CD160 and KLRG1 on exhausted HCV-specific CD8+T cells is linked to antigen recognition and T cell differentiation. *PLoS Pathog* 2010;**6**(6):e1000947.
197. Raziorrouh B, Ulsenheimer A, Schraut W, et al. Inhibitory molecules that regulate expansion and restoration of HCV-specific $CD4^+$ T cells in patients with chronic infection. *Gastroenterology* 2011;**141**(4):1422–31.
198. Yamamoto T, Price DA, Casazza JP, et al. Surface expression patterns of negative regulatory molecules identify determinants of virus-specific $CD8^+$ T-cell exhaustion in HIV infection. *Blood* 2011;**117**(18):4805–15.
199. Lipson EJ, Drake CG. Ipilimumab: an anti-CTLA-4 antibody for metastatic melanoma. *Clin Cancer Res* 2011;**17**(22):6958–62.
200. Danielli R, Ridolfi R, Chiarion-Sileni V, et al. Ipilimumab in pretreated patients with metastatic uveal melanoma: safety and clinical efficacy. *Cancer Immunol Immunother* 2012; **61**(1):41–8.

201. Brahmer JR, Drake CG, Wollner I, et al. Phase I study of single-agent anti-programmed death-1 (MDX-1106) in refractory solid tumors: safety, clinical activity, pharmacodynamics, and immunologic correlates. *J Clin Oncol* 2010;**28**(19):3167–75.
202. Kline J, Gajewski TF. Clinical development of mAbs to block the PD1 pathway as an immunotherapy for cancer. *Curr Opin Investig Drugs* 2010;**11**(12):1354–9.
203. Hodi FS, Mihm MC, Soiffer RJ, et al. Biologic activity of cytotoxic T lymphocyte-associated antigen 4 antibody blockade in previously vaccinated metastatic melanoma and ovarian carcinoma patients. *Proc Natl Acad Sci USA* 2003;**100**(8):4712–17.
204. Phan GQ, Yang JC, Sherry RM, et al. Cancer regression and autoimmunity induced by cytotoxic T lymphocyte-associated antigen 4 blockade in patients with metastatic melanoma. *Proc Natl Acad Sci USA* 2003;**100**(14):8372–7.
205. Hryniewicz A, Boasso A, Edghill-Smith Y, et al. CTLA-4 blockade decreases TGF-β, IDO, and viral RNA expression in tissues of SIVmac251-infected macaques. *Blood* 2006;**108**(12):3834–42.
206. Cecchinato V, Tryniszewska E, Ma ZM, et al. Immune activation driven by CTLA-4 blockade augments viral replication at mucosal sites in simian immunodeficiency virus infection. *J Immunol* 2008;**180**(8):5439–54.

Chapter 4

Costimulation Immunotherapy in Allergies and Asthma

INTRODUCTION

Allergic diseases affect individuals of all ages from infancy to old age and have become one of the epidemics of the twenty-first century in developed countries. The prevalence and severity of allergic diseases and asthma have increased dramatically over the past decades, affecting an estimated 20% of the population in developed countries. Different hypotheses have been postulated to explain this increase in prevalence. The "hygiene hypothesis" is one of the main propositions that suggest improved hygiene, with improved public health measures and the use of vaccines and antibiotics, has reduced the incidence of infections that would normally stimulate the immune system. These infections would "mature" the immune system thereby protecting against the development of allergic responses against innocuous environmental substances[1]. Several epidemiologic studies support the hygiene hypothesis and have clearly shown that modifications of the pattern of microbial exposure represent a critical factor underlying the rise in prevalence of atopic disorders but the immunological mechanism associated with the hygiene hypothesis has been controversial. Initial interpretations concluded that a lack of shifting from the T-helper-2 (Th2) to the Th1 phenotype (missing immune deviation) because of the reduced microbial burden was responsible.[1] A Th2 phenotype favors the development of asthma and allergy, whereas Th1 immune responses protect against asthma. However, several observations challenge the paradigm of missing immune deviation; therefore, an alternative interpretation of the hygiene hypothesis has been proposed that states that a reduced activity of regulatory T cells (Treg cells; reduced immune deviation) may be the explanatory mechanism for the hygiene hypothesis.[2] Treg cells are essential for the induction and maintenance of tolerance and tightly regulate both Th1 and Th2 immune responses. A high pathogen burden is instrumental for the development of Treg cells and thereby for a balanced development of the immune system.

Developing Costimulatory Molecules for Immunotherapy of Diseases.
DOI: http://dx.doi.org/10.1016/B978-0-12-802585-7.00004-2

Allergic diseases arise as a result of aberrant immune responsiveness against innocuous environmental proteins (antigens). Although we are all continuously being exposed to harmless antigens, only a certain percentage of the individuals experience adverse immunological reactions to these antigens. This is due to the fact that the normal immune response to allergens is associated with the induction of tolerance. Abrogation of tolerance or failure to induce tolerance may lead to the induction and perpetuation of active immune responses. Allergen-specific T-helper (Th) cells play a pivotal role in the pathogenesis of allergic hypersensitivity reactions and in the development of asthma.[3,231] Activated allergen-specific T cells are present in high frequency in the peripheral blood of allergic patients. The allergen-specific CD4+ T cells involved in the initiation of allergic reactivity have a distinct cytokine profile, characterized by the enhanced production of interleukin (IL)-4, IL-5, IL-9, and IL-13 (Th2 cytokines).[4,5] The presence of high levels of Th2 cytokines contributes to the clinical features of allergic pathophysiology. Although the most important determinant for the development of allergy and asthma is a genetic predisposition, environmental factors, such as exposure to allergens, infections, and air pollution, also play an important role in the development of allergic and asthmatic inflammatory responses. These Th cells activate a complex immune reaction that triggers the release of potent mediators and enhances the recruitment of inflammatory cells, which in turn elicit an inflammatory response that leads to the clinical symptoms of allergic disease.

The current therapies for allergic diseases focus primarily on control of symptoms and suppression of inflammation, without affecting the underlying cause. However, the knowledge about the pathophysiology of allergic diseases has substantially increased, offering new opportunities for therapeutic intervention. In this review, we will focus on current insights into the mechanism of allergic reactions. Advances in basic immunology research have enhanced our understanding of the cellular and molecular basis of the allergic response.

IMMUNOLOGY OF ALLERGY AND ASTHMA

Hypersensitivity reactions have been classified into four different types, characterized by different immunological mechanisms.[6,231] Briefly type I hypersensitivity refers to immediate hypersensitivity responses against foreign proteins that are common (pollen, grass, animal dander, etc.). It can be observed in allergic rhinitis and allergic asthma. This type of hypersensitivity is characterized by immunoglobulin (Ig) E production during the sensitization phase, which will bind to high-affinity IgE receptor (FcεRI) on mast cells and basophils. Upon renewed contact, the allergen will bind cellular IgE. Crosslinking of FcγRI receptors will lead to degranulation of mast cells and basophils.[6,7] Mediators released that way will lead to immediate and, sometimes, delayed immune responses. Type II hypersensitivity is a humoral response mediated by IgG or IgM that are produced against surface antigens on body cells. An example of type II hypersensitivity is drug-induced cytopenia caused by penicillin, cephalosporin, or transfusion reactions. In drug allergic subjects, IgG or IgM will be formed in response to drugs or their metabolites, which accumulate in membrane structures. This binding will allow the killing of the target cells by three different ways.[8–10] The first one is the activation of the classic complement pathway, which will lead to cytolysis. The second one is the antibody-dependent cell-mediated cytotoxicity, which will lead to lysis of target cells by natural killer cells. The last one is the recognition of Fc fragments of IgG and IgM by phagocytic cells, which will lead to opsonization of the target cells. Type III hypersensitivity involves the formation of immune complexes that are not well cleared by innate immune cells as in malaria, rheumatoid arthritis, or farmer's lung. This response can occur within 4–6 h. The accumulation of immune complexes (antigens bound to antibodies) in vessels and tissues can be caused by antigen excess for subjects with immunosuppression or insufficient antibody production. It can also be caused by repeated antigen exposure, which will lead to excess IgG antibody production. The presence of those persistent immune complexes will give rise to an inflammatory response due to leukocytes' activation.[11] Finally, type IV hypersensitivity is a delayed response principally mediated by T cells. The best-known example of type IV hypersensitivity is contact allergy. The sensitization phase lasts 10–15 days and is asymptomatic. In contact allergy, a hapten, a low molecular weight molecule, will interact with skin cells or proteins. After this contact, Langerhans and dendritic cells (DCs) will present antigen to naive T cells to stimulate their differentiation into CD4+ and CD8+ T cells and to induce production of memory T cells. A renewed contact between the skin and the antigen will stimulate sensitized memory T cells via antigen-presenting cells (APCs). Early arrival of CD4+ and CD8+ T cells and activation of keratinocytes, will all contribute to promote inflammatory reaction via cytokine secretion. Finally, this reaction will be controlled by Treg cells.[12] This classification of allergic reactions has been widely accepted.

One of the most studied allergic diseases is asthma. Asthmatic response is provoked by allergy in 75–80% of all asthmatic cases[13] According to the Global Initiative for Asthma,[14] asthma is defined as a chronic inflammatory disorder of the airways involving many cells and mediators. The principal associated symptoms are airway hyperresponsiveness and usually reversible airflow obstruction. These symptoms lead to recurrent episodes of wheezing, breathlessness, chest tightness, and coughing. Presently it is estimated that 300 million people suffer from asthma in the world and that this number will reach 400 million people by 2025. This represents a world prevalence of approximately 10% and a prevalence of 14.1% for Canada and of 10.9% for the United States.[15]

PATHOPHYSIOLOGY OF ASTHMA

Asthma is a complex trait that is influenced by several genes as well as by the environment; thus it presents heterogeneous clinical manifestations conventionally recognized as different subphenotypes.

Researchers agree that asthma is not a single disease but rather an array of disorders that share common characteristics.[13,16] These characteristics are inflammation, intermittent bronchial obstruction, bronchial hyperreactivity, mucus hypersecretion, and hypertrophy and hyperplasia of smooth muscle.[17] As mentioned above, in 75–80% of cases these phenotypes are caused by an allergic response, which triggers a Th2 immune response. It is a type I hypersensitivity reaction, that is an immediate exaggerated or harmful immune reaction.[9,10] Interestingly, only 7% of allergic people develop asthma, which can lead us to believe that they present a unique phenotype that distinguishes them from other allergic, but nonasthmatic, individuals. The main immune cells involved in asthma are CD4+ T cells, mast cells, and eosinophils.[18] When an allergen penetrates the airways, if not expulsed by the mucociliary barrier, it comes in contact with DCs, which will internalize and then digest the allergen. Some DCs then migrate toward the lymph nodes to present the antigen to naive T cells.[19,20] This presentation happens through the major histocompatibility complex (MHC) type II conjugated to the CD80 and CD86 costimulation molecules.[21] The introduction of the antigen to naive T cells triggers the differentiation of CD4+ T cells into Th1 or Th2. This differentiation is modulated by the cytokines present during the introduction of the allergen, for example, IL-12 (Figure 4.1). Evidence shows, at least for mild-to-moderate asthma, that Th2 cells predominate. Thus, after the differentiation of naive T cells in Th2 cells, the latter produce cytokines, including IL-4, which induces the production of IgE by B lymphocytes (Figure 4.2).

Response to Allergens in Asthma

When an individual has already been in contact with an allergen, its presence and the presence of IgE can activate mast cells and stimulate their degranulation just minutes after the contact with the allergen. The activation happens when the allergen binds with more than one IgE, which are linked to their high-affinity receptor (FcγRI; Figure 4.2). Mast cells are key cells in the immediate response. In fact, mast cell granules contain pro-inflammatory molecules such as histamine; tryptase, and other proteases; tumor necrosis factor (TNF); and heparin. New molecules are also produced and then released. These molecules are leukotrienes and prostaglandins, as well as cytokines, chemokines, and matrix metalloproteinases.[22] The releasing of these mediators triggers the development of immediate response symptoms such as coughing, bronchial spasms, smooth muscle contraction, edema, mucus secretion, and infiltration of immune cells. Mast cells, through these

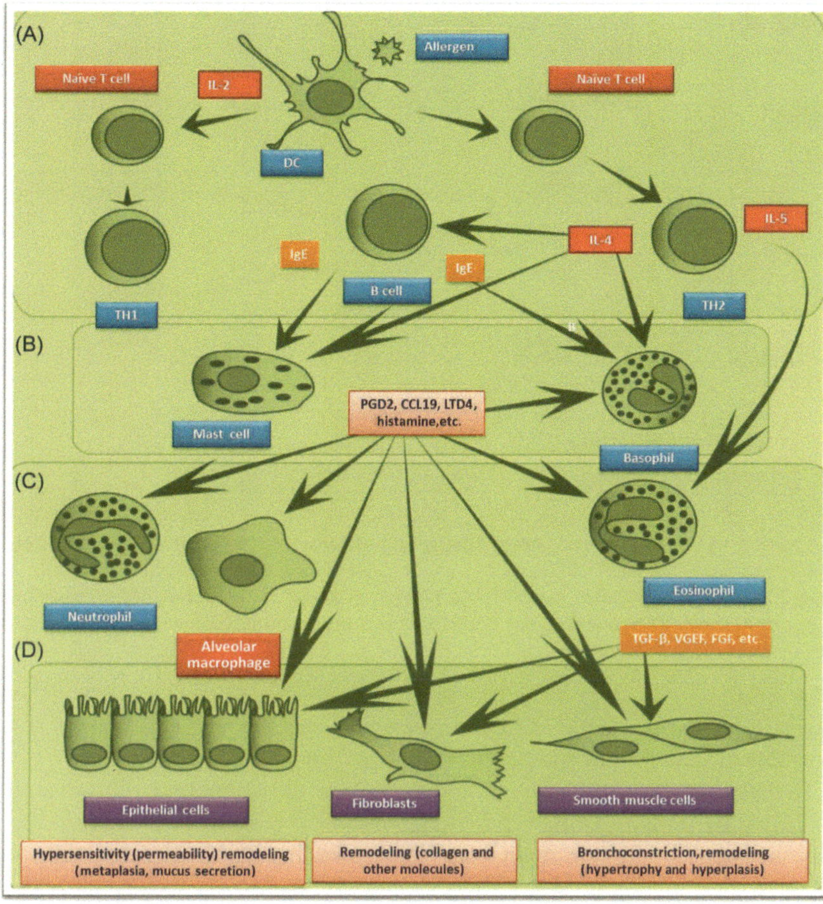

FIGURE 4.1 Innate and adaptive immune response in allergy and asthma. APCs bind with allergen, produce antigen (Ag), and display it on their surface on the MHC. This is then able to bind an antigen-specific TCR on the surface of the naive T cell (also known as signal 1). To respond to this antigen, the T cell must also be costimulated through additional receptors (costimulation, also known as signal 2). This dual stimulation can lead to a T-helper (Th)1 or Th2 response, depending on the antigen. The innate immune system plays a critical role in determining the type of T-cell differentiation and, thus, the type of adaptive immune response. A newly described subset, Th17 cells, mediates neutrophil inflammation and may play a role in asthma. Treg cells play an important role in overall regulation of the allergic response.

mediators, contribute to the recruitment and activation of immune cells in the lungs, such as eosinophils, T cells, macrophages, basophils, neutrophils, structure cells (fibroblasts, smooth muscle, and epithelial cells), and other mast cells.[23,24] Basophils, with the presence of FcγRI receptors on their surface and the expression of Th2 cytokines, histamine, and granules, can also

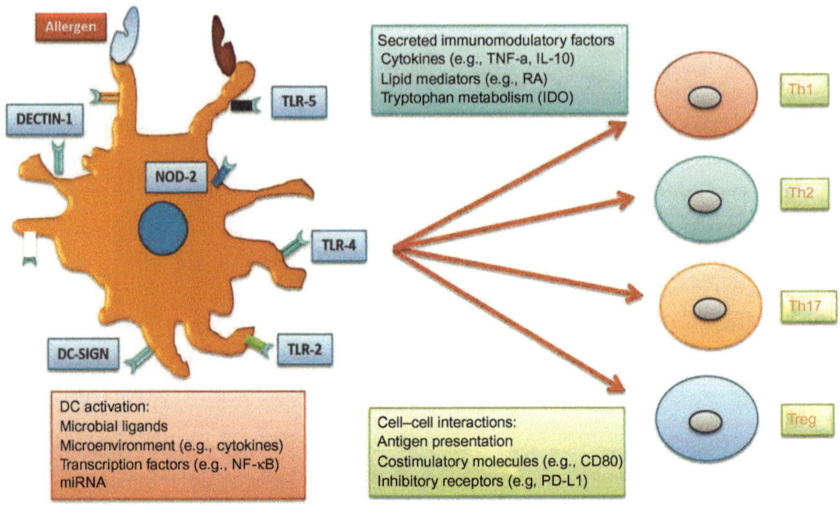

FIGURE 4.2 **Cell–cell interactions in allergy and asthma.** To respond to allergen, the T cell must be activated through TCR signal and costimulatory signal (costimulation, also known as signal 2). This dual stimulation can lead to a T-helper (Th)1 or Th2 response, depending on the antigen. A newly described subset, Th17 cells, mediates neutrophil inflammation and may play a role in asthma. Treg cells play an important role in overall regulation of the allergic response.

play a role in immediate response. However, their role in asthma is less documented than that of mast cells.[25]

Delayed, or late response, is not present in all asthmatics. It is mainly modulated by immune cells recruited by mast cells[9] (Figure 4.1). Among these cells, eosinophils are the main cells implicated in the development of this response. Eosinophils produce Th2 cytokines, leukotrienes, and proteins that cause damage to airway cells, such as major basic protein, eosinophil cationic protein, eosinophil-derived neurotoxin, and eosinophil peroxidase (EPO).[25,26]

Chronic inflammation in airways in asthma is characterized by a persisting inflammation and the presence of structure alterations in the airways (Figure 4.1). Several immune cells play a role in this response. Mast cells participate in the chronic response through mediators that have an effect on bronchoconstriction and on airway remodeling, which causes contraction, hypertrophia, and hyperplasia of smooth muscles as well as fibrogenesis.[27,28] DCs that remain in the airways after coming in contact with the allergen repeatedly present the antigen to CD4+ T cells.[29,30] These cells, as well as the activated T cells, produce pro-inflammatory cytokines and maintain the chronicity of the inflammation and the eosinophilia. Eosinophils are indirectly involved in bronchial remodeling as regards collagen deposit, fibrogenesis, angiogenesis, and hyperplasia of smooth muscles in the peripheral airways via mediators secretion and other cells activation.[31–33]

Phenotypic Variability in Asthma

To complete the topic asthmatic allergic response, the phenotypic heterogeneity has to be taken into consideration. Indeed, apart from allergic asthma, which is the most common form, other types of asthma have been described.[9,34] However, as with allergic asthma, the scientific community recognizes that IgE could be implicated in an inflammatory cascade, as well as CD4+ and CD8+ T cells, eosinophils, and mast cells. A second type of asthma is characterized by sensitivity to aspirin. It is estimated that approximately 10–20% of adult asthmatics suffer from this particular type.[35] Aspirin sensitization is thought to be non-IgE mediated so could be considered as a nonallergic subphenotype of asthma. A dysfunction of the eicosanoid metabolism is responsible for this type of asthma. It is estimated that 9–15% of all cases of asthma in adults are linked to the workplace and that up to 25% of new cases of adult asthma fall in the occupational asthma category. The two major hypotheses that could explain the induction of asthma after an effort are related to the augmentation of ventilation in the lungs. These two hypotheses are the osmotic hypothesis (dehydration by evaporation caused by the increase in ventilation) and the thermal hypothesis (airway cooling during exercise and rewarming after exercise).[36] These two hypotheses could better explain the phenotype rather than each one separately.

Asthma can also be classified according to inflammatory patterns. The three principal types are eosinophilic asthma, neutrophilic asthma, and paucigranulocytic asthma.[16] Paucigranulocytic asthma is defined as an asthma response without eosinophils or neutrophils. Another way to classify asthma is according to the severity of the phenotype. This classification is used in the clinical treatment, but is also used in research in order to document the molecular and cellular biology variation related to the severity of the disease. Intermittent, mild, moderate, or severe asthma are part of this classification. It is also interesting to note that a recruitment of Th1 and CD8+ T cells (cytotoxic T cells) has also been observed in the case of severe and chronic asthma and during exacerbation. Thus, other cell types involved in the Th1 response or in immune response regulation, such as alveolar macrophages (they inactivate DCs and they can be activated or inhibited through different pathways), could play a role in the inflammatory response observed in asthma.[37,38]

A prominent characteristic of the allergic response is a persistently elevated level of IgE antibodies against specific antigens (allergens) to which the affected individual is regularly exposed by inhalation, ingestion, or contact with the skin.[39] Allergic sensitization involves processing of the antigen by an APC and presentation, in association with a class II MHC protein, to a T-cell receptor (TCR). While DCs (and macrophages) predominantly act as APCs in primary immunization, B cells may also participate in secondary immune responses to allergens. Activation of T cells requires the signal from this trimolecular interaction and an additional costimulatory signal resulting from the binding of B7 (CD80/86) on an APC to CD28 or CTLA-4 on a T cell.[40] When stimulated by antigens, Th cells produce specific cytokines that have been designated as either Th1 cytokines [IL-2, interferon (IFN)-γ, and TNF-β] or Th2 cytokines (IL-4, IL-5, IL-9, IL-10, and IL-13). The state of T-cell activation depends on several factors.[40,41] The first of these factors is the strength of the interaction between the antigen and the T cell. The site of the antigen recognized by the T cell is termed the *epitope*. The affinity of a T cell for a specific epitope depends on the concentration of the antigen, the type of APC,[42] and the cytokine milieu of the T cell during antigen interaction. Thus, IFN-γ and IL-12 promote a Th1-like response, whereas IL-4 promotes a Th2-like response.[43] Additionally, host immune system genes may bias the overall immune responsiveness of an individual to favor a Th1- or Th2-like phenotype. A Th2-like cytokine profile is associated with the induction of IgE antibody (Ab) production *in vitro* and *in vivo*.[44] Specifically, IL-4 favors the development of Th2-like cells from uncommitted T cells, and both IL-4 and IL-13 play a role in IgE antibody production. Manifestation of an allergic reaction depends on the specific IgE levels and the amount of exposure at the time of the reaction. Although an allergic condition is a risk factor for asthma, 20–30% of asthmatics do not show positive skin tests to allergens. In general terms, asthma is an inflammatory disease in which not only lymphocytes but mast cells, basophils, eosinophils, and epithelial cells play a role. Studies to date suggest that Th2-like cytokines, such as IL-4 and IL-5, also play an important role in nonatopic asthma[45,46] (Figure 4.2).

ROLE OF MAST CELLS IN ALLERGY AND ASTHMA

Mast cells arise from progenitor cells in the bone marrow and full maturation of mast cells occurs in the peripheral tissue under the influence of various cytokines and other factors in the extracellular milieu. Mast cells express a great variety of stimulatory and inhibitory receptors. Antigen-specific mast cell activation can occur via IgE, IgG1, IgG2a, and IgG2b through crosslinking of the FcεRI and the FcγRI receptor.[8] Antigen-specific mast cell degranulation can also be induced by crosslinking of Ig-free light chains.[47] Further, antigen-independent mast cell activation can be established by various other receptors such as neurokinin receptors, c-kit, Toll-like receptors (TLRs), complement receptors, CD200 receptors, gp49a, or via direct interaction with G-proteins.[8,48–51] Activated mast cells release their granule content via exocytosis (anaphylactic degranulation) or via differential release of mediators without degranulation (piecemeal degranulation).[52] Furthermore mast cell activation results in the synthesis and release of lipid mediators and production of various chemokines and cytokines.[53]

Mast cells play a significant role in allergy and asthma and their role in allergic diseases has extensively been studied. Mast cell triggering plays an important role in the elicitation of the immediate phase of an allergic response leading to acute local responses such as edema formation, tissue swelling, or bronchoconstriction. By the release of chemotactic and proinflammatory mediators, mast cells can also have an effect on the late-phase responses of an allergic response.[49] Mast cells have been demonstrated to be of importance in the elicitation of a full-blown inflammatory response. Because of their close anatomical association with sensory nerves, bidirectional communication between mast cells and nerves can further influence the inflammatory responses.

In chronic asthma it has been demonstrated that multiple exposures to antigens resulted in FcRγ-dependent (via IgE and/or IgG1) and FcRγ-independent mast cell activation. This mast cell activation contributes to the induction of enhanced airway responsiveness and chronic inflammation including eosinophil and lymphocyte infiltration, goblet cell hyperplasia, and increased levels of lung collagen.[54]

In human asthmatic lungs, mast cells migrate into the airway epithelium, the airway mucous glands, and the airway smooth muscle, while virtually no mast cells were found in these regions in normal human airways. The number of mast cells infiltrated in the airway smooth muscle bundles was shown to correlate significantly with bronchial hyperresponsiveness in asthmatics, implicating their importance for the pathophysiology of asthma.[55]

IMMUNOTHERAPY TO ALLERGENS

The term "allergy" was first introduced by Clemens Freiherr von Pirquet, an Australian pediatrician, who believed that it was a pathological state of altered immune reactivity. However in 1911 Leonard Noon and John Freeman proposed the concept of allergen immunotherapy (IT). They hypothesized that toxins from grass pollen somehow accounted for symptoms seen in patients suffering from hay fever. By inoculating the patients with gradually increasing doses of the toxin itself to stimulate the immune system against the toxin, the symptoms could be reduced or even abolished.

Since then allergen IT has become a proven approach for treating allergic rhinitis and allergic asthma and has undergone significant development in the last two decades. Current allergen-specific IT (SIT) involves administering increasing doses of the causative allergen in order to reduce the clinical signs and symptoms associated with exposure to the allergen and thereby produce tolerance. As currently practiced, IT involves subcutaneous or sublingual administration of allergens, both methods of which have been extensively investigated. In addition to allergen IT, a number of additional non-SIT approaches are being used or are in phase II/phase III clinical trials. Such therapies include anti-IgE antibodies and the soluble IL-4 receptor (sIL-4R). Other experimental IT approaches are at the preclinical research stage and may also proceed to clinical trials and the clinic within the next

5–10 years. Here in this chapter we will discuss the pros and cons of recent developments in both currently practiced and experimental IT approaches with a focus on costimulation-based IT for allergy and asthma.

The allergens are administered by two different routes: parenteral or subcutaneous IT (SCIT) and sublingual IT (SLIT), which was introduced relatively recently. The current state of the art for each of these immunotherapeutic approaches is discussed below.

Subcutaneous IT

As currently practiced, SCIT has proven effective in allergic rhinitis and asthma and is Food and Drug Administration (FDA) approved and reimbursable. SCIT has been extensively studied in double-blind trials to determine effective doses, establish duration, define the mechanisms, and to investigate the persistence of efficacy after treatment ends. However, the need for multiple visits to the clinic for shots is inconvenient, only a few allergens have been standardized for SCIT, and the potential for systemic anaphylactic reactions is a serious limitation. Although allergen IT has been around for about a century, little is known about the absorption and fate of subcutaneously administered allergen. The pharmacokinetics of SCIT has been studied using leukocytes labeled with 99mTc-HMPAO on allergic patients injected intravenously in contralateral arms. Local inflammatory activity was noted in the first hour and the increase was time-dependent. The immune system responded quickly as the activity was traced in the lymphoid tissue of the upper mediastinum and anterior region of the neck. Thoracic and bowel focalization was also noted for the subcutaneous route. Factors important in SCIT include the dose of allergen being administered, the quality of the allergen extract, and the duration over which it is given.[56,57] The effects of duration of allergen dosing appear to depend on individual factors according to a review of studies performed between 1976 and 2006 in which the rate of relapse ranged from 0% to 50%.[58] The immune mechanism of SCIT has been extensively studied. SIT alters allergen-specific T-cell responses from Th2-like to Th1-like and reduces inflammatory cells and mediators in the target nasal mucosa and the airways.[59] For example, IT with house dust-mite extract induces antigen-specific suppressive activity by CD4+ CD25+ T cells in allergic subjects, which causes the regulatory/suppressor T cells to secrete IL-10 and transforming growth factor-β (TGF-β). This in turn increases IgG4 and IgA antibody production and suppression of IgE antibodies by B cells, thus mimicking a healthy immune response to environmental allergens.

Interestingly, a controlled study of traditional allergen vaccine IT to prevent asthma in atopic children demonstrated that more children in the non-treated group developed asthma than in the IT group. Moreover, it has been shown that IT in children sensitive to a single aeroallergen prevented new sensitization to other allergens.[60] Currently, only 2–3 million people of the

55 million with allergic diseases are on SCIT. The main reasons for this are that the target populations dislike injections or cannot afford the time and expense of frequent visits to a doctor's office. There is also a concern about the safety of SCIT, and it cannot be used for young children with allergy or asthma. In an effort to decrease the frequency of allergen administrations, intralymphatic allergen administration was attempted in a randomized (but not blinded) controlled trial.[61] While the results of this study are promising, it was not a blinded study and the technology of ultrasound-guided intralymphatic injection may not be available in all clinics.

Sublingual IT

SLIT consists of placement of an aqueous allergen extract (50% glycerin and 0.4% phenol) in single allergen tablets or capsules under the tongue. It has been extensively practiced in Europe,[62] and tested in clinical trials in the United States but is not yet FDA approved. Presently, SLIT is considered to have about one-tenth the risk of SCIT and has been shown to prevent new sensitization and progression from rhinitis to asthma. In addition, SLIT provides effective protection that persists for a long time after treatment is stopped. The disadvantages are that SLIT is less effective than SCIT and has not been tested for multiple allergen mixes. The pharmacokinetics of local IT by SLIT has been studied in allergic volunteers using radiolabeled allergen given in the form of soluble tablets. Plasma radioactivity was measured at different intervals using early and late sequential scintigraphic acquisition. No absorption through the oral mucosa was observed, and the plasma radioactivity, which peaks at 2 h, was increased only after swallowing. No allergen was detected in the blood stream.[63] Another study, in which the biodistribution of ^{123}I-radiolabeled Der p2 was assessed in allergic volunteers, confirmed these findings. Plasma radioactivity was only noted after the tablets were swallowed and the effect peaked at 1–2 h.[64] It was noted that in order for the IT to be successful, the allergen had to be swallowed after the tablet had dissolved sublingually. This confirms that the contact with oral mucosa is an important factor, although no allergen was absorbed through the oral mucosa. It was also found that duodenal enzymes were necessary for hydrolyzing the allergen.[65] Treatment with SLIT is initiated with a build-up phase lasting 4–6 weeks starting with the lowest concentration. The dosage is then gradually increased up to a maintenance dose. The recommended duration of the treatment is 3–4 years for optimal results.[66] SLIT can be administered coseasonally, preseasonally, or continuously.[67] The majority of SLIT studies have shown clinical efficacy in the form of improvement in symptom scores or medication scores, or both for allergic rhinitis and allergic asthma. A meta-analysis of five randomized double-blind, placebo-controlled studies on patients with allergic asthma showed significantly improved symptom scores and decreased use of rescue medication.[68]

Experimental IT Approaches

The availability of recombinant allergens makes it possible to treat allergic patients with identical, consistent vaccines. Recombinant allergens have other advantages which include (1) administration of allergens in optimal doses; (2) immunization with vaccines tailored to the major allergens to which the patient is allergic; (3) more accurate dosing; and (4) the possibility of modifying the structure of IgE-binding allergen epitopes, thereby increasing the safety of allergen IT. Recombinant allergens are not yet used in medicine since like other recombinant proteins; they must undergo rigorous clinical trials before they are available for clinical use.

Vaccination with a recombinant allergen before sensitization resulted in a state of immune deviation—a shift from a Th2, IgE response to a Th1, IgG2a response in a murine model.[69] Because the immune system of neonates and adult mice is similar in terms of their ability to develop immune deviation, and because allergic sensitization occurs predominantly in the first 2 years of human life,[70,71] using recombinant allergens for IT holds promise and needs further investigation. The recombinant allergens for IT may be used as aqueous, enteric-coated, or liposome-packaged vaccines or polymerized as recombinant allergoids using formaldehyde. Polymerized recombinant allergens are antigenic but nonallergenic and therefore may improve allergen-SIT. The problem with the available polymerized allergen vaccines is that they are not standardized and considerable batch-to-batch variation exists, making it uncertain whether all allergens have been uniformly polymerized or if some have been denatured. Recombinant allergens may also be conjugated with *n*-formyl-methionyl-leucyl-phenylalanine before being used to treat allergic patients.[72] These chemically modified recombinant allergen vaccines should provide a safer and more effective vaccine with fewer injections than are needed with current allergen vaccines. Furthermore, once the epitopes have been identified, an allergen-cDNA can be altered specifically to reduce the IgE-binding ability of the corresponding recombinant allergen without compromising its capacity to stimulate T cells. Genetically modified allergens not only appear to be safe, but also may prove to be effective agents for patient-tailored IT.

Allergen genes expressed in an appropriate host may be used as live vaccines while recombinant allergens and their corresponding cDNAs can be used to prevent allergen-specific IgE responses. Genes can be introduced via live bacteria, or viruses, or using plasmid vectors. Two models are noteworthy. First is oral immunization with *Salmonella typhimurium* expressing the cDNA coding for the major birch tree allergen, Bet v 1. This live vaccine promoted IgG2a instead of the default IgE antibody response in mice;[73] however, the Bet v 1-specific IgG2a response could be detected in only 10% of the immunized mice. Second, a live vaccine to treat allergic diseases using recombinant Bacillus Calmette-Guerin-expressing allergens has been proposed.[74]

These experimental approaches appear promising and may lead to effective prophylactic allergy vaccines. About one-quarter of the population is genetically predisposed to develop allergic disease. With advances in the identification of genes associated with asthma, it may be possible to develop methods for predicting atopic predisposition, which may then allow for the vaccination of predisposed individuals against the dominant allergens in their environments.

Alternatively, plasmids expressing allergens can be used for therapeutic vaccination. The immunization of mice with an allergen-cDNA cloned in a plasmid vehicle resulted in an allergen-specific IgG2a and Th1-like response, with no detectable IgE. Furthermore, the gene immunization induced a Th1-like response by reversing the ongoing allergen-specific Th2-like response. These studies suggest that immunization with allergen-cDNAs may provide a novel type of IT for allergic diseases; however, the application of DNA vaccines as a prophylactic may be more feasible because of the possibility of inducing anti-DNA antibodies and autoimmunity.

Peptide-Based Therapies

Because T cells play a dominant role in IgE synthesis, T-cell peptides may be useful as immunotherapeutic vaccines. T-cell peptide vaccines induce anergy in allergen-specific T cells or interfere with the formation of the trimolecular complexes involving the interaction of MHC—peptide duplexes with the appropriate TCR.[75,76] Peptide vaccines have several advantages: a defined chemical structure, simplicity of preparation, and prolonged shelf life. They also appear to be safe because, at least in mice, T-cell peptides do not bind to IgE;[77] however, human immune responses to allergens are more complex than murine immune responses. Various theoretical constraints are predictable: (1) some major allergens, particularly pollen allergens, contain several T-cell epitopes that are recognized by allergic individuals; (2) certain major allergens appear to have various isoforms containing crossreacting and noncrossreacting epitopes, which increase the repertoire of allergenic epitopes;[78] (3) allergic individuals differ with respect to their recognition of these epitopes; (4) B-cell and T-cell epitopes may be present on the same peptide, which increases the risk of systemic reactions; and (5) excessive doses of some peptides may induce autoimmune reactions. Thus, in individuals allergic to certain complex aeroallergens, treatment with peptides may not be effective or appropriate. In experimental animals, synthetic Fel d1 (cat major allergen) or Der p1 (house dust-mite major allergen) T-cell peptides induced peripheral T-cell tolerance.[79,80] The activation of allergen-specific T cells and IgE antibody synthesis was inhibited by *in vivo* administration of peptides by intranasal, oral, and subcutaneous routes.

The largest clinical study with allergen peptides was conducted using a total of four injections of 750 μg each of two peptides from the cat-allergen Fel d1 (ALLERVAX-CAT; ImmuLogic, Boston, MA) at 2-week intervals.

In a multicenter, randomized, double-blind, placebo-controlled study, 133 cat-allergic patients chronically exposed to cats or who had failed previous conventional cat IT, were given ALLERVAX-CAT as a 750 μg dose, and patients with reduced baseline forced expiratory volume in 1 s (FEV1) showed improved pulmonary function. Side effects of the treatment were considered to be of mild-to-moderate severity and were reported by 77 patients who had at least one respiratory system event including chest tightness, dyspnea, coughing, throat irritation, wheezing, and asthma aggravation. The most common dermatologic reaction presented was pruritus. Although severe adverse effects (AEs) did occur, there was no statistical difference in the frequency of their appearance between the treated and placebo group.[81] Therefore, although peptide therapy in severely cat-allergic patients was associated with some adverse effects, the therapy was found to be effective.

Allergen-Specific Therapy with Th1-Stimulating Adjuvants

Immune deviation from a Th2-like to Th1-like response may be achieved by designing vaccines with allergens or recombinant allergens in conjunction with adjuvants. The adjuvants may be cytokines or synthetic compounds, such as immunostimulatory DNA sequences containing a cytosine-phospho-guanosine (CpG) motif that induces a Th1-like cytokine response.[82,83] The adjuvant may be injected with natural allergens or genetically linked with allergen-cDNA. Among the cytokines, IFN-α and IL-12 both induce a strong Th1-like cytokine profile and therefore have the potential to convert allergen-specific Th2-like responses to Th1-like responses. IL-12 has also been suggested as an adjuvant for vaccination against diseases in which the Th2 profile predominates. IFN-τ, a type I IFN that lacks the toxicity associated with type I IFNs, inhibited IgE production in a murine allergy model and in an IgE-producing human myeloma cell line. Administration of a recombinant allergen (ovalbumin) vaccine with the IL-12 (subunit p40) fusion protein downregulated ovalbumin-specific IgE responses *in vivo*;[84] however, IL-12 may cause side effects, and its effectiveness requires IFN-α production by the target cells. Because IL-12's ability to convert an established Th2 to a Th1 response remains uncertain, the use of IL-12 as an adjuvant for allergen vaccines is unproven. Also of note are the studies involving TLR antagonists, which are based on the observation that LPS, the ligand of TLR-4, inhibits Th2 cytokine production in nasal explants of children.[85] MPL, a chemically modified derivative of LPS, was still a TLR-4 agonist and decreased combined symptom and medication scores compared to placebo in clinical trials.[86] A ragweed-TLR-9 agonist vaccine for IT was also tested in clinical trials in allergic rhinitis patients. While the results for the primary endpoint were not statistically significant, the secondary endpoints were significantly reduced. A similar study with this TLR-9 ligand in asthmatics showed a clear reduction of FEV1 and sputum eosinophils after allergen challenge.[87] Another potential form of IT involves the Fcγ1-linker-major cat-allergen, Fel d1, fusion protein, which was effective in inhibiting allergic responses in mice *in vivo* and human cells *in vitro*.[88] Gamma Fel D inhibits cat-allergen-induced degranulation of human basophils and cord blood mast cells in culture. Since results of mouse studies may not be translatable to humans, the proof-of-concept needs to be obtained in humans and the potential adverse effects need to be examined. Also, IT with mite allergen Der p1 on virus-like particles was reported to be safe and highly immunogenic in healthy adults.[89] The IgG response to dust mite allergens, particularly IgG1 and IgG3, but not IgG2 and IgG4, was significantly induced by these particles. However, this study was limited by lack of comparisons between Der p1 on virus and Der p1 without virus, lack of cellular studies and appropriate clinical endpoints relevant to human allergy and asthma.

Novel Approaches to Allergen-SIT

Although excellent drugs to control the symptoms of allergy and asthma are available, the only treatment able to cure allergy remains allergen-SIT. SIT is, however, rarely chosen as a therapeutic option by allergic patients mainly because it requires a treatment period lasting between 3 and 5 years to reach protection against the offending allergen. This unsatisfactory situation has strongly stimulated innovative research activities within the allergy field aimed at making SIT faster and safer in order to augment patient's compliance. Two main problems need to be reduced or eliminated to render SIT more attractive, and these are side effects and treatment time. Several exciting approaches to solve these issues are currently under clinical investigation. Therapy-related SIT side effects derive from the intrinsic property of allergens to crosslink high-affinity receptors for IgE on effector cells resulting in their degranulation and release of premade toxic substances, like histamine and leukotrienes, leading to local or generalized anaphylactic reactions. Allergoids, hypoallergens, and immunodominant allergen peptides are allergen surrogates with markedly reduced IgE-binding capacity, while conserving the whole and/or the immunodominant T-cell epitopes required for eliciting protective (IgG-mediated) immune responses. SIT with allergoids reached the market some time ago and has yielded results comparable to those obtained with allergen extracts with a reduced side effect profile, but it still requires a long treatment time. Peptide IT showed promising results in clinical trials with bee venom allergic and cat-allergic individuals.

Many genetically engineered hypoallergens have shown promising results in mouse models of allergy. Perhaps the more advanced form of IT with allergens showing a favorable safety profile is SLIT. SLIT still suffers from a long treatment time comparable to those of classical SCIT but is increasingly used as a therapeutic option, especially in Europe. These approaches have significant potential for improvement, particularly in combination with novel adjuvants and modified treatment regimens. Obviously, a long treatment time strongly reduces patient's compliance, and therefore many efforts have been undertaken to reduce the number of injections (currently 50–80 are required) in order to achieve protection. Four different strategies have entered phase I/IIA clinical trials and yielded promising results: peptides covalently coupled to virus-like particles,[89] A-type CpG oligodeoxynucleotides as an adjuvant,[90] direct injection of allergens into lymph nodes,[61] and modular antigen translocating vaccines, which directly target the MHC class II antigen presentation pathway.[91,92] All these therapeutic innovations have, if confirmed in larger multicenter clinical trials, the potential to turn IT into a true vaccination approach because only a few injections are required to achieve long-lasting protection. These approaches indicate that the problems related to the long treatment time of classical IT, which is mechanistically based on immunomodulation, which requires a long time to establish, can be reduced using strong adjuvants, by changing the route of application, or by direct targeting of the antigen presentation pathways. We conclude that the limited efficacy associated with classical SIT is not closely related to the potential of the immune system to mount protective responses against allergens. There is clear evidence that low amounts of antigen, such as those encountered during natural exposure to most of the environmental allergens, favor the switch of B cells toward IgE production in predisposed individuals, whereas higher doses of antigen favor the development of protective IgE antibody responses. Therefore, the most promising approaches to faster and more successful SIT treatment regimens will most likely derive from strategies aimed at increasing the therapeutic dose of the allergen in lymph nodes, while avoiding effector cell degranulation.

Current Immunomodulatory Strategies for Asthma Under Investigation

A number of anti-cytokine therapies are currently being examined. Daclizumab (an IL-2 receptor antagonist) has been examined in a phase II study in patients with moderate-to-severe asthma. Patients treated with daclizumab showed improved pulmonary function; reduced asthma symptoms and medication use; increased interval between severe exacerbations; and reduced blood eosinophils and serum eosinophil cationic protein levels.[93,94] Two humanized IL-5 monoclonal antibodies (mAbs)—reslizumab and mepolizumab—have been studied in humans. Mepolizumab decreased blood and airway eosinophils, but no significant sustained changes in FEV1, asthma symptom scores, sputum eosinophils, or physician-evaluated overall condition were noted with mepolizumab or reslizumab compared with placebo.[95,96] In order to neutralize the activity of IL-4, recombinant human sIL-4R has been examined.[97] Patients with moderate, persistent asthma had significant improvement in asthma symptom scores, rescue β-agonist use, and exhaled nitric oxide levels compared with those receiving placebo.[63] However, a follow-up study revealed that only asthma patients receiving the highest dose of sIL-4R maintained their lung function.[98] Blocking TNF-α using neutralizing antibodies improved lung function and quality of life and reduced exacerbation frequency in patients with asthma in some studies but not in all studies.[99–101] It is likely that additional cytokines (e.g., chemokines) will also be targeted in the near future for patients with allergy and asthma. Several humanized mAb that bind to the Fc portion of the IgE molecule have been used in clinical studies, and one (omalizumab) is currently available for treatment of allergic asthma. Anti-IgE in combination with allergen-SIT resulted in a greater reduction in seasonal allergic rhinitis symptoms and rescue medication scores compared to allergen-SIT alone.[102] Importantly, the addition of omalizumab to a rush SIT protocol significantly reduced the risk of anaphylaxis.[103]

Anti-histamine compounds that target the histamine receptor 1 (H1R) have been used for some time. However, the discovery of a new histamine receptor, H4R, has provided a new target for drug development. Thus far, only animal model data are available that demonstrate proof of the efficacy for H4R antagonists in models of asthma, allergic rhinitis, and pruritis.[104] Candidate molecules have been identified, which are expected to enter clinical trials shortly.

Monoclonal Anti-IgE Antibody Therapy

The development of an allergic state is a gradual process, and as a genetically predisposed individual undergoes the "allergic march," he or she may develop allergies to several antigens.[105] Because IgE crosslinking on the mast cell membrane by allergens is an important first step in an allergic reaction, IgE has been an attractive therapeutic target. Although the idea of anti-IgE as a therapeutic agent was conceived during the 1970s, the use of anti-IgE as a therapeutic strategy failed because the antibodies initially employed caused mast cell degranulation. With the advances in recombinant DNA technology, it has become possible to engineer mAbs that reduce unbound IgE levels in the serum by binding to circulating serum IgE antibodies but not to IgE antibodies bound to FcεRI or to FcεRII.[106]

Two mouse monoclonal anti-IgE antibodies, TES-C21 and MAE11, have been humanized[107] and MAE11 (rhuMAb E25) has been evaluated in clinical studies. In humanizing MAE11, a framework derived from consensus sequences of human VL and VH chains was used, and the critical amino acids responsible for binding IgE were engrafted onto a consensus human IgG1 framework.[89] Several clinical studies have been conducted to evaluate the safety and effectiveness of using anti-human IgE antibodies to treat allergic asthma and allergic rhinitis. The results of these studies show that anti-IgE therapy reduces allergic symptoms, is well tolerated by patients, and does not cause any severe AEs.[107] The two monoclonal anti-IgE antibodies, rhuMAb E25 and CGP51901, have been shown in a number of clinical trials including subjects with asthma or allergic rhinitis to be safe and effective in generating tolerance. The anti-IgE antibody CGP51901, which is a chimeric version of the mouse monoclonal anti-IgE TES-C21, has been evaluated in patients with seasonal allergic rhinitis.[108] These studies have shown a decrease in free serum IgE but an increase in total IgE levels. The slow clearance of IgE–anti-IgE complexes explains the increase, with complexed IgE having a half-life of 11–13 days. The reduction in free serum IgE levels was dependent upon anti-IgE doses and was reversible. It was necessary to sustain 85% or greater reduction in free serum IgE levels to achieve improved clinical symptoms, and an 85% reduction in IgE required a serum CGP51901 concentration of 5000 ng/mL. The treatment was safe, with no serum sickness and only one case of urticarial among 153 evaluated patients.[109]

The anti-IgE antibody rhuMAb E25 has been evaluated in both allergic rhinitis and asthma. It decreased free serum IgE in a dose-dependent fashion in patients with seasonal allergic rhinitis;[232,233] however, in this study, it was not possible to evaluate its clinical efficacy because only 11 subjects had undetectable IgE levels. To achieve undetectable IgE concentrations, the dose of rhuMAb E25 was 0.005 mg/kg/week for each international unit per milliliter of baseline IgE. There were no AEs related to this treatment. The rhuMAb E25 antibody has also been studied in asthma, but asthma symptoms, rescue medication use, or FEV1 did not improve; however, there was improvement in the allergen early- and late-asthmatic response, methacholine reactivity, and some inflammatory parameters in induced sputum. The evaluated patients had mild asthma, which may have limited the potential for improvement. The administration of rhuMAb E25 significantly increased the allergen doses required to cause a 15% decrease in FEV1, with a correlation between the decrease in free serum IgE and the protection against inhaled allergen.[110,111] The same study also showed that a higher dose of methacholine was necessary to reduce FEV1 by 20% after administration of rhuMAb E25. Another study showed rhuMAb E25 reduced maximal bronchoconstriction by 60% during the late asthmatic response following allergen challenge. Reduction of the early response after bronchial allergen challenge was less affected.[71] The late asthmatic response following allergen challenge correlates with airway hyperresponsiveness, airway inflammation, and improvement of asthma symptoms, suggesting rhuMAb E25 may have a clinical benefit. Additional studies support this possibility with rhuMAb E25 administration reducing the number of asthmatic exacerbations and facilitating a 50% dose reduction in use of inhaled and oral steroids.[112,113]

Among all of these reports, only minimal toxicity was observed with one case of urticaria. Recently, however, more side effects have been noted including local injection site irritation, upper respiratory infection, headache, and urticaria.[114] Among the total of 118 cases of anaphylaxis found by the

FDA AE reporting system, 19 had anaphylaxis within the first hour, 32 had reaction after receiving the first dose, while 14 reacted after the second dose, and 77 patients required hospitalization. These patients were treated with epinephrine or corticosteroids, and had anti-IgE withheld or discontinued. The vaccine was given subcutaneously every 2 or 4 weeks and the dose was determined by body weight and total pretreatment serum IgE levels. Absorption is slow from the inoculation site and the mean half-life of the drug is 26 days,[115] while the evidence shows that anti-IgE is a safe and effective immunotherapeutic treatment for asthma, it is noteworthy that anti-IgE antibodies also aid with allergen IT and reduce the risk of adverse reactions. Casale et al.[103] reported that anti-IgE reduces acute allergic reactions with SCIT rush IT, which reduces the frequency of hospital visits inherent with classical SCIT. In addition to the new treatments described above, several other potential approaches are being explored. Most of these are aimed at modulating the allergic immune response and inflammation in murine models using either soluble receptors or antibodies that alter cytokines, immunocyte coreceptors, IgE receptor binding, and cellular adhesion.

IgE-Binding Receptors

The IgE antibody binds to the FcεRI and CD23 on mast cells and basophils and to CD23 on monocytes and eosinophils. Both receptor and ligand are potential therapeutic targets. Antibodies attached to CD23 may be able to facilitate antigen presentation to T cells, but IgE regulation was not affected. Transgenic mice that overexpress CD23 on T and B cells exhibit decreased IgE production,[116] which suggests that enhancing CD23 expression on B cells before activation can effectively inhibit IgE production. Conversely, a decrease in CD23 levels with a metalloprotease resulted in an increase in IgE.[117] The administration of anti-CD23 antibodies inhibits eosinophil airway recruitment and reduces airway hyperresponsiveness.[118,119] This observation suggests that anti-CD23 antibodies may be used to block the interaction between IgE and CD23, reducing eosinophil recruitment and inflammation. More studies are necessary before IgE receptors can be viewed as important therapeutic targets for allergic disease.

Anti-IgE Monoclonal Antibodies

The anti-IgE antibody omalizumab has so far only been studied as a treatment for severe allergic asthma. There are well-documented effects on risk of asthma exacerbation.[120] The drug is expensive and requires injections at monthly or biweekly intervals. A reduction in free IgE levels following the anti-IgE therapy could lead to reduction in FcεRI expression on mast cells, basophils, and DCs.[121] One could speculate that treatment with anti-IgE in high-risk children could prevent allergic sensitization and delay or prevent development of allergic asthma. On this premise, an observational study has shown that after stopping prolonged treatment with omalizumab, asthma control can persist as a residual effect, possibly indicating a modifying effect on the natural history of asthma.[122] The results of the XPORT trial (NTC01125748), a double-blind placebo-controlled withdrawal study of moderate-to-severe asthmatic adult patients who received omalizumab for ≥5 years, have been recently disclosed. Patients were randomized to either continue receiving omalizumab, or switch to placebo for one additional year. At the end of that period, whereas the proportion of patients receiving the active treatment who had not suffered an asthma exacerbation was 67%, this only happened in 48% of patients in the placebo group. However, this would suggest that in about half of patients the effect of omalizumab would persist at least for 1 year after it was stopped.[123] Furthermore, omalizumab reduces airway remodeling by modulating bronchial reticular basement membrane thickness and eosinophil infiltration.[124] New immune modulator interventions are being developed to improve the immune response to viral infections in children with impaired innate immunity, as shown by decreased levels of IFN-γ or impaired function of TLRs.[125] Examples are inhaled IFN-β and a TLR agonist. They are being evaluated for treatment, but they may potentially have a preventive activity.

In summary, there are still no drugs to be used for primary prevention of asthma. There are, however, treatment possibilities for tertiary prevention of deterioration and exacerbations although effects on the long-term prognosis are still uncertain. Prevention of rhinovirus infections may provide a major step forward in primary prevention; immune modulators improve the innate immunity and response to virus infections; and there are other potential approaches.

sIL-4R Therapy

IL-4 is one of the most important cytokines in a variety of allergic diseases, including asthma.[126] IL-4 is produced primarily by CD4 Th2 cells but also by CD8 T cells, eosinophils, mast cells, and basophils. The role of IL-4 in human asthma has been established in several studies. The proof of the importance of IL-4 includes the following: (1) characterization of T-cell clones producing IL-4 in allergic and nonallergic individuals;[127] (2) *in situ* localization of IL-4-producing cells in bronchial biopsies;[234] (3) expression of IL-4R mRNA and protein in epithelium, subepithelium, and endothelial cell layers in bronchial biopsies of atopic asthmatics compared with controls;[128] and (4) analysis of mutations of the IL-4R and their association with asthma.[129] The importance of IL-4 in the regulation of the allergic response, coupled with the identification of the soluble receptor, suggested that the sIL-4R might be effective as a therapeutic agent. Soluble IL-4R inhibited the IL-4-induced proliferation of B cells; the expression of low-affinity IgER and MHC class II; and the secretion of both IgE and IgG1 antibodies in mice.[130] In a murine model of allergen sensitization, soluble murine IL-4R inhibited polyclonal and particularly antigen-specific IgE and IgG1 production following restimulation with these allergens.[131] In addition to inhibiting Ig class switching and IgE production, murine sIL-4R reduces allergen-induced airway reactivity, vascular cell adhesion molecule-1 (VCAM-1) expression; allergen-induced eosinophilia in bronchoalveolar lavage (BAL); and allergen-induced pulmonary infiltration and airway occlusion by inflammatory cells. The safety of sIL-4R therapy is demonstrated by transgenic mice that produce a 100-fold greater sIL-4R concentration than nontransgenic littermates. Mice with increased sIL-4R compared with controls have similar numbers of B and T lymphocytes, lymphocyte surface marker expression, and antigen-specific antibody responses.[132]

In clinical studies, soluble IL-4R blocked CD8 T-cell-mediated IgE production in allergic patients, suggesting that sIL-4R may be useful for treating allergic diseases.[133] Studies on the effects of recombinant humanized sIL-4R (rhusIL-4R) on IL-4/staphylococcal enterotoxin B-stimulated peripheral blood mononuclear cells from patients with eczema suggested that rhusIL-4R may be an immunomodulatory drug for atopic eczema.[134] In another study of human asthmatics, rhusIL-4R, was nebulized and given to 62 patients with moderate asthma at doses of 0.75, 1.5, or 3 mg. The study was double-blinded and placebo-controlled, and corticosteroid therapy was discontinued at entry. The results showed that sIL-4R was well tolerated, and the group treated with 3 mg sIL-4R demonstrated less labile FEV1 and improved asthma symptom scores compared to the placebo group.[63] In an open-label, randomized, dose-ranging study, the safety and tolerability of sIL-4R was evaluated in 16 adult patients with mild atopic asthma (FEV1 $>70\%$ of predicted). A single nebulized dose (50–100 μg) was generally well tolerated and pulmonary function improved.[135] In a phase I/II randomized, placebo-controlled trial,[63] 25 patients with moderate, inhaled corticosteroid-dependent asthma were randomly assigned to receive a single nebulized dose of IL-4R or placebo after discontinuing inhaled corticosteroids. The results indicate that sIL-4R is effective with once-weekly inhalation. The treatment is generally well tolerated and prevents a decline in FEV1, improves asthma symptom scores, and reduces β2-agonist rescue following discontinuation of inhaled corticosteroids. Pulmonary inflammation, as assessed by exhaled nitric oxide, was significantly lower in the sIL-4R treated group compared to the placebo group. The treated group had nonstatistically decreased levels of VCAM-1, intercellular adhesion molecule-1, and EPO and increased CD23 expression compared to the placebo group. These results support the potential use of sIL-4R as a therapy for asthma and other allergic diseases, but additional studies are needed.

Targeting Tregs for IT of Allergy and Asthma

The fundamental role of Treg cells in maintaining immune tolerance has been demonstrated in a wide range of animal models, in which the adoptive transfer or deliberate expansion of Treg cells was shown to prevent or cure several T-cell-mediated diseases, which include allergy, asthmatic lung inflammation, autoimmune diseases, and allograft rejection, by restoring immune tolerance to allergens, self-antigens, or alloantigens. Multiple molecular mechanisms for Treg-mediated immunosuppression have been described with secretion of IL-10 being of particular importance.[136] Absence or defective function of Treg cells has also been correlated with hyper-IgE syndrome, hypereosinophilia, and autoimmunity in humans, whereas their presence has been associated with immune tolerance.[137]

Studies on the mechanisms by which immune responses to nonpathogenic environmental antigens lead to either allergy or nonharmful immunity have demonstrated that allergen-specific IL-10 producing Tregs (TR1 cells) are the dominant T cell subset in healthy individuals.[138,139] Repeated exposure of nonallergic healthy beekeepers to bee venom antigens during the beekeeping season represents a valuable *in vivo* model to ascertain mechanisms of immune tolerance to venom antigens.[140] After multiple bee stings, venom antigen-specific Th1 and Th2 cells switch toward IL-10-secreting TR1 cells. This occurs in parallel to the suppression of cutaneous late-phase responses to allergens and inhibition of allergen-specific Th1 and Th2 cells. The response is observed as long as venom exposure persists and returns to initial levels within 2–3 months after the end of the beekeeping season. In the same model, the upregulation of H2R on specific Th2 cells suppressed allergen-stimulated T cells and increased IL-10 production. Various strategies, which are designed to enhance Treg function *in vivo*, are currently under investigation. These include the adoptive transfer of inducible or constitutive Treg cells and their induction by specific adjuvants or immunomodulators. These approaches are attractive compared to conventional treatments, as the antigen-specific suppressor capacity of Treg cells does not result in general immunosuppression and may actually lead to long-lasting antigen-specific regulation *in vivo*. Moreover, individual patient-specific treatments are possible with limited side effects. Many immunomodulators that have been developed or are under development, such as rapamycin, the CD80/CD86:CD28 costimulation blocker abatacept (Orencia; Bristol–Myers Squibb, Co., Uxbridge, Middlesex, UK), nonmitogenic anti-CD3 mAbs, and T-cell depletion and anti-TNF-α mAbs, display direct or indirect effects on Treg cells, which may enhance or suppress their function.[141–143]

There is a selective advantage to expand a population of Treg cells that can target the organ (or the lymph nodes that drain the organ) by recognition of an allergen or an autoantigen expressed in inflamed organs in mouse models.[144] Thus, transfer of organ-specific Treg cells can be effective at suppressing ongoing disease, although those Treg cells do not necessarily need to recognize exactly the same autoantigen as the autoaggressive effector T cells.[145] This observation has implications for therapeutic strategies aimed at targeting the Treg cell arm of immune tolerance against allergens, autoantigens, or transplantation antigens. Possibilities of adoptive transfer of Treg cells or small molecular compounds that induce Treg cells in the tissue are being investigated,[144] but no double-blind, placebo-controlled studies have been reported so far. To date, allergen-SIT is the only antigen-specific approach that induces Treg cell production and activation in humans. Allergen-SIT induces Treg and IL-10-secreting TR1-like cells, and treatment with glucocorticoids and β2-adrenergic agonists seems to promote the number and activity of these cells.[146–148] The essential transcriptional elements regulating expression of the Foxp3 promoter have been recently reported, and these will provide new targets for the development of novel therapeutics.[149]

COSTIMULATION IN ALLERGY AND ASTHMA

The activation of T lymphocytes in the airways, which leads to production of the inflammatory cytokines and mediators characteristic of asthma, is clearly dependent on the presence of inhaled allergen *in situ*. However, allergen by itself is not sufficient to initiate this cascade of events. It is well established that the deleterious allergic response is initiated by T-cell recognition of MHC class II–peptide complexes at the surface of APCs. While this first signal gives antigen specificity to the adaptive immune response, a second nonspecific costimulatory signal is required by T cells to become fully activated. This signal is provided by interactions between APCs and T cells through molecules borne at the surfaces of the two cell types. Depending on the type of molecules involved, this secondary signal can promote the development of an inflammatory allergic reaction or may favor immune regulation. Several molecules of the B7 family [CD80, CD86, programmed death-1 (PD-1), inducible costimulatory antigen (ICOS), CTLA-4] and TNF receptor (TNFR) family (OX40, CD30, 4-1BB, Fas, CD27, CD40) play an important role in delivering costimulatory signals in early and late phases of allergic response (Figure 4.3). Therefore, costimulatory molecules involved in promotion or prevention of allergic immune responses are potential targets for the development of novel therapeutic approaches. In order to become fully activated, T lymphocytes also require a so-called "second signal," or "costimulatory" signal, which is provided to the T lymphocytes through interaction with cells specialized in antigen capture, or APCs, found in lymphoid organs as well as at mucosal surfaces such as the airway and lung.[150] In the absence of costimulatory signals, the T-dependent immune response is greatly diminished, or even eliminated altogether. Two costimulatory molecules expressed on the surface of APCs have so far been identified, termed CD80 and CD86. Both CD80 and CD86 mediate their function by binding a receptor on T lymphocytes termed CD28. Constitutive and induced expression of CD80 and CD86 varies on different APC types, and the reasons why APCs have two different versions of the same CD28 binding molecule are unclear. However, there have been some intriguing observations that atopic Th2-type immune

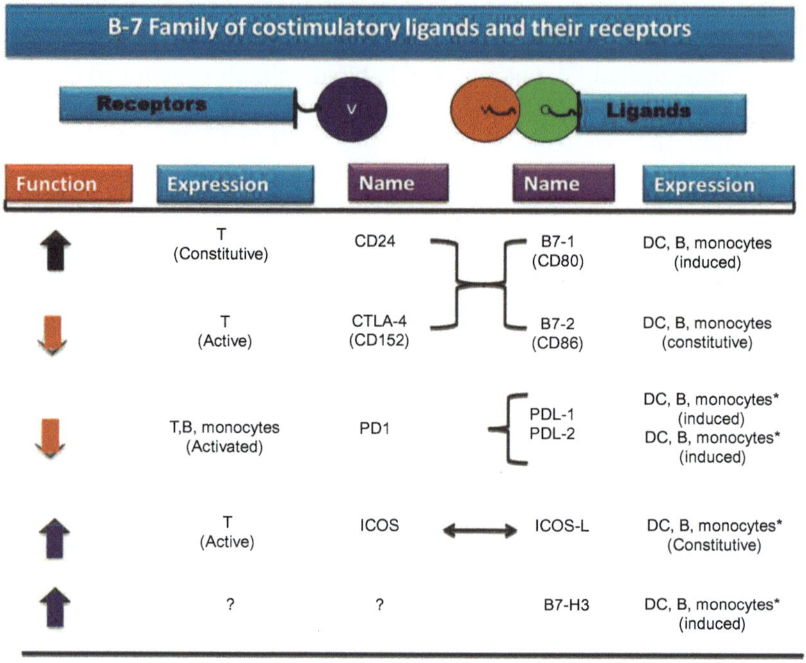

FIGURE 4.3 **Summary of B7 family ligands and their receptors.** The names of receptors and ligands are indicated, as well as a brief summary of predominant expression patterns for each. The conserved structure of a single IgV extracellular domain for receptors and IgV and IgC extracellular domains for ligands is depicted at the top. Function arrows indicate whether the pathway is thought predominantly to costimulate or inhibit the response of the receptor-bearing cell. Integration of signals through this family of costimulatory and inhibitory receptors and their ligands is critical for activation of immune responses and tolerance.

responses may be preferentially activated by CD86 while Th1-type immune responses are regulated by CD80.[151] DCs in the lung and airway express both CD80 and CD86, as do pulmonary macrophages, although at much reduced levels.[152] These cells therefore provide an effective source of costimulatory signals for the optimal activation of T lymphocytes locally.

Costimulation in Asthma

T-cell activation and cytokine secretion are important mediators of inflammation in allergic asthma.[153,154] Recent studies indicate that the costimulatory pathway CD28/CD80/CD86 plays an important role in allergic asthma. The effect of other costimulatory molecules on allergic responses (e.g., OX40L) is under scrutiny. The roles of CD80 and CD86 have been examined by selective inhibition of either CD80 or CD86 in a murine model of allergic pulmonary inflammation.[155] Inhibition of costimulation by antibodies to either CD80 or

CD86 showed decreased allergic responses. Specifically, blockade of either CD80 or CD86 in allergen ovalbumin-sensitized and challenged mice resulted in a decrease in airway eosinophilia serum IgE production, airway hyperresponsiveness (AHR), and IL-4 and IL-2 production, with an enhanced IFN-γ production. Studies using mice with germline deletions of the CD80 and/or CD86 molecules showed that mice lacking both CD80 and CD86 had no elevation of serum IgE, airway eosinophilia, or AHR.[156] These same allergic parameters were also reduced in mice lacking either CD80 or CD86. Absence of CD80 and/or CD86 resulted in increased Th1 cytokine production. In humans, costimulatory molecule expression (CD28, CD80/CD86) is increased in allergic asthmatics.[157] These observations support a role for both CD80- and CD86-mediated costimulation in allergic pulmonary inflammation.

The costimulatory molecule OX40L, a member of the TNF superfamily, has been shown to be important in T-cell priming and cytokine production. In a murine model of allergic inflammation with OX40L-deficient mice, total serum IgE, pulmonary eosinophils, cytokines, and pulmonary inflammation were significantly decreased compared with wild-type controls.[158] Levels of eotaxin messenger RNA, an eosinophil-specific chemoattractant, were also markedly reduced, paralleling the significant reduction in pulmonary eosinophils. Levels of allergen-induced Th1 as well as Th2 cytokines were also significantly reduced. Together, the data support a critical role for OX40L signals in allergic responses.[159]

Families of costimulatory molecules are involved in the regulation of most inflammatory diseases by finely controlling the intensity of the immune response. Costimulatory molecules are implicated in the development and control of allergic inflammation characterized by the establishment of an acute Th2 polarization. Elucidation of the role of costimulation pathways in the development of new subsets of Th cells has just begun, and most of the mechanisms underlying the regulation of atopic diseases by costimulatory molecules are unknown and require further investigation. With an increased understanding of these immunological mechanisms, new therapeutic strategies in the treatment of allergic airway diseases can be created by analyzing the role of costimulatory molecules that are critically involved in the induction and maintenance of allergen-induced airway diseases. Taken together, recent studies have begun to provide insight into the role of costimulatory molecules and give us new clues to design more efficient therapies to fight the increasing public health problem that allergies represent.

Recent studies have addressed the role of the costimulatory signal in animal models of asthmatic inflammation.[160] The simultaneous blockade of the signals delivered by CD80 and CD86 to T lymphocytes has dramatic effects on lung immune responses: infiltration of T lymphocytes is significantly diminished, and migration of eosinophils to the lung tissue and into the BAL fluid is also eliminated. Importantly, blockade of CD80 and CD86 only at the time of intranasal allergen challenge is sufficient to completely eliminate the lung inflammatory response, which indicates this approach could be effective even after prolonged exposure to a specific allergen has taken place.

Unfortunately, as is the case for many other immunosuppressive treatments, the effect of blockade of CD80 and CD86 is not restricted to the lung, but also has systemic effects on antibody production and other unrelated immune responses in separate organs, which essentially induces a state of generalized immune suppression. The usefulness of this approach would therefore be limited to only the most severe cases of atopic asthma. In an attempt to address this concern, recent studies in our laboratory have examined the effect of selective blockade of the CD80 costimulatory molecule by using specific reagents that inhibit CD80 but leave CD86-dependent costimulation completely functional.[160] Rather surprisingly, selective blockade of CD80 costimulation has a dramatic effect on the lung inflammatory response and appears to almost completely block the local infiltration of eosinophils that is characteristic of asthmatic inflammation.[161] At the same time, anti-CD80 treatment has no apparent effects on systemic immune responses, which leaves specific antibody responses intact, and also fails to inhibit the elevation of blood eosinophilia that is associated with allergen exposure. However, these eosinophils fail to migrate into the lung tissue upon antigen challenge, which implies that local mechanisms have been severely impaired due to unavailability of the CD80-dependent costimulatory pathway. The molecular mechanism of this finding has not yet been established, and is currently being addressed in our laboratory. We hypothesize that CD80 may provide additional costimulation, which is critical for the expression of mucosal immune responses, thereby acting as a safeguard against inappropriate immune activation. In this scenario, lack of CD80-dependent costimulation would result in incomplete activation of T cells in the lung, diminished production of IL-5 and/or other chemokines involved in the chemotaxis and migration of eosinophils into the tissues, and in turn, failure to activate a local inflammatory response.

Costimulation and T-Cell Reactivity to Allergens

The activation of T cells first requires a signal from the antigen in the context of the human leukocyte antigen (HLA) molecule and then an additional costimulatory signal involving the binding of B7 on APCs (CD80/86) to CD28 or CTLA-4 on T cells. Without costimulation, T cells become anergic. Thus, the costimulatory molecules have become targets for developing drugs that will modulate an allergic immune response. The chimeric CTLA-4-Ig molecule, which consists of the extracellular domain of CTLA-4 and the hinge, CH2, and CH3 regions of IgG, blocks the costimulatory signal that T cells receive through the interaction of CD28 with the counter-receptors CD80 or CD86 expressed on the APC membrane. CTLA-4-Ig is able to downregulate or suppress the mucosal immune response in allergic rhinitis.[162] CTLA-4-Ig inhibits airway eosinophilia and hyperresponsiveness by enhancing Th1-like cell activity. IgE formation is enhanced by the Th2 cytokine IL-4. Therefore, it is expected that downregulating Th2 activity will decrease IgE formation, as has been demonstrated in CTLA-4-Ig-treated mice.[163] The combination of antibodies to CD80/CD86 with the ligand for CTLA-4, blocks the development of allergic airway inflammation, whereas only a partial reduction occurs using either of these antibodies alone. However, only the anti-CD86 antibody inhibits the production of IgE.[164] Therefore, the CD28–CD80/CD86 complex is a potential target for developing new strategies of allergy treatment.

The first costimulatory molecules described were the ligands of CD28: CD80 (B7-1) and CD86 (B7-2). The CD28 costimulation pathway is an important factor for the promotion of an effective antigen-specific immune response. Costimulatory molecules are involved in the fine tuning of the T-cell response by mediating both stimulatory as well as inhibitory signals. In many recent studies, numerous new costimulatory molecules have been described leading to the recognition that costimulation pathways are more complex than the classical two-signal model. In general, costimulatory molecules are divided into two main families: molecules from the B7:CD28 family, such as CTLA-4 or PD-L1, and from the TNFR superfamily, such as OX40 or CD27.[165] All these costimulatory molecules have particular effects on T-cell activation, function, and survival (Table 4.1) and are implicated in nearly all inflammatory diseases. Studies to better characterize the specific role of these molecules in allergy and asthma are still ongoing. Recent investigations have uncovered the importance of a second costimulatory molecule on T cells termed CTLA-4 or CD152 that is also activated by CD80 and CD86 expressed on APCs.[165] In contrast to CD28, CTLA-4 delivers a negative signal to T cells, but because CTLA-4 is not normally expressed on the surface of T cells until 48 h after activation it is seen as a late-acting component that serves to shut off an immune response. Intriguingly, in experiments when this negative CTLA-4 signal was neutralized during an *in vivo* Th2 immune response, the level of Th2 cytokine production was greatly enhanced and the timing of production was advanced.[166] Preliminary investigations looking at T cells from atopic patients have also indicated that CTLA-4 is not expressed as highly as in healthy controls, as well as being delayed in its appearance after T-cell activation.[167] Such differences in CTLA-4 expression, between atopic and normal, may indicate an underlying genetic abnormality. These observations could indicate that T cells from atopic patients are not as sensitive to the normal inhibitory controls, which leads to prolonged immune responses with the potential for provoking disease. Even if the association between individual variation of CTLA-4 expression and atopy does not hold, it would certainly be worthwhile to explore the development of agonists of CTLA-4 activity attempt to terminate unwelcome atopic T-cell immune responses.

TABLE 4.1 The Role of Various Costimulatory Molecules in Allergic Diseases and Asthma

Costimulatory Family	APC	Effector Cell	Functions and Characteristics
B7 family	CD80 CD86	CTLA-4	Contributes to the suppressive activity of allergen-specific regulatory cells during sensitization
			Polymorphism in CTLA-4 promoter and gene favors allergic diseases
		CD28	CD80 and CD86 expression is upregulated on the surface of various cells of allergic patients
			Soluble CD86 is increased in the sera of allergic patients
	ICOS-L	ICOS	Regulates Th2-effector cell function and their infiltration in the lungs, production of Th2 cytokine
			Promotes B-cell differentiation and IgE production
			Expression on iNKT cells contributes to airway hyperreactivity
			Contributes to the differentiation of regulatory cells in pulmonary lymph nodes
	PD-L1	PD-1	Drives the differentiation of Foxp3+ CD4+ T cells
			Downregulates contact hypersensitivity reaction
	PD-L2	PD-1	Regulates asthma by an IFN-dependent mechanism
			Downregulates airway hyperreactivity, prevents eosinophil infiltration in the lungs, and prevents IgE production
	B7-H3	Unknown receptor	Promotes Th2 differentiation, eosinophil infiltration, and development of airway hyperreactivity
			Decreases the severity of allergic conjunctivitis

Costimulatory Family	APC	Effector Cell	Functions and Characteristics
TNFR family	OX40L	OX40	Promotes the development of Th2 cells
			Prevents differentiation of Treg cells
			Abrogates mast cell degranulation
	CD30L	CD30	CD30 is expressed by Langerhans cells, CD4+, and CD8+ T cells of atopic patients
			Soluble CD30 is increased in the sera of allergic patients
	4-IBB-L	4-IBB	Promotes airway hyperreactivity, eosinophil infiltration, and IgE production
			Upregulates Th2 cell proliferation and mast cell cytokine production
	Fas	FasL	Delays resolution of airway hyperresponsiveness
			Promotes eosinophil apoptosis in the lungs
	CD27	CD70	Increases production of IgE by B cells
	CD40	CD40L	Contributes to isotype class switching toward IgE
			Enhances development of airway inflammation
			Increases production of Th2 cytokine and decreases number of Treg cells
Other costimulators	CD2	CD58	Promotes differentiation of Th2 cells and the production of IgE
			Expressed on monocytes of allergic patients

The expression of CD28 ligands (CD80 and CD86) has been extensively studied in clinical samples from asthmatic patients. It is well known that B lymphocytes from asthmatic patients exposed to allergens express higher levels of surface CD86, but not CD80, compared with those from asthmatic patients not exposed to allergen or with those from healthy individuals.[168] Another study demonstrated that CD80 and, to a lesser extent, CD86 were upregulated at the surface of alveolar macrophages from allergic patients compared with those from pulmonary sarcoidosis, extrinsic allergic alveolitis patients, or from normal subjects.[169] CD86 can also be expressed in a soluble form, where the transmembrane domain is deleted. This form is mostly produced by circulating monocytes and, like membrane-bound CD86, crosslinks CD28 or CTLA-4 and activates T lymphocytes.[170] In patients with acute asthma, the level of soluble CD86 has been shown to be increased relative to that in patients with stable asthma or in healthy individuals. Monocytes from allergic patients produce more soluble CD86 compared with those of healthy individuals.[171] It was also observed that the level of soluble CD86 is correlated with the severity of the airway hyperresponsiveness (AHR). These results are consistent with studies that show that the concentrations of soluble CD80 and soluble CD86 are elevated in asthmatic patients. Interestingly, the administration of a glucocorticoid (e.g., prednisolone), used to reduce airway inflammation in allergic patients, reduces the level of circulating CD86.[172] Recently, it has been shown that the topical administration of a silencer RNA specific to the CD86 gene reduced local inflammation in a mouse model of atopic dermatitis by decreasing the recruitment of DCs into the skin, production of antigen-specific IL-4, and induction of serum IgE and IgG1.[173] It has also been reported that pulmonary tolerogenic DCs stimulated by allergen exposure express high levels of both CD80 and CD86.[174] Taken together, these studies suggest that overexpression of CD80 and/or CD86 is correlated with the development of allergic disease and asthma.

WHAT MAKES COSTIMULATORY MOLECULES A PROMISING TARGET IN ALLERGY AND ASTHMA?

From studies in murine models of allergen-mediated airway inflammation, as well as from experiences of other immune modulators in allergy and asthmatic patients, some baseline conclusions may be drawn that characterize specific costimulatory molecules as optimal targets for therapeutic intervention (Table 4.2).

T-Cell Specificity

When targeting T cells, T-cell specificity is a major criterion, as simultaneous expression of the target molecule on anything other than T cells may lead to unforeseen side effects. An example of this was experienced in early

TABLE 4.2 Criteria for Optimal Targets in Allergic Diseases Through Costimulatory Molecules

Criteria	BTLA	CD27	CD28	CD30	CVTLA-4	HVEM	ICOS	OX40	PD-1	SLAM	4-1BB
T-cell specificity	–	–	+	–	+	–	+	+	–	–	–
Nonconstitutive expression	–	–	–	+	+	–	+	+	+	+	+
Predominance for secondary immune reaction	–	–	–	+	–	–	+	+	+	–	–
Positive regulatory role	–	+	+	+	–	+	+	+	–	+	+
Th2 basis	–	–	–	+	–	ND	+	+	–	–	–

Note: BTLA: B- and T-lymphocyte attenuator; CTLA: cytotoxic T-lymphocyte-associated antigen; HVEM: herpes virus entry mediator; ICOS: inducible costimulatory antigen; OX40: CD134; PD: programmed death; SLAM: signaling lymphocyte activation molecule; Th2: type-2 T-helper cell; ND: not determined.

clinical trials blocking the CD40 ligand (CD40L) with mAbs. Blocking of CD40L in murine models was shown to attenuate IgE production,[175] although it had no effect on cellular infiltration of the airways. In patients, a mAb directed against CD40L (Ruplizumab) was first used for the treatment of systemic lupus erythematosus. However, the trials had to be discontinued because of life-threatening prothrombotic side effects due to expression of CD40L on activated platelets.[176] Therefore, T-cell restricted expression should be considered critical when identifying targets with which to modulate T-cell function. To date, this criterion is not met by the costimulatory molecules CD27, CD30, B- and T-lymphocyte attenuator (BTLA), and PD-1.

Expression on T Cells

Targeting a molecule that is expressed constitutively on T cells implies targeting all T cells unselectively. Nonselective depletion of T cells bears the risk of long-lasting lymphopenia and immune suppression, as experienced in clinical trials using anti-CD3 mAbs for immune suppression after organ transplantation.[177] Nonselective and strong stimulation of all T cells via a constitutively expressed costimulatory molecule can lead to cytokine release syndrome as seen recently with the anti-CD28 antibody TGN1412.[178] As these are unacceptable side effects in the treatment of allergic inflammation, the constitutively expressed costimulatory molecules CD27, CD28, BTLA, and herpes virus entry mediator do not qualify as optimal targets.

Predominant Involvement in Secondary Immune Reactions

In patients with bronchial asthma, allergic airway disease is an ongoing secondary immune response triggered by reexposure to specific allergens. A therapeutic intervention against asthma would preferably interfere with these secondary inflammatory reactions, while leaving primary immune reactions—critical in mounting a host defense against pathogens—unaffected. CD28, for instance, is the major costimulatory factor for the activation of naive T cells, and is therefore critical for the initiation of primary immune responses. In murine models, CD28 blockade was most effective when administered during allergen sensitization. This would render CD28 blockade an improper treatment strategy for human allergies because the time-point of sensitization is impossible to determine in the course of human allergic disease. However, blocking CD28 during secondary immune responses has shown some anti-inflammatory effects in mice. Moreover, clinical trials for the treatment of rheumatoid arthritis, employing the blockade of the CD28/B7 pathway with a CTLA-4-Ig fusion protein, have shown little apparent toxicity and good anti-inflammatory properties.[179,180] In fact, this CTLA-4-Ig fusion protein, abatacept, is the first approved anti-costimulatory drug on the market.[181] Two costimulatory molecules predominantly involved in secondary immune reactions are ICOS and OX40. In contrast to CD28, ICOS expression is limited to currently activated T cells.[182,183] In murine studies, ICOS-blocking reagents were most effective during secondary immune responses. Targeting OX40 in animal models of allergic airway disease was revealed to be effective during sensitization, as well as during rechallenge with allergen.

Positive Regulatory Signal

One major concern, besides compromising primary physiological immune reactions, is that negative signals delivered by costimulatory molecules would also be compromised by this approach. Blocking negative signals bears the risk of autoreactive immune responses and increased development of autoimmune diseases as a consequence of a disrupted negative feedback mechanism of immune balance. Therefore, this may disqualify negative costimulatory factors, such as BTLA and CTLA-4, as optimal treatment targets.

Th2 T-Cell Bias

The allergic airway inflammation is a Th2-dominated process, although recently, evidence for the involvement of Th1 cytokines, especially in established airway disease, has arisen. The predominant involvement of Th2-cytokines in airway inflammation makes these molecules a preferable target in the therapy of allergic reaction. This criterion is only met by the costimulatory molecules CD30, ICOS, and OX40. CD30, however, does not meet the criteria of T-cell specificity. ICOS is expressed on Th1 as well as on Th2 T cells, but only Th2-mediated airway inflammation is affected by ICOS-blockade. However, during an established inflammatory response like allergic asthma, this situation might be more complex than it appears in murine models of acute airway inflammation. ICOS is also expressed on Treg cells and may be important for the production of the immune suppressive cytokine, IL-10.[184] Even though a further study using a murine colitis model demonstrated that ICOS blockade had minimal effect on Treg function,[185] it remains to be determined how the immune balance is affected by long-term blockade of ICOS. A complete lack of ICOS expression in humans is associated with a loss of B-cell memory,[186] a side effect that may be desirable concerning local memory for IgE, but is definitely intolerable for any other systemic immune response. Therefore, the route of application and the place of deposition are important factors that need to be considered when targeting costimulatory molecules.

TARGETING COSTIMULATORY MOLECULES FOR TREATMENT OF ALLERGEN-INDUCED AIRWAY INFLAMMATION

Keeping in view the role played by costimulatory molecules in the regulation of immune response to allergens, costimulatory molecules have become targets for developing drugs that will modulate an allergic immune response. The chimeric CTLA-4-Ig molecule, which consists of the extracellular domain of CTLA-4 and the hinge, CH2, and CH3 regions of IgG, blocks the costimulatory signal that T cells receive through the interaction of CD28 with the counter-receptors CD80 or CD86 expressed on the APC membrane. CTLA-4-Ig is able to downregulate or suppress the mucosal immune response in allergic rhinitis. CTLA-4-Ig inhibits airway eosinophilia and hyperresponsiveness by enhancing Th1-like cell activity. IgE formation is enhanced by the Th2 cytokine IL-4. Therefore, it is expected that down-regulating Th2 activity will decrease IgE formation, as has been demonstrated in CTLA-4-Ig-treated mice. The combination of antibodies to CD80/CD86 with the ligand for CTLA-4, blocks the development of allergic airway inflammation, whereas only a partial reduction occurs using either of these antibodies alone. However, only the anti-CD86 antibody inhibits the production of IgE. Therefore, the CD28–CD80/CD86 complex is a potential target for developing new strategies of allergy treatment.

Even though not fully applicable to human disease, animal models provide valuable insight into the processes involved and are the basis for further research in humans. Due to the lack of human studies on costimulatory molecules in allergic airway disease, the present discussion is based on current knowledge as gained from animal models. In general, it is obvious from the experimental data that early blocking of allergic sensitization effectively inhibits the development of specific IgE, cytokine production by type-2 T-helper cells (Th2; mostly determined in BAL fluids), airway hyperresponsiveness (AHR), and inflammation (Table 4.3). The role of costimulatory molecules in allergen-induced airway inflammation may be classified according to the time of intervention as (1) primary intervention that targets the induction phase of the allergic sensitization; (2) secondary prevention, which targets the induction of airway inflammation in already sensitized animals; or (3) treatment of animals after sensitization and airway allergen challenges. The most intensively studied molecules in this context are CD28, ICOS, and CD134 (OX40), and because only preliminary data is available regarding other costimulatory pathways, these molecules are discussed in detail. See Table 4.3, which provides an overview of the available data regarding the role of costimulatory molecules in allergen-induced airway disease.

Targeting B7-CD28 Costimulatory Pathway

The role of CD28 in models of allergic airway inflammation has been extensively studied in allergen-induced airway inflammation murine models (Table 4.3). Although the primary goal of these studies was to analyze the impact of costimulatory molecules on different aspects of the inflammatory process, for example, eosinophilic airway inflammation, Th2 cytokine production, and AHR and systemic IgE synthesis, these data can also be used to

TABLE 4.3 Experimental Evidence from Blocking of Costimulatory Signaling in Allergen-Induced Airway Disease in Murine Models

Approach	Target	Outcome			
		Eosinophilia in BAL	Pulmonary Infiltration	AHR	IgE
Prevention of sensitization	CD80/CD86	↓	ND	↓	↓
	CD80/CD86	ND	↓	↓	ND
	CTLA-4	↑	ND	↑	↑
	ICOSL	ND	↓	ND	ND
	ICOS	ND	↓	ND	↑
	ICOS	(↓)	↔	↔	(↓)
	OX40L	↓	↓	↓	↓
	CD30L	ND	↓	↓	↓
	CD30	ND	↓	↓	↓
Prevention of airway inflammation	CD80/CD86	↓	↓	ND	↓
	CD80/CD86	↓	ND	↓	↓
	CD80/CD86	↓	ND	↓	↓
	CD80/CD86	↓	ND	↓	↓
	CD80/CD86	↓	ND	↓	
	CD80/CD86	↔	ND	↔	↔
	CD80/CD86	↓	↓	ND	↔
	CTLA-4	(↓)	ND	↔	↓
	ICOS-L	↓	↓	↓	ND
	ICOS-L	↓	↓	ND	ND
	ICOS	↓	↓	↓	↓
	OX40L	↔	↔	↔	ND
	OX40L	↓	↓	↓	↓
Treatment of established airway inflammation	CD80/CD86	↓	ND	ND	↓
	ICOS-L	ND	↔	ND	↔
	CD30	ND	↔	↔	↔
	CD30-L	ND	↔	↔	↔

Note: BAL: bronchoalveolar lavage; AHR: airway hyperresponsiveness; Ig: immunoglobulin; ND: not determined; CTLA: cytotoxic T-lymphoctye-associated antigen; ICOS: inducible costimulator antigen; ICOS-L; ICOS ligand; OX40: CD134; OX40L: OX40 ligand; ↓: decreased; ↑: increased; (↓): weak increase; ↔: unchanged.

assess the suitability of CD28 as a therapeutic target in the treatment of allergic airway inflammation. Systemic administration of the fusion protein cytotoxic T-lymphocyte-associated antigen-4 (CTLA-4)-Ig inhibits the ligation of CD28 with its ligands, CD80 and CD86. When given during the course of allergen sensitization, a drastic effect on airway inflammation and AHR was observed; however, the production of the Th1 cytokine interferon (IFN-c) was unaltered.[187] Some of these effects may be explained by the complete inhibition of the germinal center reaction after blockade of the CD28/CD86 signal during the primary immune response.[188] When CTLA-4-IgG was applied after the initial T-cell sensitization, that is, during the phase of allergen rechallenge, this treatment also led to a marked reduction in the inflammatory response.[189] Only one report has shown contrasting results with no effect on AHR and cellular infiltration following the administration of CTLA-4-Ig at the time of allergen challenge.[190] Thus, interruption of the CD28 costimulatory signal also inhibits secondary immune responses, in at least some protocols of murine allergen-induced airway inflammation, but has the strongest impact on primary immune responses upon the first exposure to allergen.

In other studies, mAbs against the two ligands of CD28, CD80, and CD86 were administered independently to delineate the role of these molecules. Overall analysis of these studies reveals that CD86 appears to be the major ligand responsible for CD28-dependent immune responses observed during allergen-induced airway inflammation (Table 4.3). This is also implied by the observation that a combination of antibodies against both ligands was not superior to anti-CD86 treatment alone in two out of three studies. The question of a differentiated role of the two CD28 ligands was further addressed by the use of a fusion protein, Y100F. This molecule blocks CD28–CD80 interactions, leaving CD28 signaling via CD86 intact. Similar to CTLA-4-Ig, application of Y100F reduced eosinophilic infiltration into the lungs, mainly due to decreased IL-5 productions by allergen-specific T cells. In contrast to blocking all CD28 signals, Y100F had no effect on the number of eosinophils in peripheral blood or on systemic IgE production, indicating a major role of CD86 signals in local immune responses. In somewhat different experimental settings, ligation of CD28 by the CD28 ligand CD80 has been shown to have either no, an increasing, or a decreasing effect on allergen-induced airway responses.[160,191–193] Thus, the precise role of this CD28 ligand in the T-cell differentiation remains an unanswered question.

CTLA-4 has been described to be an important regulator of T-cell activation and is constitutively and exclusively expressed by T lymphocytes in both mice and humans. Contribution of CTLA-4 in the regulation of the immune system is demonstrated by the development of multiple organ autoimmune pathologies and lympho-proliferative disease in CTLA-4-deficient mice.[194,195] Blockade of CTLA-4 activity abolishes the suppressive function of CD4+ CD25+ T cells.[196] In inflammatory bowel disease, the effect of transfer of a population of CD4+ CD45RB low Treg cells in decreasing intestinal inflammation is abrogated by the coadministration of a blocking anti-CTLA-4 antibody.[197] This suggests that the engagement of CTLA-4 at the surface of Treg cells by its ligands CD80 or CD86 contributes to the regulation of suppressive functions of Treg cells. Polymorphism in CTLA-4 gene is also considered a risk factor for allergy and asthma. Four single nucleotide polymorphisms have been related to allergic and asthma phenotypes.[198] They demonstrated that these specific polymorphisms alone or in combinations are correlated with an elevated IgE titer or bronchial hyperresponsiveness in patients with asthma. Interestingly, in the same study, no correlation between allergic phenotype and single nucleotide polymorphisms for CD28 was observed. The polymorphism at the level of the promoter was correlated to asthma severity while the +49 C/G polymorphism is associated with airway hyperresponsiveness.[199,200] Interestingly, CTLA-4 seems to play a more important role in the sensitization phase than in established allergy. In a model of mice sensitized with grass pollen, the administration of a blocking anti-CTLA-4 or a blocking anti-CD154 (anti-CD40L) antibody during the sensitization phase prevents the production of allergen-specific antibody. These findings confirm that CTLA-4 is indeed involved in the course of allergic diseases.

Targeting PD-1, PD-L1/PD-L2 Costimulatory Pathway

The other B7:CD28 family of receptors includes the PD-1 receptor and its ligands PD-L1 (B7-H1) and PD-L2 (B7-DC). The PD-1 receptor was initially discovered in T cells undergoing cell death. The inhibitory signal provided by engagement of PD-1 was demonstrated by the development of autoimmune diseases in PD-1-deficient mice.[201] Since then several groups have reported that engagement of PD-1 by PD-L1 or PD-L2 results in inhibition of proliferation and polarized or altered cytokine production.[202,203] In asthma it has been demonstrated that PD-L2 is highly expressed on pulmonary DCs and macrophages of sensitized mice. Moreover, administration of blocking antibody against PD-L2, but not PD-1 or PD-L1, during challenge enhances the airway hyperresponsiveness and production of Th2 cytokines. This effect is mediated by IFN-γ, given that no improvement is observed in IFN-γ-deficient mice following treatment with anti-PD-L2.[204,205] The administration of the sHIgM12 antibody (an antibody inducing reverse signaling through PD-L2) in a mouse model of allergic asthma blocks the development of AHR.[206] An additional study demonstrates that administration of PD-L2-Fc in a mouse model of allergic asthma resulted in elevated levels of serum IgE and increased eosinophilic and lymphocytic infiltration into the BAL fluid.[207] These studies emphasize the pivotal role of PD-L2 in the development of allergic asthma. In addition, in a model of experimental allergic conjunctivitis, treatment with anti-PD-L2 blocking antibody during the effector phase enhanced infiltration of eosinophils into the conjunctiva without change in the systemic response.[208] Finally, using PD-L2-deficient mice, it was reported that this molecule is dispensable for Th2 differentiation and required for the induction of mucosal tolerance.[209] Taken together, these reports strongly suggest that PD-L2 is involved in the downregulation of Th2-allergic immune response.

Only preliminary data exist on manipulation of the negative regulatory molecule PD-1: an analysis of the distinctive contribution of its two ligands, PD-L1 and PD-L2, in the development of allergen-induced murine airway inflammation showed that a substantial number of pulmonary DCs, macrophages, and B cells isolated from the lungs of naive mice expressed PD-L1, which was further enhanced after allergen sensitization and airway challenge.[205] In contrast, PD-L2 expression was detectable at very low levels in lymphocytes of unchallenged mice and was only moderately enhanced in DCs and macrophages after allergen challenge of sensitized mice. Although PD-L1 was abundantly expressed on various APCs in the inflamed lung tissues, treatment with a blocking antibody did not alter the allergic airway response, whereas treatment with anti-PD-L2 mAb (TY25) during allergen challenge significantly increased the development of AHR, and lung eosinophilia increased levels of IL-5 and IL-13 in BAL fluid.[207] When PD-L2 was only blocked during sensitization, no effect on the inflammatory response was demonstrated, indicating that the inhibitory function of PD-L2 was limited to the effector phase (airway challenge) of the airway response.

Anti-PD-L1 blocking antibody enhanced contact hypersensitivity reaction, possibly by increasing the proliferative response of T cells in response to hapten-pulsed APCs. This suggests a unique role of PD-L1 in the regulation of inflammatory responses.[210] During allergen-SIT, the expression of PD-L1 on both monocytes and B lymphocytes is increased relative to that in the untreated control group. So PD-L1 could be used as a marker to monitor the effect of allergen-SIT and could also be targeted to enhance immunosuppression.[211] Upon stimulation by a TLR-4 ligand, PD-L1-positive tolerogenic Langerhans cells in the sublingual mucosa in humans release a higher level of IL-10 compared with untreated control cells. These Langerhans cells have decreased capacity to stimulate T cells and are able to support the differentiation of Treg cells expressing Foxp3, producing IL-10 and TGF-β.[212,213] These sublingual tolerogenic Langerhans cells stimulated via their TLR-4 expressed higher levels of the coinhibitory molecules PD-L1 and B7-H3, while CD86 expression is lowered. Consequently, the expression of these molecules by APCs seems to be linked with tolerogenic properties. These studies represent a body of evidence that suggests that PD-L1 is involved in the maintenance of the peripheral tolerance and may contribute to the induction of allergy. Clearly, further work is required to understand the role of PD-1 and its ligands in allergic diseases and asthma.

Targeting ICOS

In contrast to blocking CD28, blockade of ICOS by the application of ICOS-Ig or anti-ICOS mAbs at the time of allergen sensitization, showed only little effect on the development of airway inflammation (Table 4.3). However, blockade of ICOS in sensitized mice significantly reduced signs of allergic airway inflammation, such as increased IgE and Th2 cytokine production.[190] Using a model of adoptive transfer, it was further demonstrated that blockade of ICOS distinctively inhibited Th2-mediated lung eosinophilia and AHR, but did not abrogate Th1-mediated neutrophilic airway inflammation.[214] Similarly, the Th2-associated airway inflammatory response to *Schistosoma mansoni* eggs was attenuated by ICOS blockade, whereas the priming of T cells toward the Th2 cell direction was abolished by this approach.[215] The differential role of ICOS in Th1- versus Th2-biased immune reactions was further analyzed in a model of allergen-induced primary immune reactions induced by the local application of Th1 and Th2 cytokines. In this model, blockade of ICOS inhibited the early inflammatory cell influx and IL-5 production in the lungs in the Th2, but not in the Th1, model.[216] Taken together these results render ICOS a promising target to interfere with secondary immune responses, and suggest a predominant involvement of ICOS in Th2-type responses.

Targeting OX40

Utilizing OX40 knock-out mice, it was demonstrated that OX40 plays an important role in effector cell expansion and the formation and reactivation of memory T cells. Blocking the OX40 signal with mAb against OX40L in a model of *Leishmania major* infection resulted in decreased synthesis of Th2 cytokines (IL-4, IL-10 and IL-13) as well as reduced production of IgE.[217] In mouse models of allergen-induced airway inflammation there are somewhat controversial results regarding the time-point of OX40 action. Blockade of OX40L abolished the development of airway inflammation only when the anti-OX40L mAb was applied during allergen sensitization but not when given to already sensitized mice prior to allergen airway challenge.[218] In contrast, another study demonstrated that OX40L blockade of sensitized mice during allergen airway challenges abolished inflammatory responses, also at very late time-points of the experimental protocol.[219]

Targeting BTLA-4

Very limited information is available on the effects of blocking other costimulatory molecules in murine models of allergen-induced airway disease. To date, no studies investigating the blockade of BTLA or B7-H3 have been published. Recently, it was shown that a single injection of mAb against the costimulatory factor CD137 (4-1BB) prevented the development of AHR, eosinophilic airway inflammation, and elevated IgE production. This treatment was also able to reverse previously established airway disease. The inhibitory effect was most likely due to reduced Th2 cytokine production and increased secretion of IFN-c by CD8+ T cells. Recently, blockade of CD30 and its ligand CD153 with mAbs was shown to significantly reduce airway inflammation, AHR, and the production of allergen-specific IgE when the blocking antibody was administered before and after sensitization.[220,221] However, neither blocking reagent had any effect when administered during established allergic airway disease.

TOOLS FOR MODULATION OF COSTIMULATORY SIGNALS

Not only is the identification of the optimal target molecule a prerequisite for effective treatment by interfering with costimulatory molecules, but also careful considerations need to be made about the tools, administration, and the immunological aim of successful intervention into an ongoing inflammatory process.

Blocking costimulatory signals can either be achieved using mAbs or fusion proteins containing the counter-receptor. Half-life and tissue distribution of the blocking reagent within the human body are critical variables that will determine the duration of the blocking effect and the frequency required for application. The first insights in the human system have been gained by the use of anti-CD3 mAbs in organ transplantation and the CTLA-4 fusion protein for rheumatoid arthritis. Data from these and other studies show that using humanized mAbs is, in general, safe and does not bear the risk of anaphylactic side effects. Due to the complexity of the allergic immune-response and the asthmatic airway-response it is highly likely that targeting a single molecule may not be sufficient to gain complete control of allergen-mediated inflammation. For murine models of allograft rejection, it was shown that dual blockade with mAbs was more effective than blockade of a single molecule.[222] In this respect, a feasible approach may be to target not only one, but two (e.g., ICOS and OX40), or even more costimulatory molecules to treat asthma (Figure 4.2). However, such studies are still outstanding for allergic disease models. The consequences of using agonistic mAbs may be far more difficult to predict than those with blocking reagents. While dosing antagonists is stoichiometric, the action of agonists is a function of the strength of the agonist, the cascade it induces and the consequences of that cascade.[223] In-depth knowledge of receptor distribution and action, as well as intensive animal testing, are critical, as demonstrated by the TeGenero fiasco with an agonistic anti-CD28 antibody.

Administration of Immune Modulators

Besides systemic administration of an immune modulator, local deposition of a blocking reagent in the lungs should be considered a feasible route of application. During allergic airway inflammation, the number of T cells producing Th2 cytokines is increased in the pulmonary compartment.[224] Therefore, it seems reasonable to directly target this process in the lung to avoid systemic side effects. Indeed, in mouse models of allergen-induced airway disease, local application of mAbs or fusion proteins into the airways was shown to control allergic airway inflammation, as demonstrated for the IL-13 receptor, a fusion protein, and anti-IL5 mAbs.[225,226] In humans, one study showed that administration of an inhaled monoclonal anti-IgE antibody (E25) was generally well tolerated and led to detectable levels of the antibody in both BAL and serum.[227] However, the aerosolized antibody did not attenuate the airway response to inhaled allergen as it did when applied intravenously. The authors speculated that the aerosol route of application did not lead to sufficient concentrations of the antibody in the critical tissue compartments surrounding IgE effector cells. Furthermore, one subject developed IgG and IgA antibodies against E25, suggesting that lung deposition of the antibody may be more immunogenic than the parental route. Therefore, local deposition, tissue penetration, serum levels and half-life, as well as immunogenicity, are critical variables that need to be considered when evaluating this route of application.

Blockade Versus Elimination of Allergen-Specific T Cells

An interesting alternative to continuous application of a blocking agent would be the permanent elimination of allergen-specific T cells from the immune system.[228] This would require a target that is T-cell specific and not expressed on naıve or quiescent memory T cells, but rather is expressed on recently activated T-effector or reactivated memory cells. From the group of costimulatory molecules, ICOS and OX40 meet these criteria. Elimination of all ICOS- and OX40-positive T cells during an ongoing allergic reaction may remove the allergen-specific T-effector and reactivated memory T cells, subsequently leading to downregulation of humoral responses and inflammatory cell infiltration, which both depend on T-cell help. The aspired benefits of such an approach would be a long-lasting therapeutic effect achieved by only a short-term treatment. Furthermore, this sort of treatment would be available and effective for allergic sensitization against all possible allergens, in contrast to SIT. However, the feasibility of this approach remains to be tested in appropriate animal models.

The underlying immune mechanisms of allergic airway disease have been untangled via the use of mouse models and clinical studies. The time has now come to widen the repertoire of therapeutic tools and to initiate immunological and pathogenesis-related approaches to treatment. One of the most promising new strategies is based on the blockade of costimulation, a critical and early event in the induction and maintenance of allergen-induced airway diseases such as bronchial asthma. So developing costimulatory molecules for the intervention in allergic and asthmatic diseases holds the promise for treatment in the future.

REFERENCES

1. Strachan DP. Hay fever, hygiene, and household size. *BMJ* 1989;**299**:1259–60.
2. Yazdanbakhsh M, Kremsner PG, van Ree R. Allergy, parasites, and the hygiene hypothesis. *Science* 2002;**296**:490–4.
3. Romagnani S. The role of lymphocytes in allergic disease. *J Allergy Clin Immunol* 2000;**105**:399–408.
4. Romagnani S. Coming back to a missing immune deviation as the main explanatory mechanism for the hygiene hypothesis. *J Allergy Clin Immunol* 2007;**119**:1511–13.
5. Umetsu DT, DeKruyff RH. TH1 and TH2 CD4+ cells in human allergic diseases. *J Allergy Clin Immunol* 1997;**100**:1–6.
6. Gell PGH, Coombs RRA. The classification of allergic reactions underlying disease. In: Coombs RRA, Gell PGH, editors. *Clinical aspects of immunology* 1963.
7. Averbeck M, Gebhardt C, Emmrich F, Treudler R, Simon JC. Immunologic principles of allergic disease. *J Dtsch Dermatol Ges* 2007;**5**(11):1015–28.
8. Gilfillan AM, Tkaczyk C. Integrated signalling pathways for mast-cell activation. *Nat Rev Immunol* 2006;**6**(3):218–30.
9. Verstraelen S, Bloemen K, Nelissen I, Witters H, Schoeters G, Van Den Heuvel R. Cell types involved in allergic asthma and their use in in vitro models to assess respiratory sensitization. *Toxicol In Vitro* 2008;**22**(6):1419–31.
10. Male D. Hypersensitivity (type II). In: Male D, Brostoff J, Roth DB, Roitt I, editors. *Immunology*. 7th ed. Philadelphia, PA: Elsevier; 2006. . p. 449–60.
11. Hay F, Westwood OMR. Hypersensitivity (type III). In: Male D, Brostoff J, Roth DB, Roitt I, editors. *Immunology*. 7th ed. Philadelphia, PA: Elsevier; 2006. . p. 461–76.
12. Britton W. Type IV hypersensitivity. In: Male D, Brostoff J, Roth DB, Roitt I, editors. *Immunology*. 7th ed. Philadelphia, PA: Elsevier; 2006. . p. 477–91.
13. Holgate ST. Pathogenesis of asthma. *Clin Exp Allergy* 2008;**38**(6):872–97.
14. Global Initiative for Asthma. Global strategy for asthma management and prevention; 2008.
15. Masoli M, Fabian D, Holt S, Beasley R. Global burden of asthma. Developed for the Global Initiative for Asthma, Medical Research Institute of New Zealand, Wellington, New Zealand, and University of Southampton, Southampton, United Kingdom; 2004.
16. Wenzel SE. Asthma: defining of the persistent adult phenotypes. *Lancet* 2006;**368**(9537): 804–13.
17. Kiley J, Smith R, Noel P. Asthma phenotypes. *Curr Opin Pulm Med* 2007;**13**(1):19–23.
18. Kay AB. The role of eosinophils in the pathogenesis of asthma. *Trends Mol Med* 2005;**11**(4): 148–52.
19. Constant SL, Brogdon JL, Piggott DA, Herrick CA, Visintin I, Ruddle NH, et al. Resident lung antigen presenting cells have the capacity to promote Th2 T cell differentiation in situ. *J Clin Invest* 2002;**110**(10):1441–8.
20. Julia V, Hessel EM, Malherbe L, Glaichenhaus N, O'Garra A, Coffman RL. A restricted subset of dendritic cells captures airborne antigens and remains able to activate specific T cells long after antigen exposure. *Immunity* 2002;**16**(2):271–83.
21. Riese RJ, Chapman HA. Cathepsins and compartmentalization in antigen presentation. *Curr Opin Immunol* 2000;**12**(1):107–13.
22. Platts-Mills TAE. Immediate hypersensitivity (Type I). In: Male D, Brostoff J, Roth DB, Roitt I, editors. *Immunology*. 7th ed. Philadelphia, PA: Elsevier; 2006. p. 423–47.
23. Ogawa Y, Calhoun WJ. The role of leukotrienes in airway inflammation. *J Allergy Clin Immunol* 2006;**118**(4):789–98. quiz 799–800.

24. Bradding P, Holgate ST. Immunopathology and human mast cell cytokines. *Crit Rev Oncol Hematol* 1999;**31**(2):119–33.
25. Frigas E, Motojima S, Gleich GJ. The eosinophilic injury to the mucosa of the airways in the pathogenesis of bronchial asthma. *Eur Respir J Suppl* 1991;**13**:123s–135ss.
26. Jacobsen EA, Taranova AG, Lee NA, Lee JJ. Eosinophils: singularly destructive effector cells or purveyors of immunoregulation? *J Allergy Clin Immunol* 2007;**119**(6): 1313–20.
27. Kaur D, Saunders R, Berger P, Siddiqui S, Woodman L, Wardlaw A, et al. Airway smooth muscle and mast cell-derived CC chemokine ligand 19 mediate airway smooth muscle migration in asthma. *Am J Respir Crit Care Med* 2006;**174**(11):1179–88.
28. Bradding P, Walls AF, Holgate ST. The role of the mast cell in the pathophysiology of asthma. *J Allergy Clin Immunol* 2006;**117**(6):1277–84.
29. Lipscomb MF, Masten BJ. Dendritic cells: immune regulators in health and disease. *Physiol Rev* 2002;**82**(1):97–130.
30. Wills-Karp M, Luyimbazi J, Xu X, Schofield B, Neben TY, Karp CL, et al. Interleukin-13: central mediator of allergic asthma. *Science* 1998;**282**(5397):2258–61.
31. Nissim Ben Efraim AH, Levi-Schaffer F. Tissue remodeling and angiogenesis in asthma: the role of the eosinophil. *Ther Adv Respir Dis* 2008;**2**(3):163–71.
32. Humbles AA, Lloyd CM, McMillan SJ, Friend DS, Xanthou G, McKenna EE, et al. A critical role for eosinophils in allergic airways remodeling. *Science* 2004;**305**(5691):1776–9.
33. Munitz A, Bachelet I, Levi-Schaffer F. Reversal of airway inflammation and remodeling in asthma by a bispecific antibody fragment linking CCR3 to CD300a. *J Allergy Clin Immunol* 2006;**118**(5):1082–9.
34. Carlsen KH, Kowalski ML. Asthma, allergy, the athlete and the Olympics. *Allergy* 2008;**63**(4): 383–6.
35. Szczeklik A, Sanak M. The broken balance in aspirin hypersensitivity. *Eur J Pharmacol* 2006;**533**(1–3):145–55.
36. Anderson SD. Is there a unifying hypothesis for exercise-induced asthma? *J Allergy Clin Immunol* 1984;**73**(5 Pt 2):660–5.
37. Bissonnette E. Alveolar macrophages in the pathogenesis of asthma. *Recent Res Devol Allergy Clin Immunol* 2000;**1**:129–41.
38. Peters-Golden M. The alveolar macrophage: the forgotten cell in asthma. *Am J Respir Cell Mol Biol* 2004;**31**(1):3–7.
39. Marsh DG. *Genetics of asthma and other atopic diseases. Post-graduate education course.* New Orleans, LA: American Academy of Allergy and Immunology; 1996. pp. 1–5.
40. Healy JI, Goodnow CC. Positive versus negative signaling by lymphocyte antigen receptors. *Annu Rev Immunol* 1998;**16**:645–70.
41. Wills-Karp M. Immunologic basis of antigen-induced airway hyperresponsiveness. *Annu Rev Immunol* 1999;**17**:255–81.
42. Tsitoura DC, Verhoef A, Gelder CM, O'Hehir RE, Lamb JR. Altered T cell ligands derived from a major house dust mite allergen enhance IFN-alpha production but not IL-4 production by human CD4 T cells. *J Immunol* 1996;**157**:2160–5.
43. Constant SL, Bottomly K. Induction of TH 1 and TH 2 CD4+ T cell responses: the alternative approaches. *Annu Rev Immunol* 1997;**15**:297–322.
44. Romagnani S. Lymphokine production by human T cells in disease states. *Annu Rev Immunol* 1994;**12**:227–57.
45. Bochner BS, Undem BJ, Lichtenstein LM. Immunological aspects of allergic asthma. *Annu Rev Immunol* 1994;**12**:295–335.

46. Pereira C, Botelho F, Tavares B, Lourenço C, Baeta C, Palma-Carlos AG, et al. Kinetics and dynamic evaluation of specific immunotherapy. *Eur Ann Allergy Clin Immunol* 2004;**36**: 375–86.
47. Redegeld FA, van der Heijden MW, Kool M, Heijdra BM, Garssen J, Kraneveld AD, et al. Immunoglobulin-free light chains elicit immediate hypersensitivity-like responses. *Nat Med* 2002;**8**:694–701.
48. McCurdy JD, Olynych TJ, Maher LH, Marshall JS. Cutting edge: distinct Tolllike receptor 2 activators selectively induce different classes of mediator production from human mast cells. *J Immunol* 2003;**170**:1625–9.
49. Metz M, Grimbaldeston MA, Nakae S, Piliponsky AM, Tsai M, Galli SJ. Mast cells in the promotion and limitation of chronic inflammation. *Immunol Rev* 2007;**217**:304–28.
50. Mortaz E, Redegeld FA, Nijkamp FP, Wong HR, Engels F. Acetylsalicylic acid-induced release of HSP70 from mast cells results in cell activation through TLR pathway. *Exp Hematol* 2006;**34**:8–18.
51. Van der Heijden MW, Van der Kleij HPM, Roecken M, Redegeld FA. Mast cells. In: Bos JD, editor. *The skin immune system*. 3rd ed. Boca Raton, FL: CRC Press; 2005. pp. 237–61.
52. Theoharides TC, Kempuraj D, Tagen M, Conti P, Kalogeromitros D. Differential release of mast cell mediators and the pathogenesis of inflammation. *Immunol Rev* 2007;**217**:65–78.
53. Brown JM, Wilson TM, Metcalfe DD. The mast cell and allergic diseases: role in pathogenesis and implications for therapy. *Clin Exp Allergy* 2008;**38**:4–18.
54. Yu M, Tsai M, Tam SY, Jones C, Zehnder J, Galli SJ. Mast cells can promote the development of multiple features of chronic asthma in mice. *J Clin Invest* 2006;**116**:1633–41.
55. Brightling CE, Bradding P, Symon FA, Holgate ST, Wardlaw AJ, Pavord ID. Mast cell infiltration of airway smooth muscle in asthma. *N Engl J Med* 2002;**346**:1699–705.
56. Bousquet J, Lockey R, Malling HJ. Allergen immunotherapy: therapeutic vaccines for allergic diseases. A WHO position paper. *J Allergy Clin Immunol* 1998;**102**:558–62.
57. Crameri R. Allergy diagnosis, allergen repertoires, and their implications for allergen-specific immunotherapy. *Immunol Allergy Clin North Am* 2006;**26**:179–89.
58. Cox L, Cohn JR. Duration of allergen immunotherapy in respiratory allergy: when is enough, enough? *Ann Allergy Asthma Immunol* 2007;**98**:416–26.
59. Nelson H. Does allergen immunotherapy have a role in the treatment of bronchial asthma? *Allergy Asthma Proc* 1997;**18**:157–62.
60. Des Roches A, Paradis L, Menardo J-L, Bouges S, Daures JP, Bousquet J. Immunotherapy with a standardized *D. pteronyssinus* extract: specific therapy prevents the onset of new sensitizations in children. *J Allergy Clin Immunol* 1997;**99**:450–3.
61. Senti G, Prinz Vavricka BM, Erdmann I, Diaz MI, Markus R, McCormack SJ, et al. Intralymphatic allergen administration renders specific immunotherapy faster and safer: a randomized controlled trial. *Proc Natl Acad Sci USA* 2008;**105**:17908–12.
62. Canonica GW, Bousquet J, Casale T, Lockey RF, Baena-Cagnani CE, Pawankar R, et al. Sub-lingual immunotherapy: World Allergy Organization position paper 2009. *Allergy* 2009;**64**(Suppl. 91):1–59.
63. Borish LC, Nelson H, Lanz M, Claussen L, Whitmore JB, Agosti JM, et al. Interleukin-4 receptor in moderate atopic asthma: a phase I/II randomized, placebo-controlled trial. *Am J Respir Crit Care Med* 1999;**160**:1816–23.
64. Bagnasco M, Altrinetti V, Pesce G, Caputo M, Mistrello G, Falagiani P, et al. Pharmacokinetics of Der p 2 allergen and derived monomeric allergoid in allergic volunteers. *Int Arch Allergy Immunol* 2005;**138**:197–202.

65. Einarsson R, Renck B, Taudorf E. In vitro studies of degradation of birch and timothy pollen allergen preparations by human duodenal juice. *Allergy* 1988;**43**:469–72.
66. Frati F, La Grutta S, Bernardini R, Zampogna S, Scurati S, Puccinelli P, et al. Sublingual immunotherapy: administration, dosages, use. *Int J Immunopathol Pharmacol* 2009;**22**: 13–16.
67. Lombardi C, Incorvaia C, Braga M, Senna G, Canonica GW, Passalacqua G. Administration regimens for sublingual immunotherapy to pollen allergens: what do we know? *Allergy* 2009;**64**:849–54.
68. Compalati E, Passalacqua G, Bonini M, Canonica GW. The efficacy of sublingual immunotherapy for house dust mites respiratory allergy: results of a GA2LEN meta-analysis. *Allergy* 2009;**64**:1570–9.
69. Mohapatra SS. An integrated approach to immune deviation and prevention of allergies and asthma. *Allergy Clin Immunol Int* 1996;**8**:164.
70. Barres MP, Einarsson R, Bjorksren B. Serum levels of interleukin-4, soluble CD23, and IFNgamma in relation to the development of allergic disease during the first 18 months of life. *Clin Exp Allergy* 1995;**25**:543–8.
71. Holt PG. A potential vaccine strategy for asthma and allied atopic diseases during early childhood. *Lancet* 1994;**344**:456–8.
72. Wheeler AW, Whittall N, Cook RM, Spackman VM, Moran DM. T cell reactivity of conjugates of *N*-formyl-methionyl-leucyl-phenylalanine and rye grass pollen allergens. *Int Arch Allergy Appl Immunol* 1987;**84**:69–73.
73. Vrtala S, Grote M, Ferreira F, Susani M, Stocker B, Kraft D, et al. Humoral immune responses to recombinant tree pollen allergens (Bet v 1 and Bet v 2) in mice: construction of a live oral allergy vaccine. *Int Arch Allergy Appl Immunol* 1995;**107**:290–4.
74. Kumar M, Behera AK, Matsuse H, Lockey RF, Mohapatra SS. A recombinant BCG vaccine generates a Th1-like response and inhibits IgE synthesis in BALB/c mice. *Immunology* 1999;**97**:515–21.
75. Rolland J, O'Hehir R. Immunotherapy of allergy: anergy, deletion, and immune deviation. *Curr Opin Immunol* 1998;**10**:640–5.
76. Sloan-Lancaster J, Allen PM. Altered peptide ligand-induced partial T cell activation: molecular mechanisms and role in T cell biology. *Annu Rev Immunol* 1996;**14**:1–27.
77. Rogers BL, Bond JF, Craig SJ, Nault AK, Segal DB, Morgenstern JP, et al. Potential therapeutic recombinant proteins comprised of peptides containing recombined T cell epitopes. *Mol Immunol* 1994;**31**:955–66.
78. Sparholt SH, Larsen JN, Ipsen H, Schou C, van Neerven RJ. Crossreactivity and T-cell epitope specificity of Bet v 1-specific T cells suggest the involvement of multiple isoallergens in sensitization to birch pollen. *Clin Exp Allergy* 1997;**27**:932–41.
79. Briner TJ, Kuo MC, Keating KM, Rogers BL, Greenstein JL. Peripheral T cell tolerance induced in naive and primed mice by subcutaneous injection of peptides from the major cat allergen Fel d1. *Proc Natl Acad Sci USA* 1993;**90**:7608–12.
80. Hoyne GF, O'Hehir RE, Wraith DC, Thomas WR, Lamb JR. Inhibition of T cell and antibody responses to house dust mite allergens by inhalation of the dominant T cell epitopes in naive and sensitized mice. *J Exp Med* 1993;**178**:1783–8.
81. Maguire P, Nicodemus C, Robinson D, Aaronson D, Umetsu DT. The safety and efficacy of ALLERVAX-CAT in cat allergic patients. *Clin Immunol* 1999;**93**:222–31.
82. Jahn-Schmid B, Wiedermann U, Bohle B, Repa A, Kraft D, Ebner C. Oligodeoxynucleotides containing CpG motifs modulate the allergic TH 2 response of BALB/c mice to Bet v 1, the major birch pollen allergen. *J Allergy Clin Immunol* 1999;**104**:1015–23.

83. Parronchi P, Mohapatra S, Sampognaro S, Giannarini L, Wahn U, Chong P. Effects of interferon-alpha on cytokine profile, T cell receptor repertoire and peptide reactivity of human allergen-specific T cells. *Eur J Immunol* 1996;**26**:697–703.
84. Kim TS, De Kryff RH, Rupper R, Maecker HT, Levy S, Umetsu DT. An ovalbumin-IL-12 fusion protein is more effective than ovalbumin plus free recombinant IL-12 in inducing a helper T cell type 1 dominated immune response and inhibiting antigen-specific IgE production. *J Immunol* 1997;**158**:4137–44.
85. Tulic MK, Fiset PO, Manoukian JJ, Frenkiel S, Lavigne F, Eidelman DH, et al. Role of tolllike receptor 4 in protection by bacterial lipopolysaccharide in the nasal mucosa of atopic children but not adults. *Lancet* 2004;**363**:1689–97.
86. Drachenberg KJ, Urban E, Pröll S, Woroniecki SR. Sublingual specific immunotherapy for adults and children: a post-marketing surveillance study. *Allergol Immunopathol (Madr)* 2004;**32**:76–81.
87. Gauvreau GM, Boulet LP, Cockcroft DW, Baatjes A, Cote J, Deschesnes F, et al. Antisense therapy against CCR3 and the common beta chain attenuates allergen-induced eosinophilic responses. *Am J Respir Crit Care Med* 2008;**177**:952–8.
88. Zhu D, Kepley CL, Zhang K, Terada T, Yamada T, Saxon A. A chimeric human-cat fusion protein blocks cat-induced allergy. *Nat Med* 2005;**11**:446–9.
89. Kündig TM, Senti G, Schnetzler G, Wolf C, Prinz Vavricka BM, Fulurija A, et al. Der p 1 peptide on virus-like particles is safe and highly immunogenic in healthy adults. *J Allergy Clin Immunol* 2006;**117**:1470–6.
90. Senti G, Johansen P, Haug S, Bull C, Gottschaller C, Müller P, et al. Use of A-type CpG oligodeoxynucleotides as an adjuvant in allergen-specific immunotherapy in humans: a phase I/IIA clinical trial. *Clin Exp Allergy* 2009;**39**:562–70.
91. Crameri R, Kündig TM, Akdis CA. Modular antigen translocation as a novel vaccine strategy for allergen-specific immunotherapy. *Curr Opin Allergy Clin Immunol* 2009;**9**:568–73.
92. Senti G, Johansen P, Kündig TM. Intralymphatic immunotherapy. *Curr Opin Allergy Clin Immunol* 2009;**9**:537–43.
93. Casale TB, Stokes JR. Immunomodulators for allergic respiratory disorders. *J Allergy Clin Immunol* 2008;**121**:288–96.
94. Busse WW, Israel E, Nelson HS, Baker JW, Charous BL, Young DY, Daclizumab Asthma Study Group, et al. Daclizumab improves asthma control in patients with moderate to severe persistent asthma: a randomized, controlled trial. *Am J Respir Crit Care Med* 2008;**178**:1002–8.
95. Flood-Page PT, Manzies-Gow AN, Kay AB, Robinson DS. Eosinophil's role remains uncertain as anti-interleukin-5 only partially depletes numbers in asthmatic airway. *Am J Respir Crit Care Med* 2003;**167**:199–204.
96. Kips JC, O'Connor BJ, Langley SJ, Woodcock A, Kerstjens HA, Postma DS, et al. Effect of SCH55700, a humanized anti-human interleukin-5 antibody, in severe persistent asthma: a pilot study. *Am J Respir Crit Care Med* 2003;**167**:1655–9.
97. Andrews AL, Holloway JW, Holgate ST, Davies DE. IL-4 receptor alpha is an important modulator of IL-4 and IL-13 receptor binding: implications for the development of therapeutic targets. *J Immunol* 2006;**176**:7456–61.
98. Borish LC, Nelson HS, Corren J, Bensch G, Busse WW, Whitmore JB, IL-4R Asthma Study Group, et al. . Efficacy of soluble IL-4 receptor for the treatment of adults with asthma. *J Allergy Clin Immunol* 2001;**107**:963–70.
99. Morjaria JB, Chauhan AJ, Babu KS, Polosa R, Davies DE, Holgate ST. The role of a soluble TNFalpha receptor fusion protein (etanercept) in corticosteroid refractory asthma: a double blind, randomised, placebo controlled trial. *Thorax* 2008;**63**:584–91.

100. Berry MA, Hargadon B, Shelley M, Parker D, Shaw DE, Green RH, et al. Evidence of a role of tumor necrosis factor alpha in refractory asthma. *N Engl J Med* 2006;**354**: 697–708.
101. Wenzel SE, Barnes PJ, Bleecker ER, Bousquet J, Busse W, T03 asthma investigators, et al. A randomized, double-blind, placebo-controlled study of TNF-alpha blockade in severe persistent asthma. *Am J Respir Crit Care Med* 2009;**179**:549–58.
102. Kuehr J, Brauburger J, Zielen S, Schauer U, Kamin W, Von Berg A, et al. Efficacy of combination treatment with anti-IgE plus specific immunotherapy in polysensitized children and adolescents with seasonal allergic rhinitis. *J Allergy Clin Immunol* 2002;**109**: 274–80.
103. Casale TB, Busse WW, Kline JN, Ballas ZK, Moss MH, Townley RG, Immune Tolerance Network Group, et al. Omalizumab pretreatment decreases acute reactions after rush immunotherapy for ragweed-induced seasonal allergic rhinitis. *J Allergy Clin Immunol* 2006;**117**:134–40.
104. Engelhardt H, Smits RA, Leurs R, Haaksma E, de Esch IJ. A new generation of anti-histamines: histamine H4 receptor antagonists on their way to the clinic. *Curr Opin Drug Discov Devel* 2009;**12**:628–43.
105. Cookson W. The alliances of genes and environment in asthma and allergy. *Nature* 1999;**402**:B5.
106. Presta LG, Lahr SJ, Shields RL, Porter JP, Gorman CM, Fendly BM, et al. Humanization of an antibody directed against IgE. *J Immunol* 1993;**151**:2623–32.
107. Kolbinger F, Saldanha J, Hardman N, Bendig MM. Humanization of a mouse anti-human IgE antibody: a potential therapeutic for IgE-mediated allergies. *Protein Eng* 1993;**6**: 971–80.
108. Corne J, Djukanovic R, Thomas L, Warner J, Botta L, Grandordy B, et al. The effect of intravenous administration of a chimeric anti-IgE antibody on serum IgE levels in atopic subjects: efficacy, safety, and pharmacokinetics. *J Clin Invest* 1997;**99**:879–88.
109. Racine-Poon A, Botta L, Chang TW, Davis FM, Gygax D, Liou RS, et al. Efficacy, pharmacodynamics, and pharmacokinetics of CGP 51901, an antiimmunoglobulin E chimeric monoclonal antibody, in patients with seasonal allergic rhinitis. *Clin Pharmacol Ther* 1997;**62**:675–90.
110. Boulet L-P, Chapman KR, Cote J, Kalra S, Bhagat R, Swystun VA, et al. Inhibitory effect of an anti-IgE antibody E25 on allergen-induced early asthmatic response. *Am J Respir Crit Care Med* 1997;**155**:1835–40.
111. Fahy JV, Fleming HE, Wong HH, Liu JT, Su JQ, Reimann J, et al. The effect of an anti-IgE monoclonal antibody on the early- and late-phase responses to allergen inhalation in asthmatic subjects. *Am J Respir Crit Care Med* 1997;**155**:1828–34.
112. Fick RB, Simon SJ, Su JQ. Anti-IgE (rhumAb) treatment of the symptoms of moderate to severe allergic asthma [abstract]. *Ann Asthma Allergy Immunol* 1998;**80**:80.
113. Metzger WJ, Fick RB. The E25 Asthma Study Group. Corticosteroid (CS) withdrawal in a study of recombinant humanized monoclonal antibody to IgE (RhumAb E25) [abstract]. *J Allergy Clin Immunol* 1998;**101**:S231.
114. Berger W, Gupta N, McAlary M, Fowler-Taylor A. Evaluation of long-term safety of the anti-IgE antibody, omalizumab, in children with allergic asthma. *Ann Allergy Asthma Immunol* 2003;**91**:182–8.
115. Lin RY, Rodriguez-Baez G, Bhargave GA. Omalizumab-associated anaphylactic reactions reported between January 2007 and June 2008. *Ann Allergy Asthma Immunol* 2009;**103**: 442–5.

116. Payet M, Woodward EC, Conrad DH. Humoral response suppression observed with CD23 transgenics. *J Immunol* 1999;**163**:217–23.
117. Christie G, Barton A, Bolognese B, Buckle DR, Cook RM, et al. IgE secretion is attenuated by an inhibitor of proteolytic processing of CD23 (Fc-epsilonRII). *Eur J Immunol* 1997;**27**:3228–35.
118. Coyle AJ, Wagner K, Bertrand C, Tsuyuki S, Bews J, Heusser C. Central role of immunoglobulin (Ig) E in the induction of lung eosinophil infiltration and T helper 2 cell cytokine production: inhibition by a non-anaphylactogenic anti-IgE antibody. *J Exp Med* 1996;**183**: 1303–10.
119. Dasic G, Juillard P, Graber P, Herren S, Angell T, Knowles R, et al. Critical role of CD23 in allergen-induced bronchoconstriction in a murine model of allergic asthma. *Eur J Immunol* 1999;**29**:2957–67.
120. Busse WW, Morgan WJ, Gergen PJ, Mitchell HE, Gern JE, Liu AH, et al. Randomized trial of omalizumab (anti-IgE) for asthma in inner-city children. *N Engl J Med* 2011;**364**:1005–15.
121. Nakamura T, Kloetzer WS, Brams P, Hariharan K, Chamat S, Cao X, et al. In vitro IgE inhibition in B cells by anti-CD23 monoclonal antibodies is functionally dependent on the immunoglobulin Fc domain. *Int J Immunopharmacol* 2000;**22**:131–41.
122. Nopp A, Johansson SG, Ankerst J, Palmqvist M, Oman H. CD-sens and clinical changes during withdrawal of Xolair after 6 years of treatment. *Allergy* 2007;**62**:1175–81.
123. Busse WW, Trzaskoma B, Omachi TA, Canvin J, Rosen K, Chipps BE, et al. Evaluating Xolair persistency of response after long-term therapy (Xport). *Am J Respir Crit Care Med* 2014;**189**:A6576. [abstract].
124. Riccio AM, Dal Negro RW, Micheletto C, De Ferrari L, Folli C, Chiappori A, et al. Omalizumab modulates bronchial reticular basement membrane thickness and eosinophil infiltration in severe persistent allergic asthma patients. *Int J Immunopathol Pharmacol* 2012;**25**:475–84.
125. Jackson DJ, Sykes A, Mallia P, Johnston SL. Asthma exacerbations: origin, effect, and prevention. *J Allergy Clin Immunol* 2011;**128**:1165–74.
126. Ohara J, Paul WE. Production of a monoclonal antibody to and molecular characterization of B cell stimulatory factor-1. *Nature* 1985;**315**:23.
127. Wierenga EA, Snoek M, De Groot C, Chrétien I, Bos JD, Jansen HM, et al. Evidence for compartmentalization of functional subsets of CD4+ T lymphocytes in atopic patients. *J Immunol* 1990;**144**:4651–6.
128. Kotsimbos TC, Ghaffar O, Minshall EM, Humbert M, Durham SR, Pfister R, et al. Expression of the IL-4 receptor subunit is increased in bronchial biopsy specimens from atopic and nonatopic asthmatic subjects. *J Allergy Clin Immunol* 1998;**102**:859–66.
129. Mitsuyasu H, Izuhara K, Mao XQ, Gao PS, Arinobu Y, Enomoto T, et al. Ile50Val variant of the IL-4R up regulates IgE synthesis and associates with atopic asthma. *Nat Genet* 1998;**19**:119–20.
130. Maliszewski CR, Sato TA, Vanden Bos T, Waugh S, Dower SK, Slack J, et al. Cytokine receptors and B cell functions. I: recombinant soluble receptors specifically inhibit IL-1 and IL-4-induced B cells activities in vitro. *J Immunol* 1990;**144**:3028–33.
131. Renz H, Enssle K, Lauffer L, Kurrle R, Gelfand EW. Inhibition of allergen-induced IgE and IgG1 production by soluble IL-4 receptor. *Int Arch Allergy Immunol* 1995;**106**:46–54.
132. Maliszewski CR, Morrissey PJ, Fanslow WC, Sato TA, Willis C, Davison B. Delayed allograft rejection in mice transgenic for a soluble form of the IL-4 receptor. *Cell Immunol* 1992;**143**:434–48.

133. Meissner N, Kussebi F, Jung T, Ratti H, Baumgarten C, Werfel T, et al. A subset of CD8+ T cells from allergic patients produce IL-4 and stimulate IgE production in vitro. *Clin Exp Allergy* 1997;**27**:1402–11.
134. Sperhake K, Neuber K, Enssle K, Ring J. Effects of recombinant human soluble interleukin-4 receptor on interleukin-4/staphylococcal enterotoxin B-stimulated peripheral mononuclear cells from patients with atopic eczema. *Br J Dermatol* 1998; **139**:784–90.
135. Borish LC, Nelson H, Nathan B. Phase I nebulization study of recombinant human IL-4 receptor (rhuIL-4R) in adult patients with mild atopic asthma. *J Allergy Clin Immunol* 1997;**99**:S413.
136. Taylor A, Akdis M, Joss A, Akkoc T, Wenig R, Colonna M, et al. IL-10 inhibits CD28 and ICOS costimulations of T cells via src homology 2 domain-containing protein tyrosine phosphatase 1. *J Allergy Clin Immunol* 2007;**120**:76–83.
137. Chatila TA. Role of regulatory T cells in human diseases. *J Allergy Clin Immunol* 2005;**116**:949–59.
138. Akdis M, Verhagen J, Taylor A, Karamloo F, Karagiannidis C, Crameri R, et al. Immune responses in healthy and allergic individuals are characterized by a fine balance between allergen-specific T regulatory 1 and T helper 2 cells. *J Exp Med* 2004;**199**(11):1567–75.
139. Akdis M. Healthy immune response to allergens: T regulatory cells and more. *Curr Opin Immunol* 2006;**18**:738–44.
140. Meiler F, Zumkehr J, Klunker S, Rückert B, Akdis CA, Akdis M. In vivo switch to IL-10-secreting T regulatory cells in high dose allergen exposure. *J Exp Med* 2008;**205**: 2887–98.
141. Hendrikx TK, Velthuis JH, Klepper M, van Gurp E, Geel A, Schoordijk W, et al. Monotherapy rapamycin allows an increase of CD4(þ) CD25(brightþ) FoxP3(þ) T cells in renal recipients. *Transpl Int* 2009;**22**:884–91.
142. Utset TO, Auger JA, Peace D, Zivin RA, Xu D, Jolliffe L, et al. Modified anti-CD3 therapy in psoriatic arthritis: a phase I/II clinical trial. *J Rheumatol* 2002;**29**:1907–13.
143. Ehrenstein MR, Evans JG, Singh A, Moore S, Warnes G, Isenberg DA, et al. Compromised function of regulatory T cells in rheumatoid arthritis and reversal by anti-TNFalpha therapy. *J Exp Med* 2004;**200**:277–85.
144. O'Connor RA, Anderton SM. Multi-faceted control of autoaggression: Foxp3þ regulatory T cells in murine models of organ-specific autoimmune disease. *Cell Immunol* 2008;**251**:8–18.
145. Roncarolo MG, Battaglia M. Regulatory T-cell immunotherapy for tolerance to self antigens and alloantigens in humans. *Nat Rev Immunol* 2007;**7**:585–98.
146. Peek EJ, Richards DF, Faith A, Lavender P, Lee TH, Corrigan CJ, et al. Interleukin-10-secreting "regulatory" T cells induced by glucocorticoids and beta2-agonists. *Am J Respir Cell Mol Biol* 2005;**33**:105–11.
147. Karagiannidis C, Akdis M, Holopainen P, Woolley NJ, Hense G, Rückert B, et al. Glucocorticoids upregulate FOXP3 expression and regulatory T cells in asthma. *J Allergy Clin Immunol* 2004;**114**:1425–33.
148. Akdis M, Akdis CA. Mechanisms of allergen-specific immunotherapy. *J Allergy Clin Immunol* 2007;**119**:780–91.
149. Klunker S, Chong MM, Mantel PY, Palomares O, Bassin C, Ziegler M, et al. Transcription factors RUNX1 and RUNX3 in the induction and suppressive function of Foxp3þ inducible regulatory T cells. *J Exp Med* 2009;**206**:2701–15.
150. Lenschow DJ, Walunas TL, Bluestone JA. CD28/B7 system of T cell costimulation. *Annu Rev Immunol* 1996;**14**:233–58.

151. Kuchroo VK, Das MP, Brown JA, et al. B7-1 and B7-2 costimulatory molecules activate differentially the Th1/Th2 developmental pathways: application to autoimmune disease therapy. *Cell* 1995;**80**:707–18.
152. Masten BJ, Yates JL, Pollard Koga AM, Lipscomb MF. Characterization of accessory molecules in murine lung dendritic cell function: roles for CD80, CD86, CD54, and CD40L. *Am J Respiratory Cell Mol Biol* 1997;**16**:335–42.
153. Krinzman SJ, De Sanctis GT, Cernadas M, Kobzik L, Listman JA, Christiani DC, et al. T cell activation in a murine model of asthma. *Am J Physiol* 1996;**271**:L476–83.
154. Krinzman SJ, De Sanctis GT, Cernadas M, Mark D, Wang Y, Listman J, et al. Inhibition of T cell costimulation abrogates airway hyperresponsiveness in a murine model. *J Clin Invest* 1996;**98**:2693–9.
155. Mark DA, Donovan CE, De Sanctis GT, Krinzman SJ, Kobzik L, Linsley PS, et al. Both CD80 and CD86 co-stimulatory molecules regulate allergic pulmonary inflammation. *Int Immunol* 1998;**10**:1647–55.
156. Mark DA, Donovan CE, De Sanctis GT, He HZ, Cernadas M, Kobzik L, et al. B7-1 (CD80) and B7-2 (CD86) have complementary roles in mediating allergic pulmonary inflammation and airway hyperresponsiveness. *Am J Respir Cell Mol Biol* 2000;**22**:265–71.
157. Holgate ST. Genetic common ground between allergic and autoimmune disease: the role of cytotoxic T-lymphocyte antigen 4. *J Allergy Clin Immunol* 2004;**114**:277–9.
158. Sayegh MH, Akalin E, Hancock WW, Russell ME, Carpenter CB, Linsley PS, et al. CD28-B7 blockade after alloantigenic challenge in vivo inhibits Th1 cytokines but spares Th2. *J Exp Med* 1995;**181**:1869–74.
159. Arestides RS, He H, Westlake RM, Chen AI, Sharpe AH, Perkins DL, et al. Costimulatory molecule OX40L is critical for both Th1 and Th2 responses in allergic inflammation. *Eur J Immunol* 2002;**32**:2874–80.
160. Harris N, Peach R, Naemura J, Linsley PS, Le Gros G, Ronchese F. CD80 costimulation is essential for the induction of airway eosinophilia. *J Exp Med* 1997;**185**:177–82.
161. Bradley BL, Azzawi M, Jacobson M, Assoufi B, Collins JV, Irani AA, et al. Eosinophils, T-lymphocytes, mast cells, neutrophils, and macrophages in bronchial biopsy specimens from atopis subjects with asthma: comparison with biopsy specimens from atopic subjects without asthma and normal control subjects and relationship to bronchial hyperresponsiveness. *J Allergy Clin Immunol* 1991;**88**:661–74.
162. Sato J, Asakura K, Murakami M, Uede T, Kataura A. Topical CTLA4-Ig suppresses ongoing mucosal immune response in presensitized murine model of allergic rhinitis. *Int Arch Allergy Immunol* 1999;**19**:197–204.
163. Padrid PA, Mathur M, Li X, Herrmann K, Qin Y, Cattamanchi A, et al. CTLA4Ig inhibits airway eosinophilia and hyperresponsiveness by regulating the development of TH 1/TH 2 subsets in a murine model of asthma. *Am J Respir Cell Mol Biol* 1998;**18**:453–62.
164. Mathur M, Herrmann K, Qin Y, Gulmen F, Li X, Krimins R, et al. CD28 interactions with either CD80 or CD86 are sufficient to induce allergic airway inflammation in mice. *Am J Respir Cell Mol Biol* 1999;**21**:498–509.
165. Krummel MF, Allison JP. CD28 and CTLA-4 have opposing effects on the response of T cells to stimulation. *J Exp Med* 1995;**182**:459–65.
166. McCoy K, Camberis M, Gros GL. Protective immunity to nematode infection is induced by CTLA-4 blockade. *J Exp Med* 1997;**186**:183–7.
167. Edmead CE, Lamb JR. Altered CTLA-4 expression on T cells from atopic patients. European Immunology Society Meeting—Conference Abstracts; 1997 (P.5.02.12).

168. Hofer MF, Jirapongsananuruk O, Trumble AE, Leung DY. Upregulation of B7.2, but not B7.1, on B cells from patients with allergic asthma. *J Allergy Clin Immunol* 1998;**101**:96–102.
169. Agea E, Forenza N, Piattoni S, Russano A, Monaco A, Flenghi L, et al. Expression of B7 co-stimulatory molecules and CD1a antigen by alveolar macrophages in allergic bronchial asthma. *Clin Exp Allergy* 1998;**28**:1359–67.
170. Jeannin P, Magistrelli G, Aubry JP, Caron G, Gauchat JF, Renno T, et al. Soluble CD86 is a costimulatory molecule for human T lymphocytes. *Immunity* 2000;**13**:303–12.
171. Shi HZ, Xie ZF, Deng JM, Chen YQ, Xiao CQ. Soluble CD86 protein in serum samples of patients with asthma. *Thorax* 2004;**59**:870–5.
172. Deng JM, Shi HZ, Qin XJ, Xie ZF, Huang CP, Zhong XN. Effects of allergen inhalation and oral glucocorticoid on concentrations of serum-soluble CD86 in allergic asthmatics. *Clin Immunol* 2005;**115**:178–83.
173. Ritprajak P, Hashiguchi M, Azuma M. Topical application of cream-emulsified CD86 siRNA ameliorates allergic skin disease by targeting cutaneous dendritic cells. *Mol Ther* 2008;**16**:1323–30.
174. Akbari O, DeKruyff RH, Umetsu DT. Pulmonary dendritic cells producing IL-10 mediate tolerance induced by respiratory exposure to antigen. *Nat Immunol* 2001;**2**:725–31.
175. Hogan SP, Mould A, Kikutani H, Ramsay AJ, Foster PS. Aeroallergen-induced eosinophilic inflammation, lung damage, and airways hyperreactivity in mice can occur independently of IL-4 and allergen-specific immunoglobulins. *J Clin Invest* 1997;**99**:1329–39.
176. Kawai T, Andrews D, Colvin RB, Sachs DH, Cosimi AB. Thromboembolic complications after treatment with monoclonal antibody against CD40 ligand. *Nat Med* 2000;**6**(2):114.
177. Hesse UJ, Wienand P, Baldamus C, Pollok M, Pichlmaier H. The risk of infection following OKT3 and antilymphocyte globulin treatment for renal transplant rejection: results of a single center prospectively randomized trial. *Transpl Int* 1992;**5**(Suppl. 1):S440–3.
178. Suntharalingam G, Perry MR, Ward S, Brett SJ, Castello-Cortes A, Brunner MD, et al. Cytokine storm in a phase 1 trial of the anti-CD28 monoclonal antibody TGN1412. *N Engl J Med* 2006;**355**:1018–28.
179. Kremer JM, Westhovens R, Leon M, Giorgio ED, Alten R, Steinfeld S, et al. Treatment of rheumatoid arthritis by selective inhibition of T-cell activation with fusion protein CTLA4Ig. *N Engl J Med* 2003;**349**:1907–15.
180. Abrams JR, Kelley SL, Hayes E, Browna MJ, Kangc S, Lebwohl MG, et al. Blockade of T lymphocyte costimulation with cytotoxic T lymphocyte-associated antigen 4-immunoglobulin (CTLA4Ig) reverses the cellular pathology of psoriatic plaques, including the activation of keratinocytes, dendritic cells, and endothelial cells. *J Exp Med* 2000;**192**:681–94.
181. Bluestone JA, St Clair EW, Turka LA. CTLA4Ig: bridging the basic immunology with clinical application. *Immunity* 2006;**24**:233–8.
182. Hutloff A, Dittrich AM, Beier KC, Eljaschewitsch B, Kraft R, Anagnostopoulos I, et al. ICOS is an inducible T-cell co-stimulator structurally and functionally related to CD28. *Nature* 1999;**397**:263–6.
183. Yoshinaga SK, Whoriskey JS, Khare SD, Sarmiento U, Guo H, Horan T, et al. T-cell costimulation through B7RP-1 and ICOS. *Nature* 1999;**402**:827–32.
184. Akbari O, Freeman GJ, Meyer EH, Greenfield EA, Chang TT, Sharpe AH, et al. Antigen-specific regulatory T-cells develop via the ICOS-ICOS-ligand pathway and inhibit allergen-induced airway hyperreactivity. *Nat Med* 2002;**8**:1024–32.
185. de Jong YP, Rietdijk ST, Faubion WA, Abadia-Molina AC, Clarke K, Mizoguchi E, et al. Blocking inducible co-stimulator in the absence of CD28 impairs Th1and CD25+ regulatory T-cells in murine colitis. *Int Immunol* 2004;**16**:205–13.

186. Grimbacher B, Hutloff A, Schlesier M, Glocker E, Warnatz K, Dräger R, et al. Homozygous loss of ICOS is associated with adult-onset common variable immunodeficiency. *Nat Immunol* 2003;**4**:261–8.
187. Keane-Myers A, Gause WC, Linsley PS, Chen SJ, Wills-Karp M. B7-CD28/CTLA-4 costimulatory pathways are required for the development of T helper cell 2-mediated allergic airway responses to inhaled antigens. *J Immunol* 1997;**158**:2042–9.
188. Han S, Hathcock K, Zheng B, Kepler TB, Hodes R, Kelsoe G. Cellular interaction in germinal centers. Roles of CD40 ligand and B7-2 in established germinal centers. *J Immunol* 1995;**155**:556–67.
189. Van Oosterhout AJ, Hofstra CL, Shields R, Chan B, Van Ark I, Jardieu PM, et al. Murine CTLA4-IgG treatment inhibits airway eosinophilia and hyperresponsiveness and attenuates IgE upregulation in a murine model of allergic asthma. *Am J Respir Cell Mol Biol* 1997;**17**:386–92.
190. Gonzalo JA, Tian J, Delaney T, Corcoran J, Rottman JB, Lora J, et al. ICOS is critical for T helper cell-mediated lung mucosal inflammatory responses. *Nat Immunol* 2001;**2**:597–604.
191. Tsuyuki S, Tsuyuki J, Einsle K, Kopf M, Coyle AJ. Costimulation through B7-2 (CD86) is required for the induction of a lung mucosal T helper cell 2 (TH2) immune response and altered airway responsiveness. *J Exp Med* 1997;**185**:1671–9.
192. Keane-Myers AM, Gause WC, Finkelman FD, Xhou XD, Wills-Karp M. Development of murine allergic asthma is dependent upon B7-2 costimulation. *J Immunol* 1998;**160**: 1036–43.
193. Harris NL, Peach RJ, Ronchese F. CTLA4-Ig inhibits optimal T helper 2 cell development but not protective immunity or memory response to *Nippostrongylus brasiliensis*. *Eur J Immunol* 1999;**29**:311–16.
194. Tivol EA, Borriello F, Schweitzer AN, Lynch WP, Bluestone JA, Sharpe AH. Loss of CTLA-4 leads to massive lymphoproliferation and fatal multiorgan tissue destruction, revealing a critical negative regulatory role of CTLA-4. *Immunity* 1995;**3**:541–54.
195. Waterhouse P, Penninger JM, Timms E, Wakeham A, Shahinian A, Lee KP, et al. Lymphoproliferative disorders with early lethality in mice deficient in CTLA-4. *Science* 1995;**270**:985–8.
196. Takahashi T, Tagami T, Yamazaki S, Uede T, Shimizu J, Sakaguchi N, et al. Immunologic self-tolerance maintained by CD25(+)CD4(+) regulatory T cells constitutively expressing cytotoxic T lymphocyte-associated antigen 4. *J Exp Med* 2000;**192**:303–10.
197. Read S, Malmstrom V, Powrie F. Cytotoxic T lymphocyte-associated antigen 4 plays an essential role in the function of CD25(+)CD4(+) regulatory cells that control intestinal inflammation. *J Exp Med* 2000;**192**:295–302.
198. Howard TD, Postma DS, Hawkins GA, Koppelman GH, Zheng SL, Wysong AK, et al. Fine mapping of an IgE-controlling gene on chromosome 2q: analysis of CTLA4 and CD28. *J Allergy Clin Immunol* 2002;**110**:743–51.
199. Lee SY, Lee YH, Shin C, Shim JJ, Kang KH, Yoo SH, In KH. Association of asthma severity and bronchial hyperresponsiveness with a polymorphism in the cytotoxic T lymphocyte antigen-4 gene. *Chest* 2002;**122**:171–6.
200. Hizawa N, Yamaguchi E, Jinushi E, Konno S, Kawakami Y, Nishimura M. Increased total serum IgE levels in patients with asthma and promoter polymorphisms at CTLA4 and FCER1B. *J Allergy Clin Immunol* 2001;**108**:74–9.
201. Nishimura H, Nose M, Hiai H, Minato N, Honjo T. Development of lupus-like autoimmune diseases by disruption of the PD-1 gene encoding an ITIM motif-carrying immunoreceptor. *Immunity* 1999;**11**:141–51.

202. Freeman GJ, Long AJ, Iwai Y, Bourque K, Chernova T, Nishimura H, et al. Engagement of the PD-1 immunoinhibitory receptor by a novel B7 family member leads to negative regulation of lymphocyte activation. *J Exp Med* 2000;**192**:1027–34.
203. Tseng SY, Otsuji M, Gorski K, Huang X, Slansky JE, Pai SI, et al. B7-DC, a new dendritic cell molecule with potent costimulatory properties for T cells. *J Exp Med* 2001;**193**: 839–46.
204. Matsumoto K, Fukuyama S, Eguchi-Tsuda M, Nakano T, Matsumoto T, et al. B7-DC induced by IL-13 works as a feedback regulator in the effector phase of allergic asthma. *Biochem Biophys Res Commun* 2008;**365**:170–5.
205. Matsumoto K, Inoue H, Nakano T, Tsuda M, Yoshiura Y, Fukuyama S, et al. B7-DC regulates asthmatic response by an IFNgamma-dependent mechanism. *J Immunol* 2004;**172**: 2530–41.
206. Radhakrishnan S, Iijima K, Kobayashi T, Rodriguez M, Kita H, Pease LR. Blockade of allergic airway inflammation following systemic treatment with a B7-dendritic cell (PD-L2) cross-linking human antibody. *J Immunol* 2004;**173**:1360–5.
207. Oflazoglu E, Swart DA, Anders-Bartholo P, Jessup HK, Norment AM, et al. Paradoxical role of programmed death-1 ligand 2 in Th2 immune responses in vitro and in a mouse asthma model in vivo. *Eur J Immunol* 2004;**34**:3326–36.
208. Fukushima A, Yamaguchi T, Azuma M, Yagita H, Ueno H. Involvement of programmed death-ligand 2 (PD-L2) in the development of experimental allergic conjunctivitis in mice. *Br J Ophthalmol* 2006;**90**:1040–5.
209. Gajewska BU, Tafuri A, Swirski FK, Walker T, Johnson JR, et al. 7RP-1 is not required for the generation of Th2 responses in a model of allergic airway inflammation but is essential for the induction of inhalation tolerance. *J Immunol* 2005;**174**:3000–5.
210. Tsushima F, Iwai H, Otsuki N, Abe M, Hirose S, Yamazaki T, et al. Referential contribution of B7-H1 to programmed death-1-mediated regulation of hapten-specific allergic inflammatory responses. *Eur J Immunol* 2003;**33**:2773–82.
211. Piconi S, Trabattoni D, Saresella M, Iemoli E, Schenal M, Fusi A, et al. Effects of specific immunotherapy on the B7 family of costimulatory molecules in allergic inflammation. *J Immunol* 2007;**178**:1931–7.
212. Allam JP, Novak N, Fuchs C, Asen S, Berge S, Appel T, et al. Characterization of dendritic cells from human oral mucosa: a new Langerhans' cell type with high constitutive FcepsilonRI expression. *J Allergy Clin Immunol* 2003;**112**:141–8.
213. Allam JP, Peng WM, Appel T, Wenghoefer M, Niederhagen B, Bieber T, et al. Toll-like receptor 4 ligation enforces tolerogenic properties of oral mucosal Langerhans cells. *J Allergy Clin Immunol* 2008;**121**:368–74.
214. Coyle AJ, Lehar S, Lloyd C, Tian J, Delaney T, Manning S, et al. The CD28-related molecule ICOS is required for effective T cell-dependent immune responses. *Immunity* 2000;**13**(1):95–105.
215. Tesciuba AG, Subudhi S, Rother RP, Faas SJ, Frantz AM, Elliot D, et al. Inducible costimulator regulates Th2-mediated inflammation, but not Th2 differentiation, in a model of allergic airway disease. *J Immunol* 2001;**167**:1996–2003.
216. Wiley RE, Goncharova S, Shea T, Johnson JR, Coyle AJ, Jordana M. Evaluation of inducible costimulator/B7-related protein-1 as a therapeutic target in a murine model of allergic airway inflammation. *Am J Respir Cell Mol Biol* 2003;**28**:722–30.
217. Akiba H, Miyahira Y, Atsuta M, Takeda K, Nohara C, Futagawa T, et al. Critical contribution of OX40 ligand to T helper cell type 2 differentiation in experimental leishmaniasis. *J Exp Med* 2000;**191**:375–80.

218. Hoshino A, Tanaka Y, Akiba H, Asakura Y, Mita Y, Sakurai T, et al. Critical role for OX40 ligand in the development of pathogenic Th2 cells in a murine model of asthma. *Eur J Immunol* 2003;**33**:861–9.
219. Salek-Ardakani S, Song J, Halteman BS, Jember AG, Akiba H, Yagita H, et al. OX40 (CD134) controls memory T helper 2 cells that drive lung inflammation. *J Exp Med* 2003;**198**:315–24.
220. Polte T, Foell J, Werner C, Hoymann HG, Braun A, Burdach S, et al. CD137-mediated immunotherapy for allergic asthma. *J Clin Invest* 2006;**116**:1025–36.
221. Polte T, Behrendt AK, Hansen G. Direct evidence for a critical role of CD30 in the development of allergic asthma. *J Allergy Clin Immunol* 2006;**118**:942–8.
222. Larsen CP, Elwood ET, Alexander DZ, Ritchie SC, Hendrix R, Tucker-Burden C, et al. Long-term acceptance of skin and cardiac allografts after blocking CD40 and CD28 pathways. *Nature* 1996;**381**:434–8.
223. Sheridan C. TeGenero fiasco prompts regulatory rethink. *Nat Biotechnol* 2006;**24**:475–6.
224. Robinson DS, Bentley AM, Hartnell A, Kay AB, Durham SR. Activated memory T helper cells in bronchoalveolar lavage fluid from patients with atopic asthma: relation to asthma symptoms, lung function, and bronchial responsiveness. *Thorax* 1993;**48**:26–32.
225. Grunig G, Warnock M, Wakil AE, Venkayya R, Brombacher F, Rennick DM, et al. Requirement for IL-13 independently of IL-4 in experimental asthma. *Science* 1998;**282**:2261–3.
226. Shardonofsky FR, Venzor III J, Barrios R, Leong KP, Huston DP. Therapeutic efficacy of an anti-IL-5 monoclonal antibody delivered into the respiratory tract in a murine model of asthma. *J Allergy Clin Immunol* 1999;**104**:215–21.
227. Fahy JV, Cockcroft DW, Boulet LP, Wong HH, Deschesnes F, Davis EE, et al. Effect of aerosolized anti-IgE (E25) on airway responses to inhaled allergen in asthmatic subjects. *Am J Respir Crit Care Med* 1999;**160**:1023–7.
228. Kroczek R, Hamelmann E. T-cell costimulatory molecules:optimal targets for the treatment of allergic airway disease with monoclonal antibodies. *J Allergy Clin Immunol* 2005;**116**:906–9.
229. Flood-Page P, Menzies-Gow A, Phipps S, Ying S, Wangoo A, Ludwig MS, et al. Anti-IL-5 treatment reduces deposition of ECM proteins in the bronchial subepithelial basement membrane of mild atopic asthmatics. *J Clin Invest* 2003;**112**:1029–36.
230. Borish LC, Nelson HS, Bensch G, Phase I/II study of soluble interleukin-4 receptor (IL-4R) in adults with moderate asthma. *Proceedings of the European Respiratory Society Annual Congress*. Madrid, Spain: European Respiratory Society; 1999. Abstract P1983.
231. Mir MA, Albaradie RS. Hypersensitive allergic reactions are caused by Pollen abundantly found in air during the spring and autumn seasons. *Int J Pure Appl Biosci* 2013;**1** (3):68–80.
232. Casale TB, Bernstein IL, Busse WW, LaForce CF, Tinkelman DG, Stoltz RR, et al. Use of an anti-IgE humanized monoclonal antibody in ragweed-induced allergic rhinitis. *J Allergy Clin Immunol* 1997;**100**(1):110–21.
233. Fahy JV, Fleming HE, Wong HH, Liu JT, Su JQ, Reimann J, et al. The effect of an anti-IgE monoclonal antibody on the early- and late-phase responses to allergen inhalation in asthmatic subjects. *Am J Respir Crit Care Med* 1997;**155**(6):1828–34.
234. Bradding P, Feather IH, Howarth PH, Mueller R, Roberts JA, Britten K, et al. Interleukin 4 is localized to and released by human mast cells. *J Exp Med* 1992;**176**(5):1381–6.

Chapter 5

Costimulation in Lymphomas and Cancers

INTRODUCTION

Cancer is a major health problem worldwide and is one of the most prominent causes of morbidity and mortality in children and adults causing about 9 million deaths annually. The transformation of normal cells to cancer cells may arise due to dysregulation of oncogenes, tumor suppressors, and/or stability genes. These transformed cells are sensed by the cells of the immune system, especially T cells, through specific receptors for an effective immune response. But unfortunately even after the interaction with T cells, an effective immune response is not generated. The success of novel cancer therapies depends on the identification of functional targets that play an essential role in tumor growth and metastasis, survival, and evasion from immunosurveillance. Cancer and the immune system are fundamentally interrelated. Cancer cells express tumor-specific aberrant antigens and must therefore evade immune detection to survive, either by inducing immunosuppression or deriving survival signals from tumor-infiltrating immune cells. T-cell-mediated antitumor immunity requires recognition of cancer-associated antigen by the major histocompatibility complex (MHC), and appropriate costimulatory and repressive secondary signals arising from complex interactions with other immune, stromal, and tumor cells. Dysfunction of costimulation pathways may contribute to failed antitumor immunity.

Although many costimulatory molecules like CD80, CD86, CD40, heat stable antigen, intercellular adhesion molecule (ICAM-1), vascular cell adhesion molecule (VCAM-1), B7-DC/programmed death ligand-2 (PDL-2), B7-H1/programmed death ligand-1 (PDL-1), etc., are known to be expressed on the surface of antigen-presenting cells (APCs). But the best-defined costimulatory molecules are two structurally related proteins known as CD80 (B7-1) and CD86 (B7-2).[1] Both CD80 and CD86 have their ligands, CD28 and cytotoxic T-lymphocyte associated antigen (CTLA-4), expressed on T cells. The delivery

Developing Costimulatory Molecules for Immunotherapy of Diseases.
DOI: http://dx.doi.org/10.1016/B978-0-12-802585-7.00005-4

of costimulatory signals is necessary to ensure an effective immune response against the tumors. It has been established recently that CD80 and CD86 play a role in the activation of APCs. Stimulation via CD86 in B cells can modulate their proliferation; IgG secretion and expression of proapoptotic and antiapoptotic molecules; nuclear localization of NF-κB (p50) subunit; phosphorylation of v-rel reticulo endotheliosis viral oncogene homolog A (Rel A) (p65) and IκB-alpha; and increased octamer-binding transcription factor 2 (oct-2) expression.[2,3] It has been now established that CD80/CD86 contact with CD28 and CTLA-4 delivers signals that activate and inhibit T-cell activity, respectively. Furthermore, in the case of dendritic cells (DCs), it has been shown recently that it enhances the production of IL-6 and IFN-γ which in turn, up-regulates the expression of the immunoregulatory enzyme indolamine 2,3-dioxygenase (IDO) that results in tryptophan catabolism, suppresses T-cell responses, and promotes tumor resistance. Reverse signaling by CTLA-4 through CD80/CD86 in DCs causes the activation of the transcription factor NF-κB followed by suppressor of cytokine signaling 3 (SOCS3) down-regulation and IFN-γ release. This in turn causes the induction of IDO and tryptophan catabolism, hence its depletion, and kynurinine production, which produces the biological effect.[4–6] It has also been shown that silencing of SOCS3 by small interfering RNA (siRNA) makes CD28–Ig capable of activating IDO hence in the absence of SOCS3 CD28–Ig becomes immunosuppressive and mimics the action of CTLA-4–Ig on tryptophan catabolism. These effects appear to result from a combination of unopposed IFN-γ signaling and the occurrence of IFN-γ like actions by IL-6. However, in the case of CD80, it has been illustrated that signaling through this molecule can arrest the growth of lymphomas by upregulating expression of proapoptotic molecules and downregulating antiapoptotic molecules (see Figure 5.3 and Figure 5.4).[7–11]

Major Costimulatory and Coinhibitory Pathways in Antitumor Immunity

Costimulatory molecules belong to two major families: B7/CD28 family and tumor necrosis factor (TNF)/TNF receptor (TNFR) family (see Table 5.1). All molecules belonging to B7/CD28 family are members of the larger immunoglobulin superfamily (IGSF) and are involved in the triggering of cell-mediated immune response. Instead, the TNF/TNFR family members are involved in the later phases of T-cell activation and are induced from hours to days following the T-cell receptor (TCR) engagement. Currently the B7 family has seven members: B7.1, B7.2, ICOS-L, PD-L1, PD-L2, B7-H3, and B7-H4. While as TNFR/TNF family has six members herpes virus entry mediator (HVEM), B- and T-lymphocyte attenuator (BTLA), CD70, CD30, 4-IBBL, and OX40L.[9,10] Presence of an efficient costimulation is crucial for improving antitumor immunity. In fact, one of the mechanisms through which a tumor is able to evade immune surveillance is the lower expression

TABLE 5.1 Members of B7 and TNFR Family of Costimulatory Molecules and Ligands

Costimulatory Families	Superfamily	Expression	Costimulatory Molecule	Ligand	Signal Type
TNF/TNFR Superfamily	TNF/TNFR	Constitutive	CD27	CD70	Positive
	TNF/TNFR	Inducible	OX40 (CD134)	OX40L	Positive
	TNF/TNFR	Inducible	4-1BB (CD 137)	4-IBBL	Positive
	TNF/TNFR	Inducible	CD30	CD30L (CD153)	Positive
TNF/TNFRR, CD28/B7 Superfamily	TNF/TNFR, CD28/B7	Constitutive	HVEM	LIGHT, BTLA	Positive
	TNF/TNFR, CD28/B7	Constitutive	BTLA	HVEM	Negative
CD28/B7 Superfamily	CD28/B7	Constitutive	CD28	B7-1, B7-2 (CD80, CD86)	Positive
	CD28/B7	Inducible	CTLA-4 (CD152)	B7-1, B7-2 (CD80, CD86)	Negative
	CD28/B7	Inducible	ICOS	ICOS-L	Positive
	CD28/B7	Inducible	PD-1	PD-Ll, PDL-2	Negative
	CD28/B7	Inducible	Unknown	B7-H4	Negative
	CD28/B7	Inducible	Unknown	B7-H3	Obscure
CD2 Family	CD2	Inducible	SLAM (CD150)	SLAM (CD150)	Positive

Note: TNF, tumor necrosis factor; R, receptor; HVEM, herpes virus entry mediator; LIGHT, homologous to lymphotoxin inducible expression, competing for GpD of herpes virus, expressed on activated T lymphocytes; BLTA, B- and T-lymphocyte attenuator; ICOS, inducible costimulator; L, ligand; SLAM, signaling lymphocyte activation molecule; CTLA, cytotoxic T-lymphocyte antigen; PD, programmed death; B7-H4 and H3, B7 homologues 4 and 3.

of costimulatory molecules or the upregulation of coinhibitory molecules. The lack of costimulation in the tumor microenvironment could be responsible for the generation of anergic T cells and, consequently, the absence of an appropriate antitumor immune response.[10]

The B7 system of costimulatory molecules is one of the most important secondary signaling mechanisms and is essential in maintaining the delicate balance between immune potency and suppression of autoimmunity (summarized in Table 5.2). Potential therapeutic applications include immune-boosting adjuvants to conventional anticancer therapy, hematopoietic stem cell transplantation (HSCT), antitumor vaccines, bioengineered T cells as well as attenuation of graft-versus-host disease (GVHD). The B7 family is only one aspect of a complex signaling network (explained in Figures 5.1 and 5.2) that comprises other IGSF members, the TNF superfamily (TNFRSF), chemokines, cytokines, and adhesion molecules. However, based on a substantial evidence base and a growing therapeutic armory, the B7 family requires particular attention, as summarized in Table 5.3. Therefore manipulation of signals delivered by B7 ligands shows a great potential in treatment of cancers. So interfering with the costimulatory/inhibitory ligand-receptor network that regulates the immune response has become a promising approach in cancer immunotherapy. Thus, antagonistic antibodies directed against inhibitory receptors of the immunoglobulin-like (Ig) superfamily (e.g., CTLA-4, PD-1) and agonistic antibodies directed against costimulatory receptors of the TNFR superfamily (e.g., 4-1BB, OX40, GITR, CD127, CD40) are being evaluated in clinical trials.[10]

Targeting T Cell Costimulatory Molecules to Improve Antitumor Immunity

The tumor microenvironment is often characterized by the presence of anergic T cells, due to the lack of positive costimulatory molecules, mainly B7-1 and B7-2, on the surface of cancer cells.[27] One strategy to reverse this scenario is to force B7 expression on tumor cells, rendering them able to activate T-cell immune response. Several studies showed that the induction of B7-1 on tumor cells was sufficient to stimulate the CD8+ T-cell-mediated rejection in several tumor models, as well as a memory response, but was insufficient to mediate rejection of poorly immunogenic tumors.[10] Several phase I clinical trials evaluated the efficacy of B7-1 transfected tumor cell vaccines, with or without IL-2, with encouraging preliminary results in patients affected by metastatic renal carcinoma and nonsmall cell lung cancer[28,29] (Table 5.3). In a phase II trial, 39 patients with metastatic renal carcinoma were vaccinated with B7-1 transfected autologous tumor cells in combination with systemic IL-2. The authors observed a decrease in the cancer.[30]

TABLE 5.2 B7 Family Members Update and Their Nomenclature

B7 Designation	CD Designation	Molecule/Eponyms	Receptor	Expression Pattern	Functions
B7-1	CD80	B7-1 or B7	CD28/CTLA-4 (CD152)	DCs, activated macrophages and B cells	Activation of naive T cells, T-cell proliferation, IL-2 production, T-cell survival/inhibition of T-cell responses
B7-2	CD86	B7-2 or B7	CD28/CTLA-4 (CD152)	DCs, activated macrophages and B cells	Activation of naive T cells, T-cell proliferation, IL-2 production, T-cell survival/inhibition of T-cell responses
B7-H1	CD274	Programmed cell death Ligand-1 PDL-1	CD279 (PD-1) ?	DCs, monocytes, macrophages, B cells, activated T cells, endothelial cells and tumor cells	Effector T-cell functions, T-cell proliferation, cytokines (IL-10, IFN-γ) production, apoptosis of CTLs DCs and monocytes, inhibition of T-cell responses
B7-H2	CD275	Inducible costimulator Ligand (B7-h, B7RP-1, LICOS/ICOS-L, GL50)	ICOS (CD278)	DCs, monocytes, Langerhanss cells, B cells, fibroblasts, endothelial cells, etc.	Effector T-cell functions, T-cell proliferation, Ig isotype class switching, cytokine (IFN-γ, IL-10, IL-4) production
B7-H3	CD276	B7-Homologue 3	?? ILT-2 (orphan ligand)	Induced on DCs and monocytes	T-cell proliferation, IFN-γ production, enhancement of CTL activity

(Continued)

TABLE 5.2 (Continued)

B7 Designation	CD Designation	Molecule/Eponyms	Receptor	Expression Pattern	Functions
B7-H4	CD276	B7-Homologue 4	BTLA (??)	Induced on T cells, B cells, DCs, Macrophages	Inhibition of T-cell proliferation, cytokine production, cell cycle arrest
B7-H6	CD276	B7-Homologue 6	NKp30	NK T cells	Costimulation, NK T-cell activation
B7-DC	CD273	Programmed cell death Ligand-2 (PDL-2)	PD-1 (CD279)	DCs, monocytes, macrophages, B cells, activated T cells, endothelial cells, and tumor cells	Effector T-cell functions, T-cell proliferation, cytokines (IL-10, IFN-γ) production, apoptosis of CTLs, DCs and monocytes, inhibition of T-cell responses, regulations of DC biology
–	CD277	BT3.1, Butyrophilin SF3 Al, BTF5	?	T, B, NK, mono, DC, endothelial, CD34 + cells, tumor cell lines	T-cell activation

Expression of selected antigens expressed on the cell surface of APC or tumor cells and their costimulatory or inhibitory ligands on the surface of T cells or NK cells.
Note: ? means unknown; and ?? means evidence is contested or based on limited date.

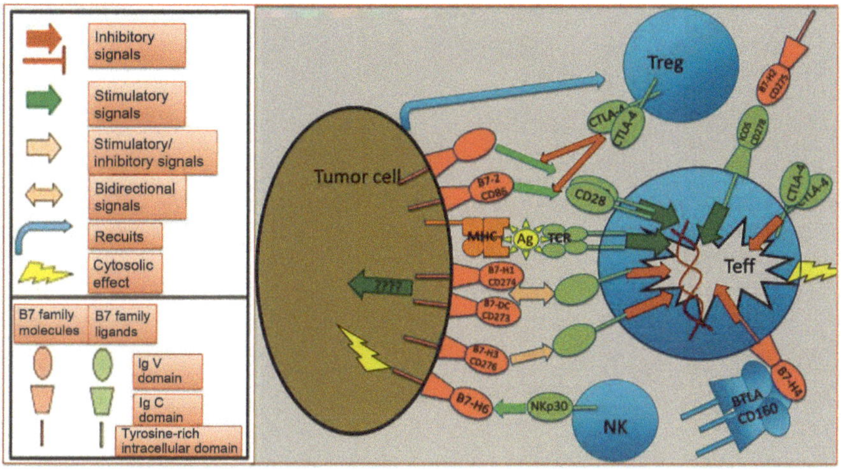

FIGURE 5.1 Expression of B7 family members and their receptors have complex interactions with the tumor immune environment.

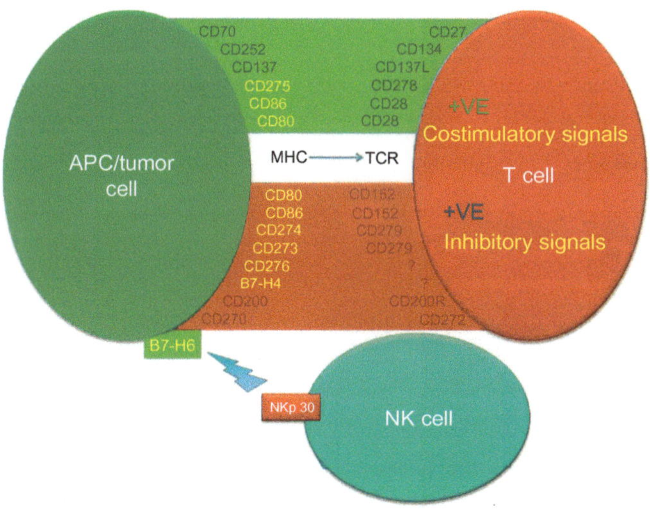

FIGURE 5.2 Expression of selected antigens expressed on the cell surface of APC or tumor cells and their costimulatory or inhibitory ligands.

B7-1 was also included in vaccine along with specific antigens, such as carcinoembryonic antigen (CEA) (Table 5.4). Recently, in a phase II trial for metastatic colorectal cancer, Kaufman et al. used a nonreplicating canarypox virus vector (ALVAC) expressing CEA and B7-1 in combination with chemotherapy. The observed objective response rate of 40.4% was similar to

TABLE 5.3 Therapeutic Potential of the B7 Family Molecules in Hematological Malignancies

B7 Target	Costimulatory Pathway	Preclinical Evidence Reference	Phase I/II Trial Agent
Augmentation of systemic antitumor immunity	CTLA-4 blockade	[13]	Ipilimumab
	PD-1/PD-L1 blockade	[14,15]	BMS936558, BMS936559, MK-3475
	ICOS pathway modulation	[16]	NA
Tumor-directed therapy against B7 targets	CD80	[13]	Galiximab
	PD-L1	[17,18]	NA
	B7-H6		NA
Augmentation of GVL	CTLA-4 blockade	[19]	Ipilimumab
	PD-1/PD-L1 blockade	[20]	NA
	ICOS pathway modulation		NA
Attenuation of GVHD	CTLA-4 stimulation		CTLA-4.Ig
	CD80/86 blockade		CD80/86 mAb
	ICOS pathway modulation	[21,22]	NA
Bioengineered T cells	CD28 CAR	[23]	Modified T cell
	CD80 CAR	[24]	Modified T cell
	NKp30 CAR		Modified NK cell
Antitumor vaccine augmentation	CTLA-4 blockade	[13]	Ipilimumab
	PD-1/PD-L1 blockade	[25,26]	NA
Treg depletion and inactivation	CTLA-4 blockade		NA

Note: mAb, monoclonal antibody; NK, natural killer; CTLA, cytolytic T-cell-associated sequence-4; PD, programmed cell death; ICOS, inducible costimulator; CAR, chimeric antigen receptor; and NA, there are currently no therapeutic agent available.

TABLE 5.4 Tumor Models and Clinical Trials of B7-CD28 Costimulatory Molecules

Tumor Model	Costimulatory Molecule	Therapeutic Strategy	Reference
Metastatic renal carcinoma	B7-1 (CD80)	Vaccination with B7-I-transfected autologous tumor cells in combination with systemic IL-2	[28–30]
Nonsmall cell lung cancer	B7-1 (CD80)	Vaccination with an adenocarcinoma cell line expressing B7-1 and human leukocyte antigen A1(HLA-A1) or A2	[29]
Metastatic colorectal cancer	B7-1 (CD80)	Vaccination with ALVAC vector expressing CEA and B7-1 in combination with chemotherapy	
CEA-expressing carcinoma, metastatic carcinoma, prostate cancer	B7-1 (CD80)	Vaccination with TRICOM vector	[31–33]
Metastatic melanoma, metastatic renal cancer, nonsmall cell lung cancer	CTLA-4	MDX-010 Ab blockade of CTLA-4 alone or in combination with vaccine, IL-2, and chemotherapy	[34,35]
Melanoma, metastatic colorectal cancer, advanced gastric cancer, and esophageal adenocarcinoma	CTLA-4	CP-675,206 Ab blockade of CTLA-4 alone or in combination with chemotherapy	[36–39]
Hematological malignancies	PD-1	CT-011 Ab blockade of PD-1	[40]
Advanced solid cancer	PD-1	MDX-1106 Ab blockade of PD-1	[41]
Solid tumors	PD-1	MK-3475	[42]
Cancers, multiple indications	PD-1	MDX-1105-01	[42]

Note: CTLA, cytotoxic T-lymphocyte antigen; PD-1, programmed death 1; B7-1 means CD80.

that reported for chemotherapy alone.[31] Improvements on new vaccine strategies led to the generation of viral vectors expressing a triad of costimulatory molecules (TRICOMs), such as B7-1, ICAM-1, and lymphocyte function-associated antigen 3 (LFA-3), along with CEA, mucin-cell-surface associated 1 (MUC-1), and prostate-specific antigen (PSA) antigens, with promising results in preclinical studies and clinical trials, both in terms of efficacy and safety[32–34] (Table 5.4). In this regard, a phase II randomized controlled trial of poxiviral-based PSA-targeted immunotherapy in patients with metastatic castration-resistant prostate cancer showed that the treatment was well tolerated and associated with 44% reduction in the death rate.[43] Recently, multitarget vaccine approaches were tested *in vitro*, resulting in enhanced antitumor immune response against hepatocellular carcinoma and glioma cell lines.[44,45] Several other preclinical evidences proved the efficacy of B7-1-based therapeutic strategy in the induction of tumor antigen-specific T-cell response.

B7 SUPERFAMILY OF COSTIMULATORY MOLECULES IN ANTITUMOR IMMUNOTHERAPY

B7-1/B7-2:CD28/CTLA-4

The B7-1/B7-2:CD28/CTLA-4 pathway is the best characterized pathway of T-cell costimulation and coinhibition and symbolizes the classical way where the ligand can bind two receptors for regulating both T-cell activation and tolerance. B7-1 (CD80) and B7-2 (CD86) are two ligands for both CD28 and CTLA-4. The balance between the activating and inhibitory signals derived from the engagement of CD28 and CTLA-4, respectively, is crucial to assure protective immunity, without falling into undesired autoimmunity. The expression of B7-1 and B7-2 is restricted to professional APCs, such as DCs, macrophages, and B cells. CD28 is constitutively expressed on the surface of T cells, whereas CTLA-4 expression is induced 24–48 h after T-cell activation, due to the action of lymphocyte cell kinase (Lck), Fyn, and resting lymphocyte kinase that phosphorylates CTLA-4, thus increasing its transport to the cell surface and preventing its internalization. CTLA-4 was shown to have higher affinity for both B7-1 and B7-2 than CD28 receptor.[10]

The B7-1/B7-2:CD28 pathway is the strongest costimulatory signal delivered by APCs to provide a full activation of T cells, promoting their proliferation and IL-2 secretion. The intracellular signaling of B7-1/B7-2:CD28 pathway occurs through the activation of phosphatidyl-inositol-3-kinase (PI3K)/Akt/nuclear factor-κappa B (NF-κB) and the mitogen-activated protein kinases (MAPKs) pathway, which support cell survival, memory development, proliferation, and cytokines production.[46] In contrast to the costimulatory signal derived from the binding of CD28 to B7-1 and B7-2, the engagement of CTLA-4 by these ligands provides a negative regulation of the immune response, as proved by the characterization of CTLA-4 deficient mice.

The tumor microenvironment is often characterized by the presence of anergic T cells, due to the lack of positive costimulatory molecules, mainly B7-1 and B7-2, on the surface of cancer cells.[27] One strategy to revert this scenario is to force B7 expression on tumor cells, rendering them able to activate T-cell immune response. Several studies showed that the induction of B7-1 on tumor cells was sufficient to stimulate the CD8 + T-cell-mediated rejection in several tumor models, as well as a memory response, but was insufficient to mediate rejection of poorly immunogenic tumors.[10] Several phase I clinical trials evaluated the efficacy of B7-1 transfected tumor cell vaccines, with or without IL-2, with encouraging preliminary results in patients affected by metastatic renal carcinoma and nonsmall cell lung cancer (Table 5.3).

Although effective as monotherapy in the treatment of small and immunogenic tumors, a combination of CTL-4 blockade with other immunotherapeutic strategies is needed to treat large and poorly immunogenic tumors. Combination of CTLA-4 blockade and irradiated tumor vaccine expressing granulocyte/macrophage colony-stimulating factor (GM-CSF) results in tumor rejection and reduction of tumor growth in the B16 melanoma model. Similar results have been reported for the poorly immunogenic SM1 mammary carcinoma line and a transgenic model of prostate carcinoma.[10,47] Moreover, the combination of anti-CTLA-4 with DNA vaccine increased T-cell immune response against melanoma-associated antigens and induced B16 tumor rejection.[48] In the same tumor model, the CTLA-4 blockade combined with CD25 + Treg depletion and vaccination was reported to be effective in inducing tyrosinase-related-protein-2-(TRP-2-) specific CD8 + T cells and in rejecting larger tumor loads.[49] An increased antitumor immunity in B16 melanoma model was reported following CTLA-4 blockade with peptide vaccine and a synthetic oligodeoxynucleotide as adjuvant.[50] The use of anti-CTLA-4 along with radiotherapy led to the improvement of survival rate in a mouse model of metastatic breast cancer, whereas CTLA-4 blockade in combination with chemotherapy provided clinical benefits in the murine myeloma model MOPC-315.[51,52]

CD80 in Lymphoma Growth Inhibition

The ability of the B cells to deliver the costimulatory signal to T cells by B7 molecules is very well established.[53,54] In contrast, whether the engagement of CD80 and CD86 molecules by CD28 and CTLA-4 affect the function of the B cells is very poorly documented.[55,56] Moreover, nothing is known precisely in the case of B-cell proliferation and differentiation by the engagement of CD80 and CD86 molecules. CD80 and CD86 serve as counter-receptors that transduce distinct signal to the APCs upon engagement by CD28 or CTLA-4. The intracellular domains of CD80 and CD86 are quite distinct and could mediate differential signal transduction. Such signaling could alter the B cells' ability to function as effector cells. However, there is

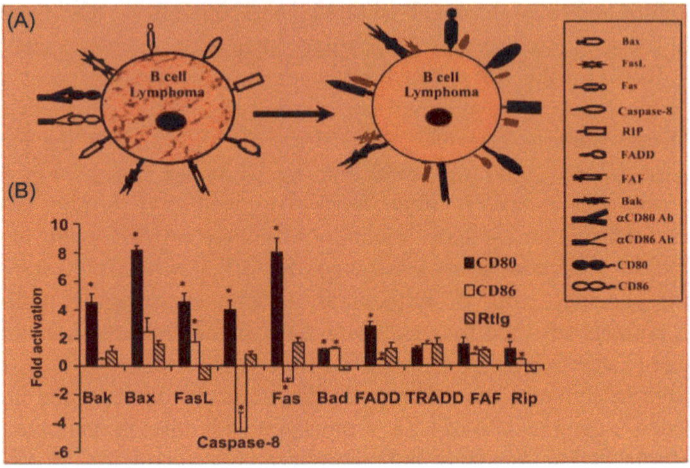

FIGURE 5.3 Modulation of the expression of proapoptotic molecules by CD80 and CD86 signaling.

indirect evidence reported earlier that CD28-CTLA-4/B7-signaling pathways may affect B-cell responses and the regulation of immunoglobulin (Ig) synthesis.[57,58] Our study was aimed to evaluate for the first time the role of CD80 and CD86 mediated signal transduction in the costimulation of B cells. The results show that triggering through CD80 specifically inhibits the proliferation and IgG secretion by LPS1-stimulated B cells. By contrast, CD86 chiefly augments the B-cell activity. Further, the growth of B-cell lymphomas could also be retarded by CD80 cross-linking. Signaling through CD80 inhibited the growth of the B-cell lymphoma by upregulating the expression of proapoptotic molecules caspase-3, caspase-8, Fas, FasL, Bak, and Bax and downregulating the levels of antiapoptotic molecule Bcl-x[L]. In contrast, triggering through CD86 augmented the level of antiapoptotic molecules Bcl-w and Bcl-x[L] and decreased the levels of caspase-8. Thus, the signals delivered by anti-B7-1 and -B7-2 antibodies can differentially regulate the activity of B cell and its lymphoma (see Figures 5.3 and 5.4).[1,2]

Costimulation signaling through CD80 in B-cell lymphomas can retard their proliferation by upregulating expression of proapoptotic molecules and downregulating antiapoptotic molecules and can therefore induce apoptosis. On the basis of our results recently, a phase I/II study of treatment with CD80-specific antibody has shown it to be quite effective in relapsed and refractory follicular lymphoma patients. Considering the importance of costimulation in the regulation of immune responses against relapsed cancer, the manipulation of this pathway to increase immunity represents a potential therapeutic approach. Furthermore, signaling by either anti-CD80 antibodies or through CD28-bearing T cells regresses the growth, augments the

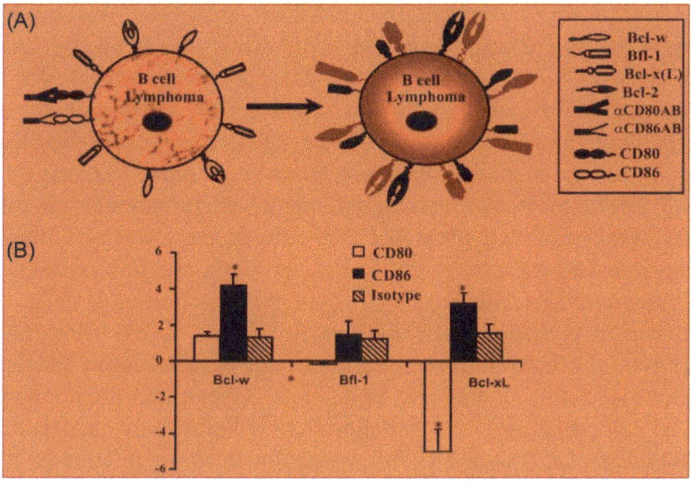

FIGURE 5.4 Modulation of the expression of antiapoptotic molecules by CD80 and CD86 signaling.

expression of proapoptotic molecules and induces apoptosis of CD80+ lymphomas. Therefore, immunotherapy utilizing anti-CD80 antibodies is a promising future treatment especially in the case of relapse and refractory lymphomas.[59,60]

The exact mechanism of sequence of signals provided by different costimulatory molecules in the stimulation and inhibition of B cells is largely unknown. We for the first time have attempted to analyze the distinct role of CD80 and CD86 costimulatory molecules in the activation and differentiation of B cells. From our study five major findings emerged which are as follows: (1) cross-linking by anti-B7-1 mAb (16-10A1) inhibited the proliferation and differentiation of B cells; (2) anti-B7-1 and CD40 mAbs acted synergistically and declined the growth of B-cell lymphomas; (3) induction of secretion of IgG isotypes by WEHI-279 cells was triggered with anti-B7-2 mAb; (4) anti-B7-2 mAb (GL1) promoted the growth and differentiation of B cells; and (5) anti-B7-1 mAbs induced apoptosis in B-cell lymphoma by enhancing the expression of caspase-3, caspase-8, Fas, FasL, Bak, and Bax and decreasing the expression of antiapoptotic molecules Bcl-x[L].[1,2,9] Our findings suggest that CD80 and CD86 costimulatory molecules are responsible for delivering the signals essential for the inhibition and expansion of B cells, respectively. To best of our knowledge, this was the first report regarding the role of CD80 and CD86 molecules in influencing the B-cell activity. To further provide weight to our findings of the regulatory capacity of anti-B7-1 and -B7-2 Abs in the activation of B cells, we utilized B-cell lymphomas, WEHI-279, which express CD80, CD86, and

CD40 molecules. More surprisingly, anti-CD80 and CD40 Abs could significantly arrest the proliferation of WEHI-279.[2] Thus it may be concluded that the signaling via CD80 and CD40 molecules may be responsible for inhibiting the growth of B-cell lymphomas. In contrast, costimulation through CD86 may help lymphomas to proliferate and secrete antibodies that may help lymphomas to evade immune surveillance. Further, triggering through CD80 and CD40 may help the regression of the lymphomas in the early stages. Although signaling through CD80 retards the growth of B-cell lymphomas by inducing the expression of Fas and FasL and in turn induces apoptosis, it fails to induce Fas and FasL or apoptosis in normal B cells.

At present, it is difficult to explain why ligation of B7-1 with anti-B7-1 has a differential effect on normal versus tumor B cells. Apart from demonstrating the expression of Fas and FasL by FACScan and their involvement in inducing apoptosis, we also monitored by ribonuclease protection assay the involvement of CD80 and CD86 molecules in the regulation of the activation of several pro- and antiapoptotic molecules in WEHI-279 B-cell lymphoma.[2] We have observed that signaling through CD80 molecule augmented the levels of proapoptotic molecules, that is, caspase-3, caspase-8, Fas, FasL, Bak, and Bax. This suggests that CD80 signaling induces apoptosis in WEHI-279 via a mechanism involving proapoptotic molecules caspase-3, caspase-8, Fas, FasL, Bak, and Bax, thus rendering WEHI-279 cells more vulnerable to apoptosis and therefore restricting the progression of the lymphoma. The T-cell costimulatory molecule CD28, which has a high and low binding affinity for CD86 and CD80, respectively, promotes T-cell survival by upregulating Bcl-x[L] and downregulating FasL expression.[2,61] Based on these results and our findings, it may be postulated that there may exist a probability that, when CD28 is ligated with CD86 it may deliver a protective signal necessary for the clonal expansion of B cells. In contrast to this, when CTLA-4 gets engaged with CD80, it may deliver a lethal signal responsible for controlling the clonal expansion of B cell and B-cell lymphomas. In contrast, signaling through CD86 increased the expression of antiapoptotic molecules Bcl-w and Bcl-x[L]. Thus, there may be a possibility that ligation of B7-2 on WEHI-279 may promote their survival by increasing the expression of antiapoptotic proteins Bcl-w and Bcl-x[L]. It has also been reported earlier that increased expression of Bcl-x[L] but not Bcl-2 could prevent the apoptosis in B-cell lymphoma WEHI-231.[62] Further, it has been reported that signaling through CD40 upregulated Bcl-x[L] and Bfl-1 and protected B-cell lymphoma from apoptosis.[63] Many studies have highlighted the lack of Costimulatory molecules as a predominant reason for the inefficient tumor rejection. Moreover, if the lymphomas express CD80, signaling through this molecule may impede their growth by inducing the expression of proapoptotic and downregulating the levels of antiapoptotic molecules and thereby facilitating apoptosis. It is important to mention here that CD80-mediated delivery of inhibitory signals may not only be responsible for apoptosis of CD80-bearing tumor cells, but may also be responsible in the regulation of immune responses and maintaining self-tolerance in B cells. Thus, in the case of tumors, ligation of B7-1 by anti-CD80 Ab may also deliver effective antitumor immunity. In conclusion, we report here that selective inhibition of B-cell proliferation and differentiation via CD80 signaling may be viewed as a novel strategy to restrict the undesired stimulation of B cell and progression of B-cell lymphomas. Moreover, costimulation through CD80 and CD86 can modulate the humoral response by transducing positive and negative signals in B cells and may control the progression of B-cell lymphomas.

Costimulation Through CD80 in Immunity Against Cancer

CD80 is a costimulatory molecule known for its role in T-cell activation and also in regulating normal and malignant B cells activity.[2] Surface CD80 is expressed transiently on activated B cells, macrophages, and DCs. Surprisingly, CD80 is downregulated on most of the cancer cells and the loss of CD80 alone is sufficient to allow them to escape the attack of the immune system and to impart anergy and apoptosis in tumor-infiltrating T cells.[64] In the absence of costimulation, recognition of antigens by T cells may not cause any response, even if tumor cells express MHC molecules and tumor-specific antigens (Figure 5.5). Hence most human malignancies that lack CD80 expression have been suggested to evade immune surveillance and therefore contribute for failure of immune recognition.[65] However, follicular lymphomas express CD80 and therefore could potentially be targeted by CD80 immunotherapies. Lack of either CD80 or MHC-I must be sufficient to allow tumor cells to evade immune response but it has been shown in some tumors that high expression of MHC-I and absence of costimulatory

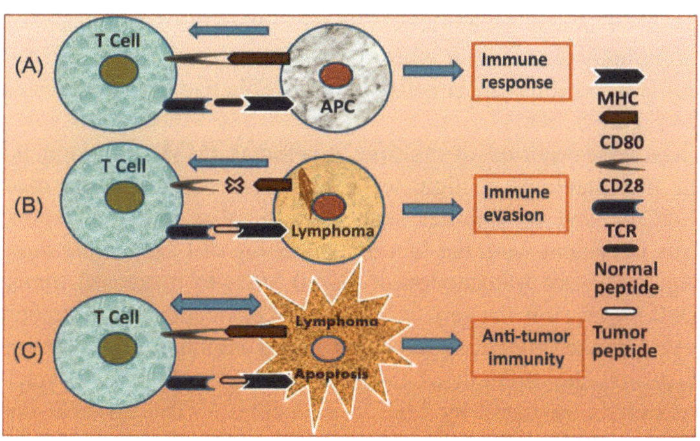

FIGURE 5.5 Reverse costimulation through CD80 in modulating the activity of cancer cells.

molecules renders them resistant to lysis by cytotoxic T lymphocytes (CTLs) (Figure 5.5A). It has been shown that high expression of MHC-I but lack of CD80 does not allow cytolysis of target cells by CTLs *ex vivo*. In contrast, CD80-transfected tumor cells become susceptible to lysis by CTLs *ex vivo*. Although priming of antitumor CTLs can also take place in absence of CD80, but the effector T cells are not produced without the expression of CD80 on tumor cells.[66] Interestingly, CD80 has also been known to enhance the memory response in CTLs.[67] This suggests that CD80 expression on a tumor is important for antitumor CTL effector function. Expression of CD80 on tumor cells confers direct presentation capacity to prime naive CTLs *in vivo*.[68] Transfection of tumor cells with CD80 will help in generating long-lasting immunity. Therefore, this approach may lead to the development of a successful vaccine against cancer.

CD80 expression is needed for the sustained predominance of CD8+ T cells within a tumor (Figure 5.5C). Transfection of CD80 cDNA into human erythro leukemia DR+ (HEL-DR+) cells induce the allogeneic response of purified T cells from both cord blood and peripheral blood of adult donors, demonstrating that CD80 expression could lead to accessory-cell-independent activation of naive T cells. Furthermore, in the P815 tumor system, CD86 was substituted for CD80, interestingly, no specific CTL activity was observed. Even though in the tumors that express CD86 there is a need for CD80 expression by host APCs for efficient eradication. Thus, it is apparent that transfection of CD80 in tumor cell serves as a co-factor for IL-2 production and in prevention of anergy by TCR ligation.[69] This suggests that expression of CD80 on cancer cells contributes towards the activation of T cells responsible for imparting anticancer immunity. The expression of CD80 on tumor cells also enhances natural killer (NK) cell recognition and lysis of tumors, which plays an important role in tumor immunity.[70] CD80 costimulation can direct the CD8 T cells to produce IL-2, proliferate and acquire cytolytic activity.[71] This helper independent generation of CTLs may have practical application in the development of tumor-specific immunotherapy.[72] So it is clear that downregulation of CD80 costimulatory molecule by various cancer cells acts as an effective immune evasion mechanism (see Figure 5.5B).

This has been reported in multiple myelomas (MM), carcinomas, leukemias, and transplantable malignancies, etc. Some of the colon carcinomas such as MC38, and melanomas such as B16, also lack the expression of CD80. This is evident from the fact that silencing of CD80 expression results in tumorigenicity and transfection of CD80 leads to decreased tumorigenicity.[73] CD80 expression triggers *in vitro* NK-cell-mediated cytotoxicity. The CD80 gene product functions as a triggering signal for NK-cell-mediated cytotoxicity and the strength of this response is such that it overrides the inhibitory signals mediated by MHC-I molecules.[74] The efficient control of solid allogeneic tumors by NK cells depends on co-delivery of both CD80 and MHC-I on the tumor cells. The co-delivery is required for optimal expansion and effector function of NK cells in response to both melanoma and plasmocytoma that express allogeneic MHC-I. The two signals required for T-cell function can also regulate NK cell immunity and reveal an important similarity between the innate NK cell response and the adaptive T-cell response. Furthermore, it has been reported that NK cells and CD8+ T cells can eliminate CD80 expressing tumors that are resistant to IL-12 gene therapy.[13,75] Hence expression of CD80 on tumor cells may also have an important bearing on NK cell effector function.

CD80 Gene Transfection of Tumor Cells to Generate Vaccine and Elicitation of Antitumor Response

The fact that CD80 plays an important role in immunity against cancer cells is now well established from the above discussion. Thus, it is apparent that expression of CD80 on cancer cells can enhance the immunity substantially (see Figure 5.5B,C). Expression of costimulatory molecule CD80 via somatic gene transfer represents one approach to improve the immunogenicity of tumor cells. Transfection of CD80 in colon cancer cells results in increased immunogenicity and tumor rejection. In contrast, silencing of CD80 expression in colon cancer cells resulted in lack of tumorigenicity.[73] The CD80 transfection into EL-4 cells, T-cell thymoma cell line, showed that CD80 plays an essential role in mediating *in vivo* antitumor rejection. Transfection of CD80 gene into various cancer cells, RMA, EL-4, P815, E6B2, B16, K1735, etc., has reduced or eliminated subsequent tumor growth in syngenic mice and can lead to the establishment of protective immunity against challenges with CD80-negative tumor cells.[68,76] The positive effects of CD80 gene transduction have also been thoroughly explored in a rapidly lethal hematopoietic leukemia cell line, which is nonimmunogenic by itself. A tumor cell engineered to provide optimal costimulation would then directly induce T-cell activation, proliferation, and differentiation in to effector cells, following recognition of the antigen. CD80 gene transfection resulted in loss of tumorigenicity and induction of protective immunity against subsequent challenges with the parental CD80 −/− cell line in immunocompetent syngenic mice. CD80 transfection has been shown to inhibit lymph node metastasis by the mechanism of enhanced immunogenicity.[77] Moreover, not only the presence but also the levels of CD80 expression can affect the tumor growth.[78] The cells generated by introduction of the CD80 gene can work as prophylactic or therapeutic vaccines against tumors that lack CD80 by means of eliciting a strong CTL and NK cell response, which is desired in antitumor immunity.[79]

The anticancer activity of the modalities, like γ-irradiation, mitomycin-C, melphalan, etc., is quite interesting that these exert their immuno-potentiating effect in tumor bearers by upregulating CD80 gene expression.[80] However, the mechanism by which surface expression of CD80 on tumor cells enhances the antitumor immunity seems to be the same as that which depends on the maturation state of DCs regulating immune response by CD80 expression, as the low expression of CD80 on immature DCs suppresses T-cell immunity in a CD80-dependent fashion and high CD80 expression by mature DCs promotes immunity.[81] Antitumor effects of CD80 expressing tumor cells can be mostly attributed to costimulatory activity resulting in activation, proliferation, and generation of CTLs. CD80 expression on tumor cells enhances their recognition by NK cells, hence causing enhanced lysis of tumor cells, which in turn makes the antigen available for the cross priming pathway, thereby generating systemic immunity to parental tumor. CD80 expression may protect T cells from activation-induced cell death upon recognition of tumor cell targets.[80] CD8+ T-cell precursors are directly primed by CD80-transfected tumors, which provide signal 1 and 2 to the T cells.[79] Indicating that, CD80-transfected cells serve directly as APCs in *in vivo* for the priming of naive CTLs.

Keeping in view the importance of the CD80 costimulatory molecule in antitumor immunity against cancer, the manipulation of this molecule to increase immunity represents a promising therapeutic and prophylactic approach. CD80 has been co-administered with various cytokine genes to elicit antitumor activity. A single intratumoral co-administration of CD80 with the IL-12 gene, by electroporation, elicited specific antitumor CTL response and eradicated the tumor from mice. This co-administration also maintains the high level of endogenous CD80 of tumor cells through STAT-1 expression.[82] The coexpression of CD80 and IL-12, administered by intratumoral injection with an adenovirus vector, effectively elicited antitumor immunity in a nonimmunogenic, therapy resistant, mouse pancreatic cancer model.[83] Recently it has been shown that primary tumor cells resected from cancer patients can be transfected effectively with CD80-SA (streptavidin) and that such transfected cells serve as APCs to induce autologous antitumor T-cell responses.[84] A dual modified tumor cell vaccine using CD80 and super antigen Staphylococcus enterotoxin A (a potent inducer of CTL activity and cytokine production) elicited significantly stronger antitumor immune responses *in vivo*.[85] When IFN-γ transfectant immunotherapy was used for cancer treatment; it promoted tumor progression. However interestingly, when a combination of IFN-γ and CD80 transfection immunotherapy was used, the cancer-promoting effect of cellular vaccination was completely abolished and instead the cancer vaccine potency to eradicate tumors increased.[86] Tumor cells transfected with CD80 and IL-7 genes induced CD28 and CD25 on tumor-infiltrating T cells and triggered strong antitumor responses. CD80 expression on tumor cells has been shown to eliminate resistance to IL-12 gene therapy. CD80+ MHC-II+-transfected tumor cells were used as a potent vaccine for stimulating tumor rejection in tumor bearing mice.[87] Transfection of CD80 gene into human hematopoietic malignant cell lines that are deficient in CD80 expression empowers their antigen presentation potency for activation of antitumor T cells. The combined expression of CD80 and IL-2 in acute myeloid leukemia blasts show increased stimulation of both allogeneic and autologous T cells. The stimulated lymphocytes secrete higher levels of Th1 cytokines and show specificity.[88] Repairing the deficiency in the CD80 costimulatory pathway in tumor cells can be a novel immunotherapeutic approach for human hematopoietic malignancies.

Use of CD80 alone or in combination with other cytokines etc. has shown healthy results in controlling the growth of tumors or their recurrence once they are removed from the body. In patients with metastatic renal cell carcinoma, the administration of CD80 gene modified autologous tumor cell vaccine in combination with systemic IL-2 in phase I clinical trials have shown promising results.[28] Apoptotic uveal melanoma cells expressing CD80 were efficient at inducing an immune response and served as potent immunogens. A tri-cistronic viral vector co-expressing IL-12 (IL-12p40 plus IL-12p35) and CD80 showed enhanced CTL and proliferative response in a myeloma tumor model.[89] This strategy could prove to be a novel adjuvant immunotherapy for the disease.[90] CD80 on tumor cells can also interact directly with CD28 on NK cells and activate them to inhibit tumor growth.[79] It has also been shown that CD80 vaccination after removal of a tumor is useful for the prevention of tumor recurrence. The model of CD80 enhancing tumor immunity is that exogenous CD80 acts as a costimulatory molecule to directly interact with CD28 on T cells, thus resulting in the activation of CD8+ T cells against tumor cells.

Costimulation through CD80 induces apoptosis via a mechanism involving proapoptotic molecules, consequently rendering the cells more vulnerable to apoptosis and therefore restricting their proliferation. It has been shown that overexpression of caspases is sufficient to cause apoptosis. The proapoptotic molecule (Bax) has been correlated with disease regression and shorter survival of B cells in chronic lymphocytic leukemia (CLL).[91–93] Resistance to apoptosis is also one of the mechanisms employed by tumor cells for evasion and it is not only relevant for tumorigenesis and resistance to chemotherapy but also influences immunosurveillance and immunotherapy. It is important to mention here that costimulatory molecule-mediated delivery of inhibitory signals may not only be responsible for the regulation of immune responses but also for apoptosis of CD80-bearing tumor cells. These studies categorically demonstrate that, tumor regression is not only the consequence of CD80-mediated activation of CTLs and NK cells but signaling through CD80 can also trigger death of lymphomas.[94,95]

Costimulatory Monoclonal Antibodies in Non-Hodgkin's Lymphoma and Chronic Lymphocytic Leukemia

The development of monoclonal antibodies, biological therapies that target tumor-associated antigens specifically, gives hope for improvement of survival in many cancers. Monoclonal antibodies make an important contribution to the therapeutic treatment of non-Hodgkin's lymphoma (NHL), CLL, breast cancer, and colorectal cancer. These antibodies can bind to their receptors on tumor cells specifically and block the binding of endogenous ligands, which leads to inhibition of phosphorylation of receptor-protein tyrosine kinases and inhibition of downstream signaling events.[96] Monoclonal antibodies that act through this mechanism include trastuzumab, which targets v-erb-b2 erythroblastic leukemia viral oncogene homolog 2(ERBB2); cetuximab, which targets EGFR; alemtuzumab a lymphocyte-depleting humanized monoclonal antibody with efficacy in the treatment of chronic lymphocytic leukemia targeting CD52;[97] and bevacizumab, which blocks angiogenic signaling by binding to and sequestering the ligand of VEGF receptor (VEGFR).[98] Rituximab is a highly specific mouse/human chimeric IgG1 antibody that targets CD20, a cell-surface protein expressed on 95% of B-cell lymphomas, has shown efficacy in patients with various lymphoid malignancies, including indolent and aggressive forms of B cell NHL and B-cell CLL. It inhibits cell proliferation and directly induces apoptosis.[99,100] It has been shown that patients can be treated safely and effectively with multiple courses of rituximab without induction of human antichimeric antibodies, cumulative myelosuppression, adverse hematological effects, and serious or opportunistic infections that are related to standard chemotherapy or radiotherapy.[99,101] Galiximab is a chimeric, anti-CD80, IgG1 antibody that targets CD80, which is constitutively expressed on a variety of lymphomas like diffuse large B-cell NHL, CLL, Hodgkin's lymphoma, and MM. Because of the favorable safety profile of galiximab and its lack of induction of myelosuppression, which is associated with typical standard chemotherapies, radiotherapy and other antibody therapies, it is an attractive agent for lymphoma therapy.[59,60] Galiximab has also shown promising results when used in combination with rituximab. These monoclonal antibodies bind to their targets specifically on the surface of cells and do not circulate in the plasma as free protein that could competitively inhibit antibody binding to lymphoma cells. Other properties of these monoclonal antibodies like long half-life, high specificity, and high safety standards compared with other cancer therapeutics together with their ability to bind to and modulate key players in signaling pathways that drive malignant transformation and enhance antitumor immune functions make them highly desirable therapeutic agents.

Anti-CD80 Antibody in Treatment of Lymphoma Patients

Over the past decade, the use of mAbs has emerged as an important component in treatment algorithms for patients with cancer, especially patients with B-cell NHL. The advantage of mAbs is that they provide targeted and effective therapy against cancer with less toxicity than standard chemotherapeutic agents. With the discovery of hybridoma technology in the 1970s the use of mAbs to treat patients with cancer has gained increasing in popularity.[102] Initial the results of preliminary clinical studies were disappointing due to limited antitumor activity. However, advances in tumor immunology and molecular biotechnology have led to the development of primatized, chimeric, and humanized mAbs with better antitumor activity and decreased immunogenicity.[103] The observation published by our laboratory on the induction of apoptosis on stimulation through CD80 has constituted a rationale for development of an anti-CD80 therapy for lymphomas. Preclinical studies indicate that targeting CD80 with anti-CD80 antibody has antitumor effects.[2,104,105] Anti-CD80 antibody therapy delays progression of lymphoma and clinical studies have shown promising results.[59,105,106] Recently, Biogene has developed an anti-CD80 antibody known as galiximab. Galiximab is a chimeric, anti-CD80, IgG1 lambda monoclonal antibody with human constant regions and primate (*Cynomolgus macaque*) variable regions. It is structurally indistinguishable from human antibodies and, therefore, is unlikely to be significantly immunogenic in humans. Some characteristics of the antibody are summarized in Table 5.5.

This indistinguishablity from human antibodies makes it more suitable for potential repeated dosing in lymphoma patients. The specificity of galiximab binding to human CD80 has been validated in competitive binding studies with several lymphoma cell lines. Preclinical *in vitro* and *in vivo* studies evaluated galiximab as a targeted therapy for lymphoma, with promising results. A phase I/II, single-agent, dose escalation, and multiple-dose study demonstrated that galiximab administration can decrease tumor burden in nearly half of all patients suffering from relapsed and refractory follicular lymphoma.[59] Treatment of relapsed/refractory follicular lymphoma with galiximab in an open-label, multicenter, phase I/II monotherapy trial in

TABLE 5.5 **Characteristics of Anti-CD80 mAb (Galiximab) in the Treatment of Lymphomas**

Characteristic Type	Property of Antibody
Antibody name	Galiximab or IDEC-114 or Anti-CD80 antibody
Type of antibody	Human–primate chimeric IgG1λ
Dose	125–500 mg/m^2 and half-life of 2–4 weeks in serum
Target	CD80 (B7-1) 60-kDa trans-membrane glyco-protein
Diseases	Follicular lymphoma, CLL, MM, etc.
Mechanism	Upregulation of proapoptotic and downregulation of antiapoptotic molecules, ADCC, complement-mediated cytotoxicity (CDC), NF-κB modulation, etc.
Side effects	Fatigue, asthenia, nausea, headache, dizziness, vomiting, etc. mostly grade 1 and 2

TABLE 5.6 Clinical Results of Patients with Relapsed or Follicular Lymphoma after Treatment with Anti-CD80 Antibody, Galiximab

Reduction in Tumor Burden		Percentage of Patients Showing Most Common Clinical AEs				
Percentage Reduction in Lesions	Number of Patients (%)	Adverse Event Type	Grade 1	Grade 2	Grade 3	Grade 4
75–100%	17 (49%)	Lymph node pain	3	3	0	0
≥50%	6 (17%)	Dyspepsia	5	0	0	0
≥50% but with disease progression	2 (6%)	Vomiting	3	3	0	0
New lesions	1 (3%)	Axillary pain	3	0	3	0
Nonmeasurable disease progression	1 (3%)	Dysguesia	5	0	0	0
Not available for measurement	4 (12%)	Loose stools	5	0	0	0
Headache			5	5	0	0

37 patients with median age of 56.5 years who received different doses of antibody has shown no dose-limiting toxicities and a favorable safety profile. The most common related adverse events (AEs) experienced were grade one or two (headache, fatigue, and nausea) with only two cases of grade three deep venous thrombosis and one case of grade 3 axillary pain. Only one (3%) of 37 patients showed cytopenias, which was also considered to be unrelated to galiximab but related to the studied disease.[107] Clinical results of this study have been summarized in Table 5.6.

Furthermore, in a study covering 242 patients receiving galiximab as part of multiple-dose psoriasis studies it has been demonstrated that its safety profile was similar to placebo: no T-cell or B-cell depletion was observed and none of the patients developed antigaliximab antibodies. Clinical results of this study have been summarized in Table 5.7.[104,106] Further a combination of galiximab and rituximab did not appear to increase the overall incidence of AEs or alter the AE profile. Studies in animal models of lymphoma have shown that a combination therapy of galiximab (anti-CD80) and rituximab

TABLE 5.7 Clinical Results of Patients with Moderate to Severe Plaque Psoriasis Showing Reduction in Psoriasis Area and Severity Index (PASI*) and Improvement in Physicians Global Psoriasis Assessment (PGA) after Treatment with an Anti-CD80 Antibody, Galiximab

Study days after treatment of patients with galiximab	15	29	36	43	50	57	71	99	127
Number of patients assessed after treatment	35	20	15	20	15	20	35	35	35
Percentage of patients showing ≥50% reduction in PASI*	3	10	7	15	20	20	23	26	29
Percentage of patients showing ≥75% reduction in PASI*	3	5	NA	10	NA	10	9	9	11

Note: *PASI is calculated in ill patients after treatment by visually assessing the extent of psoriatic involvement in four main body areas (head, trunk, upper extremities, and lower extremities) weighted by % of total body area and the severity of signs in those areas.
Taking all time points and all dose groups, 20 out of 35 patients (i.e., 57%) achieved a PGA rating of Good and seven patients (i.e., 20%) achieved a PGA rating of Excellent. NA: Not available.

(anti-CD20) has more clinical benefits, and when galiximab was combined with chemotherapeutic agents like fludarabine or doxorubicin, it enhanced the efficacy of anti-CD80 therapy significantly.[105] Recently, Leonard and co-workers have used a combination therapy of galiximab and rituximab for treatment of relapsed or refractory follicular lymphoma.[59] They found that this combination therapy does not alter the pharmacokinetics or immunogenicity but instead has the potential to avoid or delay chemotherapy or its associated toxicity or to amalgamate with other lymphoma therapies. Hence galiximab can be combined safely with a standard course of rituximab for treatment of relapsed or refractory follicular lymphoma. Based on these observations a phase III, randomized study has been initiated to evaluate the clinical benefits of rituximab therapy versus combination therapy.[107] A phase I/II study of galiximab in combination with rituximab therapy in patients with relapsed or refractory disease has shown promising preliminary results for clinical activity without added toxicity compared with single-agent rituximab alone.[60] The future plans in this direction include evaluating maintenance therapy with the combination treatment of galiximab and rituximab in follicular NHL and galiximab, rituximab, plus chemotherapy for follicular and diffused aggressive NHL.

Experimental and clinical results, make it quite evident that anti-CD80 antibody treatment is effective against relapsed and refractory follicular lymphoma. Future studies in other CD80-positive hematological malignancies (e.g., diffuse large B-cell NHL, CLL, Hodgkin's lymphoma, and MM) should also be taken under consideration.[59] Thus, anti-CD80 antibody immunotherapy may have a potent role in the treatment of CD80-bearing cancer cells because their binding can modulate the key molecules in the signaling pathway and enhance antitumor response. Considering the importance of CD80 signaling in the regulation of immune responses against cancer, the manipulation of this signaling pathway to increase immunity against cancer represents a potential therapeutic approach.

The FDA in 1997 approved rituximab an anti-Cd80 mAb for the treatment of patients with B-cell lymphoma and heralded the onset of a new era in cancer therapeutics.[108] The early use of rituximab as a single agent or in combination with systemic chemotherapy regimens has resulted in improved response rates and survival in patients with follicular lymphoma.[109,110] Prior to the incorporation of rituximab into standard antilymphoma regimens, estimated median overall survival time for follicular NHL patients was 8–10 years from initial diagnosis.[111] With the possible exception of allogeneic stem cell transplantation, there is no curative therapy for advanced follicular NHL.[112] Therapeutic options currently in use include single-agent rituximab, single-agent or combination chemotherapy ± rituximab, radio-immunotherapy, and involved-field radiotherapy (generally used for localized or chemotherapy-refractory disease). Commonly used single-agent chemotherapies include oral-alkylating agents and purine analogues. More aggressive combination drug regimens offer higher response rates than single agents, albeit at the cost of greater toxicity and no discernible improvement in long-term survival.[104,113] Historically, it has been shown that "watchful waiting" instead of immediate therapy did not adversely affect outcome in appropriately selected patients.[114] The fact that successful lymphoma therapies can be based on targeting pathways engaged in lymphomagenesis with less nonspecific toxicities than standard chemotherapy is a significant advancement in the treatment of B-cell lymphoma patients. Ongoing challenges in the treatment of patients with NHL consist not only in identifying biomarkers of response to specific "targeted" therapies, but also in the timely discovery and development of novel therapeutic agents with improved activity and decreased toxicity. In addition to rituximab, other mAbs targeting cell-surface antigen present on B-cell neoplasms are being actively studied in a large number of ongoing clinical trials.

Understanding of mechanisms by which tumor cells escape immune surveillance will help us to establish new and effective approaches to vaccination and immunotherapy. The success of novel cancer therapies depends on the identification of functional targets that play an essential role in tumor growth and metastasis, survival, and evasion from immunosurveillance. One of the most important immune evasion mechanism employed by tumor cells is the downregulation of the CD80 costimulatory molecule. Anti-CD80 therapies can be used to target tumors expressing CD80. The clinical success of anti-CD80 antibody for the treatment of refractory follicular lymphoma has stimulated great interest in the promise of antibody therapeutics for cancer. The qualities of galiximab, like long half-life and high specificity and safety compared with other cancer therapeutics, together with its ability to bind to and modulate key players in signaling pathways that drive malignant transformation and enhance antitumor immune functions, makes it a highly desirable therapeutic agent.

Most tumors do not regress but continue to grow in spite of the presence of spontaneous or antigen induced immune responses, due to downregulation of costimulatory molecules like CD80. It is now well established that T cells are rendered anergic due to the lack of costimulatory molecule(s) expression by tumor cells. Tumor cells are able to induce antigen-specific tolerance or anergy on the basis of MHC-I-restricted antigen presentation without the expression of costimulatory molecules. This unresponsiveness, however, can be reversed when tumor cells are genetically modified to express costimulatory molecules. A plethora of studies suggest that the insertion of genes encoding CD80 into tumors generally increases their immunogenicity and can be used as vaccine.

Recently, fusagene vectors were developed to encode multiple gene products like CD80 with cytokines or MHC molecules as fusion proteins from a single cistron to increase the immunogenicity of target tumor cells. The vectors generated could be used in immunotherapy for the treatment of MM, leukemias, and other cancers, as they have been shown to stimulate allogeneic mixed lymphocyte proliferation and augment increases in CTL and NK cell responses and IFN-γ release. Considering the importance of costimulation in the regulation of immune responses against relapsed cancer, the manipulation of this pathway to increase immunity represents a potential therapeutic approach. Furthermore, signaling by either anti-CD80 antibodies or through CD28-bearing T cells regresses the growth and augments the expression of proapoptotic molecules and induces apoptosis of CD80+ lymphomas. Therefore, immunotherapy utilizing anti-CD80 antibodies is a promising future treatment especially in the case of relapse and refractory lymphomas. Clinical studies have demonstrated that administration of anti-CD80 antibody can decrease tumor burden in patients suffering from lymphomas.[59] CD80 is expressed transiently on the surface of activated B cells and other APCs, including DCs, but is constitutively expressed on a variety of NHLs, including follicular lymphomas. Thus, CD80 is an attractive target for lymphoma therapy. Targeting CD80 on NHLs with anti-CD80 antibody can arrest their growth and therefore can serve as a therapeutic intervention for treating cancer.

A significant number of patients relapse or do not respond to rituximab due to intrinsic or acquired resistance. Hence, mAbs targeting other cell surface antigens on B-cell lymphomas are being studied. CD80 serves as an attractive target in the continued development of mAbs against lymphoma. Preclinical studies with galiximab, an anti-CD80 primatized mAb, have been encouraging and have demonstrated antitumor activity against various B-cell lymphoma models, both as a single agent as well as in combination with rituximab. Data were reviewed from a PubMed literature search from 1975 to 2009 and also included a review of abstracts from published proceedings of annual meetings from the American Society of Hematology and International Conference of Malignant Lymphoma, Lugano.

Galiximab (Biogen Idec, Inc., San Diego, CA) is a chimeric, primatized IgG1 1 mAb consisting of human constant and primate (*cynomolgus macaque*) variable regions targeting CD80. It binds specifically to CD80, which is transiently expressed on the surface of activated B cells and APCs, including DCs, but is constitutively expressed on a variety of NHLs, including follicular lymphoma (FL).[115] Thus, CD80 serves as an attractive target for the development of antilymphoma therapy. Galiximab is emerging as an interesting and effective therapy for the treatment of patients with NHL, especially in combination with rituximab. Its favorable toxicity profile makes it an attractive alternative to existing agents. This "primatized" antibody is structurally indistinguishable from human antibodies and, therefore, is not significantly immunogenic in humans. Although a number of *in vivo* as well as *in vitro* studies point towards possible "unique" mechanisms of action of galiximab, more studies are needed to fully understand this agent's antitumor activity, as well as to establish strategies by which to optimize its efficacy. However to further assess the therapeutic role of galiximab in the treatment of patients with follicular and other lymphoma subtypes, as monotherapy or in combination with rituximab or systemic chemotherapy, additional studies designed are under active consideration.[116,117]

FULLY HUMANIZED ANTI-CTLA-4 ANTIBODY IN TREATMENT OF TUMORS

Ipilimumab (Fully Humanized Anti-CTLA-4 Antibody) in the Treatment of Tumors

The encouraging results obtained in preclinical models led to the development of two fully humanized anti-CTLA-4 antibodies, MDX-010 (ipilimumab), and CP-675,206 (tremelimumab) (Table 5.3). Ipilimumab is an IgG1 with a plasma half-life of 12–14 days, and it was approved by the FDA in March 2011 for the treatment of advanced melanoma (Bristol-Myers Squibb, Princeton, NJ). Both agents are able to recognize human CTLA-4 and block the interaction of CTLA-4 with CD80 or CD86, but their exact mechanism of action is not fully understood. Preliminary data about an increase in antigen-specific effector T cells following ipilimumab treatment in combination with vaccine in three melanoma patients are also published.[118] Ipilimumab and tremelimumab were tested in ovarian, breast, prostate, colon carcinoma, and, mainly, in melanoma and renal cell cancer clinical trials.[119] Several early phase II studies evaluated ipilimumab in metastatic melanoma, reported an objective response rate ranging from 6% to 21% and a disease-control rate of about 30%.[34,35,120] Recently, a multicenter single-arm phase II study evaluated the efficacy and the safety of ipilimumab monotherapy in patients with pretreated advanced melanoma. Patients ($n = 155$) were treated with ipilimumab at 10 mg/kg and the authors showed that 1- and 2-year survival rates were 47.2% and 32.8%, respectively, with a median overall survival of 10.2 months.[121] Moreover, a randomized, double blind, placebo-controlled, phase II trial of ipilimumab at 10 mg/kg, with or without budesonide, in 115 patients with unresectable stage III or IV melanoma, showed that 2-year survival rate was approximately 40% in each arm.[122] In another randomized, double blind, multicenter, phase II, dose-ranging study, 217 melanoma patients were randomly assigned to receive ipilimumab at 10 mg/kg ($n = 73$), 3 mg/kg ($n = 72$), or 0.3 mg/kg ($n = 72$). The authors observed a dose-dependent antitumor effect of ipilimumab, with the best overall response of 11.1% in patients treated with 10 mg/kg.[120] Ipilimumab was also tested in combination with other therapeutic agents such as IL-2, vaccine or chemotherapy, such as dacarbazine.[123–125] In particular, interesting results came from the phase III trial by Hodi et al.; in this study, melanoma patients were randomized to receive ipilimumab 3 mg/kg, with or without a gp100 peptide vaccine, or the vaccine alone. The primary endpoint of the study was the overall survival. The median overall survival was approximately 10.0 months among patients receiving ipilimumab (with or without gp100 vaccine), as compared with 6.4 months among patients receiving gp100 alone.[126] In another phase III study, the administration of ipilimumab (at a dose of 10 mg/kg) in combination with dacarbazine was associated with a significant improvement in overall survival among patients with previously untreated metastatic melanoma.[125] Ipilimumab was also tested in other types of malignancies. In a phase II study on 61 patients affected by metastatic renal cell carcinoma, ipilimumab was administrated at a dose of 1 mg/kg or 3 mg/kg; five of 40 patients treated with 3 mg/kg had a partial response.[127] A recent phase II study compared the addition of ipilimumab to carboplatin and paclitaxel chemotherapy in nonsmall cell lung cancer patients. Ipilimumab was administered either concurrently or in a phased schedule after receiving the first two cycles of chemotherapy. Patients treated with ipilimumab plus chemotherapy, in concurrent and sequential regimens, showed an improved overall survival compared with patients receiving chemotherapy alone.[128]

Tremelimumab (Fully Humanized Anti-CTLA-4 Antibody) in the Treatment of Tumors

Tremelimumab (CP-675,206) is fully humanized anti-CTLA-4 an IgG2 antibody with a plasma half-life of approximately 22 days (Pfizer, New York, NY). Tremelimumab was first evaluated in the treatment of metastatic melanoma. A phase I clinical trials evaluating the maximum-tolerated dose of tremelimumab showed antitumor activity of this drug in melanoma patients.[36] Other phase I/II studies reported stable disease (SD) occurring in about 30% of melanoma patients treated with tremelimumab and an objective antitumor response in 10% of patients.[37,129] A phase II study evaluated the antitumor activity of 15 mg/kg tremelimumab in 246 patients affected by melanoma, and reported an objective response rate of 6.6%, with duration of response ranged from 8.9 to 29.8 months.[130] Tremelimumab was also tested in cancers others than melanoma, both as monotherapy and in combination therapy, such as metastatic renal cell carcinoma, metastatic colorectal cancer, and advanced gastric and esophageal adenocarcinoma, but not significant clinical improvements were reported.[38,39,131] The treatment with both ipilimumab and tremelimumab is associated with inflammatory AE like rash, diarrhea, colitis, and hypophysitis; this side effect profile could be linked to the potentiation of Th17 cell differentiation following CTLA-4 blockade.[132]

ICOS-L:ICOS Costimulatory Pathway

The inducible costimulator (ICOS, CD278) is a costimulatory receptor that is weakly expressed on naive T cells and quickly upregulated in activated CD4+ and CD8+ T cells. A constitutive expression of ICOS by CD25+CD4+Foxp3+ Tregs has also been reported.[133] The cognate ligand for ICOS is ICOS-L (B7h, B7RP-1, CD275), which is expressed by professional APCs and by peripheral epithelial and endothelial cells following TNF-α stimulation.[134] The ICOS:ICOS-L pathway provides a key costimulatory signal for T-cell proliferation and, mainly, for T-cell survival. Moreover, ICOS regulates development and response of T follicular helper (Tfh), Th1, Th2, and Th17 cells and plays roles in the maintenance of memory effector T cells and Tregs homeostasis.[135] Due to its role in sustaining T-cell activation and effector functions, targeting ICOS:ICOS-L could represent a plausible approach to enhance antitumor immunity. The ICOS-L costimulation, through its expression on tumor cells, was capable of inducing cancer regression in Sa1/N fibrosarcoma and J558 plasmacytoma models.[136,137] Systemic treatment with murine ICOS-L-IgG fusion protein was effective in promoting INF-γ-dependent antitumor immunity in MethA fibrosarcoma and B16F1 melanoma tumor models.[138] Recent data showed an increase of ICOShi CD4+ effector T cells percentage after CTLA-4 blockade in several cancer models. In addition, upon CTLA-4 blockade, this cell population produced greater levels of INF-γ than ICOSlo CD4+ T cells, suggesting that ICOS could be used as a marker for CD4+ effector T-cell response.[16,139,140]

A downregulation of ICOS was shown in colon cancer patients and the expression of ICOS in tumors was associated with a greater survival of melanoma patients.[141,142] A recent study investigated the role of ICOS in the Tregs in melanoma and demonstrated the selective expression of ICOS on a "hyperactivated" Treg population, which strongly inhibits T-cell response through IL-10-mediated APCs suppression.[143] Moreover, ICOS-L was expressed by both cultured and freshly isolated melanoma cells from stage IV melanoma patients and could provide costimulation through ICOS for the activation and expansion of Tregs in the tumor microenvironment, as another mechanism of escape from immune surveillance.[144] Thus, targeting costimulatory and coinhibitory molecules on Tregs might be a promising approach for modulating peripheral tolerance in cancer patients.

PD-L1/PD-L2:PD-1 Costimulatory Pathway

Programmed cell death 1 (PD-1) is a negative costimulatory receptor belonging to the B7/CD28 family. PD-1 expression is induced on activated T cells, B cells, monocytes, DCs, and, at low levels, on natural killer T cells (NKT). Negative costimulatory signals mediated via PD-1 and CTLA-4 are not redundant; in fact PD-1 mainly acts in regulating inflammatory responses in peripheral tissues, whereas CTLA-4 modulates T-cell priming in lymphoid organs. In addition, in contrast to CTLA-4, PD-1 is able to block TCR- and CD28-mediated activation through the recruitment of inhibitory phosphatases, such as SHP-2, which inhibits the induction of PI3K activity.[145] PD-1 has two known ligands belonging to the B7 family: PD-L1 (B7-H1) and PD-L2 (B7-DC). To date, one of the major differences between these ligands concerns their expression pattern. PD-L1 mRNA is broadly expressed in multiple peripheral tissues such as heart, placenta, muscle, fetal liver, spleen, lymph nodes, and thymus; PD-L1 protein has been found in activated T cells, B cells, monocytes, DCs, endothelial cells, and myocardium and can be upregulated following exposure to type I or type II interferon, providing a negative feedback mechanism to dampen immune response.[145] On the contrary, PD-L2 expression is largely restricted to activated macrophages and DCs, but only PD-L2 mRNA can also be observed in the human heart, placenta, lung, and liver.[17]

CD279 (PD-1), CD274 (PD-L1), and CD273 (PD-L2) Expression in Malignancy

Although initial *in vitro* work showed PD-L1/PD-L2.Ig transmitted stimulatory signals to activated lymphocytes binding to their ligand PD-1 conveyed potent suppressive signals.[17] Evidence for bidirectional signaling emerged from murine B-cell- and T-cell-specific gene deletion and transplantation experiments. Knock-out of T-cell-specific PD-1 or B-cell-specific PD-L2 impaired long-lived plasma cell formation, which implied a stimulatory role for reverse signaling. Receptor/ligand pairing is also more promiscuous than originally believed. A search for binding partners for CD80 using *Ctla-4*$^{-tl}$*Cd28*$^{-d2}$ activated CD4+ T cells suggested PD-1 as a candidate, with CD80 signaling through PD-1 independent of CTLA-4 or CD28, to inhibit T-cell proliferation.[146] The complexity of the B7 system is becoming clear: context and direction of signaling determines responder cell outcome.

CD279 is invariably expressed in angioimmunoblastic T-cell lymphoma, frequently in CLL, but absent in most other NHL. CD279 is expressed in the immune microenvironment of NHL, where it may have a prognostic significance.[147] Evidence for expression of CD274 in NHL is sparse and inconsistent. Immunohistochemistry and flow cytometric studies have shown expression by the malignant cell in the majority of primary mediastinal large B-cell lymphoma and anaplastic large cell lymphoma (ALCL), a minority of diffuse large B-cell lymphoma, and not at all in most other NHL. CD274 is overexpressed in the Hodgkin and Reed-Sternberg (HRS) cells of classic Hodgkin lymphoma (CHL) associated with copy number aberrations and activating translocations involving the 9p24 chromosomal region containing the CD273 and CD274 genes,[148] and upstream through the CD274 and CD273 expression-regulating JAK2 pathway.[149] Limited *in vitro* evidence suggests that there is CD274-dependent suppression of T cells in CHL, evidenced by suppressed proliferation and IFN-γ production.

There is variable expression of CD274 in myeloma with evidence for an important role in myeloma-induced immunosuppression. CTL generated *in vitro* by exposure to IFN-γ-treated myeloma cell lines show impaired cytolysis of subsequently presented target myeloma cells NK-cell trafficking, and cytotoxic potency *in vitro* is augmented by pretreatment with anti-PD-1 mAb. An autologous transplantation and costimulator/vaccine-based treatment strategy for myeloma in a cell line-based mouse model, which had showed evidence for the emergence of dysfunctional circulating CD279-expressing CD8+ T cells, is augmented by the administration of PD-L1 antibodies.[150–152] While somewhat conflicting and lacking functional corroboration, these findings suggest that therapeutic modulation of this axis in hematologic malignancy may have a role.

Therapeutic Modulation of PD-1 (CD274), PDL-1 (CD279), and PDL-2 (CD273)

The PD-1/PD-L1/PD-L2 axis has been widely demonstrated to contribute to failed antitumor immunity. *Pd-1*$^{-d-}$ mice and *Pd-1*$^{wt/wt}$ mice treated with anti-PD-L1 antibody demonstrate superior rejection of PD-L1-expressing tumors through PD-1-dependent and -independent pathways.[14,18] Growth of pancreatic cancer cells in immunocompetent B6 mice is impaired by administration of anti-PD-1 or PD-L1 mAbs.[15] Tumor-specific T cells fail to lyse melanoma cells in host 2C/*Rag2*$^{-ag}$ mice despite stimulatory IFN-γ treatment because IFN-γ also induces upregulation of immunosuppressive PD-L1.[153] PD-L1 is expressed in many tumors and cell lines and appears to be associated with poorer outcome in solid malignancy, while PD-1 expression by tumor-infiltrating lymphocytes (TILs) may also confer poorer outcomes. After treatment using a tumor vaccination strategy of murine acute leukemia, long-lived residual leukemia cells were found to upregulate PD-L1, which suggests a mechanism of leukemia persistence and relapse.[154] These cells resisted CTL-mediated cell lysis, which could be overcome by anti-PD-L1 mAbs. However, blockade using anti-PD-1 mAbs did not reverse CTL resistance, while blocking CD80 had a similar effect to a PD-L1 block. The B7 system's complexity is further illustrated by these findings: CD274 appears to have further immunosuppressive binding partners, while CD80 may be capable of mediating suppressive as well as costimulatory signals.[155]

There is sparse and conflicting evidence for CD274 (PD-L2) expression in acute leukemia,[156] although the molecule is apparently upregulated on malignant cell exposure to IFN-γ or Toll-like receptor (TLR) ligand, and at relapse. Evidence for reduced T-cell-mediated specific lysis *in vitro* correlates with CD274 expression and is reversible by blocking CD274.[157] Functional work in CLL has demonstrated a clear role for the PD-1/PD-L1 axis in mediating systemic, as well as antitumor, immune defects. Expression of CD279 by circulating T cells and CD274 by leukemia and FL cells is greater than in nonmalignant control cells, while CD274 expression is associated with poorer clinical outcome. T cells derived from patients with various malignancies have impaired *in vitro* ρ-GTPase signaling with reduced immune synapse formation This defect is reversed by treatment with anti-PD-1 and anti-PD-L1 mAbs, along with blockade of further inhibitory molecules CD200, CD270, and CD276 (B7-H3). Lenalidomide exposure also reverses this defect, coincident with downregulation of CD274 and CD276 expression.[158] These findings, along with evidence that CD80 expression is upregulated on lenalidomide-exposed CLL cells,[159] provide some insight into the drug's mechanism of action. In patients with adult T-cell leukemia/lymphoma (ATLL), CD279 expression on CD8 + T cells is upregulated compared with ATLL-free human T-cell lymphotrophic virus (HTLV1+) controls.[160]

PD-L1 aberrant expression has been reported in many human cancers, such as glioblastoma, melanoma, and cancers of the head and neck, lung, ovary, colon, stomach, kidney, and breast.[161,162] Moreover, in several follow-up studies, the expression of PD-L1 correlates with a poor prognosis of patients.[15,163–165] Based on these experimental evidences, PD-L1 blockade has been proposed for cancer immunotherapy. Two independent studies have shown that forced expression of PD-L1 in the murine myeloma cell line P815 render them more resistant to *in vitro* cytolysis and less susceptible to rejection than control when inoculated in mice.[18] In addition, the treatment with anti-PD-L1 mAbs was capable of inhibiting the growth of P815-PD-L1 *in vivo*.[14] PD-1 blockade was able to restore the antitumor immunity to accelerate tumor eradication in murine squamous cancer cell line SCCVII and in P815 cell line and to block both CT26 colon carcinoma metastasis to the lung and B16 melanoma metastasis to the liver. *In vivo* studies in these tumor models examined the combination of anti-PD-1 mAb with GM-CSF-secreting tumor cell vaccine and reported that the administration of anti-PD-1 mAb enhanced the efficacy of vaccine by increasing number and activity of tumor-specific CD8 + T cells.[166]

Recent a study reported that the combination of PD-1 blockade and NKT cell activation results in increased antitumor responses in a melanoma model.[167] A reduced number of Tregs at the tumor site was observed after the treatment with anti-PD-1 mAb and the TLR agonist CpG, which suggests that it could be another mechanism by which PD-1 blockade exerts antitumor effects.[168] The expression of PD-L1 on DCs is also able to block antitumor T-cell response; myeloid DCs expressing PD-L1 isolated from ovarian cancer poorly stimulated T cells and PD-L1 blockade could revert this scenario.[169] In addition, the anti-PD-L1 therapy was observed to revitalize "exhausted" antiviral CD8 + T cells in animals with chronic viral infections.[170] The promising results in preclinical models have led to the development of two humanized antibodies against PD-1 receptor that block its interaction with PD-L1:CT-011 and MDX-1106 (Table 5.4). A preclinical study evaluated the combination of CT-011 with low dose of cyclophosphamide and with a tumor vaccine; the authors reported the complete regression of established tumors in most of the animals treated.[171] Benson et al. reported that CT-011 enhances NK-cell migration toward malignant plasma cells in MM.[152] To date, only phase I clinical trials have been conducted to evaluate both efficacy and safety of these two agents. In a phase I trial enrolling 17 patients with advanced hematological malignancies, the treatment with CT-011 at doses ranging from 0.2 to 6 mg/kg led to clinical improvement in 33% of patients.[40] Recently, the administration of CT-011 in combination with autologous DC/myeloma fusion-vaccine was demonstrated to stimulate T-cell responses after vaccine administration.[25] The efficacy of MX-1106 was evaluated in a phase I study enrolling 39 patients with advanced solid cancers (melanoma, colorectal cancer, castrate-resistant prostate cancer, nonsmall cell lung cancer, and renal cell carcinoma) obtaining very promising results; phase II and III trials are under evaluation.[41] In particular, it will be interesting to evaluate the combination of anti-PD-1 with other agents, such as anti-CTLA-4 mAb, vaccines, and chemotherapy. Several phase II clinical trials are testing the safety and the efficacy of these two PD-1 antibodies in several types of cancer.[172] MK-3475 and MDX-1105-01 are other two antibodies against PD-1 and PD-L1, respectively, which are currently being investigated in phase I clinical trials[42] (also see Table 5.4).

Fully humanized IgG4 mAbs targeting the PD-1/PD-L1 axis have reached clinical trials. Anti-PD-L1 therapy (BMS936559) (see Table 5.4) was administered to 160 heavily pretreated patients with a diverse group of solid tumors in a phase 1 trial[173] Objective and often durable responses were observed in up to 19% of patients, along with autoimmune and infusion reactions consistent with the murine PD-L1$^{-/-}$ models. A similar clinical trial of an anti-PD-1 monoclonal antibody therapy (BMS936558) demonstrated comparable response rates in 296 patients.[174] There was an association between response and level of tumor PD-L1 expression. Further combination therapy approaches using anti-PD-1 mAbs are under way, which include combination with the anti-CTLA-4 mAb ipilimumab in melanoma (NCT01024231), with conventional combination chemotherapy in nonsmall cell lung cancer (NCT01454102) and with tyrosine kinase inhibitors sunitinib and pazopanib in renal cell carcinoma (NCT01592370). Another PD-1 antibody (MK-3475) has also shown activity in patients with advanced solid tumors.[175] A phase 1 safety and pharmacokinetic study of the anti-PD-1 mAb in advanced diverse hematologic malignancies showed a reasonable safety profile and a 33% overall response rate (ORR)[40] with further monotherapy and combination therapy trials proposed. The results are promising, but these drugs remain at an early stage of development and are likely to find their most active role as immune adjuvants to conventional therapy.

HVEM:BTLA/CD160 Costimulatory Pathway

The BTLA is another member of the B7/CD28 family acting as a negative costimulatory receptor. The constitutive expression of BTLA has been reported, at low levels, on naive B and T cells, Tfh, macrophages, DCs, NKT cells, and NK cells, but unlike CTLA-4 and PD-1, BTLA is not expressed on Tregs.[176] The HVEM, a member of TNFR superfamily, has been identified as a BTLA ligand. HVEM expression is high in naive T and B cells, but it decreases during T-cell activation. HVEM is also expressed on DCs, Tregs, monocytes, NK cells, and neutrophils, and in non-hematopoietic cells, such as parenchymal cells. In addition to BTLA, HVEM binds also CD160, another member of the B7/CD28 family. CD160 is highly expressed on CD56dimCD16 NK cells, NKT cells, $\gamma\delta$ T cells, CD8+CD28− T cells, a small subset of CD4+ cells and intestinal intraepithelial T cells.[176] HVEM also interacts with LIGHT (described below in the text) and lymphotoxin alpha (LTα) of TNFR family, as and such is a unique example of a direct interaction between the two families. Therefore, HVEM is considered a molecular switch because of its ability to regulate the immune response, which depends on which cognate ligand binds. The role of BTLA as a negative costimulatory receptor has been shown by the phenotype of BTLA deficient mice, which were more susceptible to develop autoimmune disorders, and by the *in vitro* observation that anti-BTLA agonists drive negative signals to T cells.[177] The engagement of BTLA results in the inhibition of CD3/CD28 T-cell activation. BTLA signals through the recruitment of SHP-2 phosphatase, but the downstream target of SHP-2 is unclear. Anyway, recent studies showed that triggering BTLA signaling in B cells resulted in blocking B-cell proliferation through the inhibition of phosphorylation of some transcription factors like NF-κB.[178]

The similarity between BTLA and PD-1 signaling could justify a possible use of BTLA blockade to enhance antitumor immunity. The expression of BTLA was found in CLL/small lymphocytic lymphoma.[179] Moreover, soluble BTLA seems to enhance antitumor efficacy of the HSP70 vaccine in murine TC-1 cervical cancer mice.[180] Recently, a study by Derré et al. demonstrated the potentiality of targeting BTLA for cancer immunotherapy, and reported that BTLA is expressed on tumor antigen-specific CD8 + T cells from melanoma patients and that this molecule inhibits their fully functionality; following the vaccination with CpG adjuvants, the authors observed a downregulation of BTLA, with a partial recovery of CD8 + T cells functionality.[181] BTLA-HVEM blockade showed antitumor effects in murine TC-1 cervical cancer model *in vivo*, resulting in downregulation of IL-10 and TGF-beta and in activation of DCs in IL-12- and B7-1-dependent manner.

In addition, BTLA-HVEM blockade alone was not effective in eradicating the tumor, whereas the combination with HSP70 vaccine improved antitumor immunity by increasing IL-2 and INF-γ production and decreasing IL-10, TGF-beta, and Foxp3 transcription levels in the tumor microenvironment.[180] The evidences supporting a negative costimulatory function for CD160 come from *in vitro* studies because CD160 deficient mice have not been generated. CD160 agonists strongly inhibited CD4+ T-cell proliferation and cytokines production and reduced INF-γ secretion by NK cell line.[182] Recently, Cai et al. reported a strong inhibition of CD3/CD28-induced T-cell activation after the use of CD160 agonists, but the downstream intracellular pathways involved are not known.[183] Indeed, Liu et al. reported that CD160 is expressed in B-cell CLL, in which its engagement mediates survival and growth signals. In fact, CD160 activation was associated with upregulation of antiapoptotic genes Bcl-2, Bcl-xL, and Mcl-1 and, consequently, with reduced mitochondrial membrane potential collapse and cytochrome c release. CD160 engagement also induced cell cycle progression and proliferation.[184] A recent study examined the expression of CD160 in 811 cases of B-cell lymphoproliferative disorders (B-LPD). The authors showed that CD160 was expressed in 98% of CLL cases, 100% of hairy cell leukemia cases, 15% of mantle cell lymphoma in the leukemic phase, and 16% of other B-LPD cases, whereas it was absent in the normal B-cell lineage.[185] Recently, Chabot et al. suggested a role for CD160 in tumor neoangiogenesis. CD160 was expressed on newly formed blood vessels in human colon carcinoma and mouse B16 melanoma, but not in the healthy vessels. Treatment with anti-CD160 monoclonal antibody CL1-R2 in combination with cyclophosphamide chemotherapy resulted in the regression of tumor vessels in B16 melanoma-bearing mice.[186] Further studies are needed to clarify this pathway so as to design potential CD160/BTLA-based antitumor therapeutic strategies.

B7-H3 and B7-H4 Costimulatory Pathway

B7-H3 and B7-H4 (B7x, B7S1) are two of the newer members of the B7 family. B7-H3 expression has been found to be inducible on T cells, NK cells, and APCs. B7-H3 is also broadly expressed on osteoblasts, fibroblasts, and epithelial cells, as well as in liver, lung, bladder, testis, prostate, breast, placenta, and lymphoid organs. To date, only one potential receptor of B7-H3 on activated T cells named TLT-2 has been identified.[187] There are conflicting data about the functions mediated by B7-H3, as both stimulatory and inhibitory properties have been reported. Because of these controversial results, the possible existence of additional receptors for B7-H3 has been taken into consideration.

Recently, several works reported B7-H3 expression in different human cancers, as reviewed by Loos et al. The double stimulatory and inhibitory nature of B7-H3 signaling also appeared in murine cancer models and in human cancers. The authors showed that B7-H3 expression is associated both with favorable and adverse clinic-pathologic features.[187] Due to its immunomodulatory ability, B7-H3 blockade could be a potential anticancer immunotherapy, but the controversial findings about its role remain to be elucidated.

B7-H4 mRNA is broadly expressed in the peripheral tissues, whereas protein expression is restricted to activated B cells, T cells, and monocytes. Several studies reported the expression of B7-H4 in many human cancers, such as nonsmall cell lung cancer, ovarian cancer, prostate cancer, breast cancer, and renal cancer. To date, the cognate receptor of B7-H4 on activated T cells remains unclear, although BTLA has been reported as a possible receptor. Unlike B7-H3, which shows opposite functions, B7-H4 mediates a negative costimulatory signal. B7-H4 strongly inhibited T-cell proliferation and IL-2 secretion, and its blockade with antagonistic mAbs resulted in *in vitro* enhanced T-cell response and *in vivo* exacerbation of EAE.[188,189]

Recent studies indicate that B7-H4 could be a potential diagnostic/prognostic marker and/or therapeutic target for several cancers. In fact, B7-H4 expression was found to correlate with stage, pathological types, and biological behavior of many tumors, as shown by retrospective analyses on 13 types of human cancers. Moreover, the expression of B7-H4 reverse correlated with the survival of patients in most cancer analyzed.[190] A recent study by Quandt et al. demonstrated that the overexpression of B7-H4 in melanoma cells impaired the antitumor immune response by decreasing IFN-γ, TNF-α, and IL-2 production.[191]

In ovarian cancer, the inhibitory role of B7-H4 might be due to B7-H4 expression on tumor-associated macrophages (TAMs). Kryczek et al. showed that B7-H4-expressing TAMs could block activation of T cells in the setting of ovarian cancer. B7-H4 expression in TAMs was upregulated by IL-6 and IL-10 present in the tumor microenvironment, whereas its expression was inhibited by GM-CSF and IL-4. It has been shown that Treg cells induced APCs to produces IL-10 and IL-6, providing a new mechanism by which Tregs exert their suppressive action. B7-H4 blockade by antisense oligonucleotides restored T-cell antitumor immune response and led to tumor regression *in vivo*.[192] Recently, Qian et al. reported the development of a monoclonal antibody to B7-H4 and preliminary data showed that it could effectively inhibit the activity of B7-H4, promoting the growth of T cells and the secretion of IL-2, IL-4, IL-10, and IFN-γ.[193] Based on these preliminary data, the blockade of B7-H4 could be an attractive opportunity to enhance antitumor immunity in a subset of human cancers.

TNF:TNFR SUPERFAMILY OF COSTIMULATORY MOLECULES IN ANTITUMOR IMMUNITY

CD40L:CD40 Costimulatory Pathway

CD40 receptor and its ligand CD40L (CD154) were the first members belonging to the TNF:TNFR family to be identified. CD40 expression was originally found on B cells, but it is also expressed on DCs, monocytes, platelets, macrophages as well as myofibroblasts, fibroblasts, epithelial, and endothelial cells.[194] CD40L is expressed on activated T and B cells, by platelets, monocytes, NK cells, mast cells, and basophils, where CD40L is induced following proinflammatory stimuli. CD40L:CD40 signaling in B cells is also important for the generation of long-lived plasma cells and memory B cells, as well as for their survival. CD40 intracellular signaling is mediated by the recruitment of TNFR-associated factors (TRAFs), which in turn activate different pathways, such as the canonical and noncanonical NF-κB pathway, MAPKs, PI3K, and the phospholipase Cγ pathway.[195] The engagement of CD40 by CD40L on APCs has been shown to promote cytokines production and upregulation of costimulatory molecules, crucial events for T-cell activation, and differentiation.[196]

CD40/CD40L pathway is crucial for the development of antitumor immunity. CD40L blockade resulted in lacking of protective immune response following administration of a GM-CSF-expressing B16 melanoma cells vaccine. In addition, low expression of CD40L was sufficient to induce a long-lasting antitumor immune response via CTLs in a small number of cancers.[195] Another aspect to take into consideration is the direct effect of CD40:CD40L pathway on tumor cells. Elgueta et al. reviewed that CD40 is broadly expressed in several tumors, such as melanoma, prostate cancer, lung cancer, as well as carcinoma of nasopharynx, bladder, cervix and ovary, Hodgkin's and NHL, MM, and acute myeloid leukemia. The engagement of CD40 on tumor cells can provide growth arrest and apoptosis of malignant cells, as dictated by the type of malignancies and the microenvironment.[195] The combination of CD40L expression with other immunomodulators (IL-2, GM-CSF, and INF-γ) has been found to promote antitumor immunity in several cancer models. Gene therapy approach with the use of recombinant adenovirus encoding CD40L was also effective in colorectal, lung, and melanoma cancer models. An early study reported that the use of CD40 agonistic antibodies triggered CTL-4 responses in a lymphoma system, with the consequent tumor eradication.[197] Recently, the use of activators of both adaptive and innate immunity, such as CD40 agonists and TLR agonists, induced antitumor-specific immunity in many tumor models.[198] Currently, the combination of CD40 tumor therapy with other approaches, such as cancer vaccines, chemotherapy, radiation, CTLA blockade, TLR agonists, and cytokines, is becoming overriding.[199,200]

To date, three humanized CD40 agonistic antibodies have been developed: CP-870,893, SGN-40, and HCD122 (Table 5.8). CP-870,893 is a fully human, IgG2 antibody that selectively binds to CD40. It enhances the expression of MHC class II, CD54, CD86, and CD23 on human B cells *in vitro*. CP-870,893 also enhances DC activity as demonstrated by secretion of IL-12, IL-23, and IL-8, by the upregulation of CD86 and CD83, and by the capacity to prime T cells to secrete IFN-γ.[211,212] Results from a phase I

TABLE 5.8 Tumor Models and Clinical Trials of TNF-TNFR Costimulatory Molecules

Tumor Model	Costimulatory Molecule	Therapeutic Strategy	Reference
Melanoma, advanced cancers	CD40	CP-870,893 agonistic Ab anti-CD40	[201,202]
Myeloma, B-cell lymphoma, diffuse large cell lymphoma	CD40	SGN-40 agonistic Ab anti-CD40	[203–205]
MM, B-cell CLL	CD40	HCD122 agonistic Ab anti-CD40	[195]
Solid tumors	4-1BB	BMS-663513 agonistic Ab anti-4-IBB	[206]
Metastatic prostate cancer	OX40	Agonistic Ab anti-OX40	[42]
Melanoma	GITR	TRX518	[42]
CD30-positive lymphoma	CD30	Brentuximab vedotin Ab-drug conjugates anti-CD30	[207–210]

study showed that administration of CP-870,893 was associated with early signs of clinical efficacy, especially in patients with melanoma.[201] The same authors reported that weekly infusions of this agonist CD40 antibody were associated with little clinical activity in advanced cancer patients.[202] SGN-40 (dacetuzumab) is a humanized anti-CD40 monoclonal antibody with multiple mechanisms of action. In non-Hodgkin lymphoma, Dacetuzumab activates two distinct proapoptotic signaling pathways; on the one hand, it constitutively activates the NF-κB and MAPK signaling pathways producing the sustained downregulation of the oncoprotein B-cell lymphoma 6, which loss results in c-Myc downregulation and activation of early B-cell maturation, concomitant with reduced proliferation and cell death. On the other hand, dacetuzumab induces the expression of the proapoptotic p53 family member TAp63α and downstream proteins associated with the intrinsic and extrinsic apoptotic machinery.[213] *In vitro*, dacetuzumab exhibited antitumor activity against several B-cell lymphoma and MM cell lines, and induced direct apoptosis as well as the engagement of effective antibody-dependent cell-mediated cytotoxicity (ADCC).[214]

Early clinical trials have evaluated the pharmacokinetics, safety, and efficacy of dacetuzumab in patients with relapsed/refractory B-cell lymphomas, MM, and CLL.[203–205] Dacetuzumab resulted in modest antitumor activity in B-cell lymphomas and, to a lesser extent, in MM. In CLL dacetuzumab showed modest activity as monotherapy, while better results were obtained by using combination therapy with lenalidomide.[215] Dacetuzumab is currently in multiple phase II trials for the treatment of myeloma and diffuse large cell lymphoma. HCD122 is a human IgG1 monoclonal antibody and currently in a phase I trial for the treatment of MM and B-cell CLL. In B-cell CLL, HCD122 exerts antitumor activity by killing leukemia cells through ADCC and inhibiting CD40L induced survival and proliferation of tumor cells.[216]

1BBL:4-1BB Costimulatory Pathway

4-1BB is an inducible costimulatory receptor expressed on activated CD4+ and CD8+ T cell, NKT, NK cells, DCs, macrophages, eosinophils, neutrophils, and mast cells, as well as Tregs. In the most cases, 4-1BB is induced on the cellular surface following activation, except for APCs and Tregs, where its expression is constitutive. The ligand of 4-1BB is 4-1BBL, which is expressed on activated professional APCs.[217,218] 4-1BB:4-1BBL pathway seems to amplify the existing costimulatory signals, even if the engagement of 4-1BB in the presence of a strong TCR signaling can induce IL-2 production in a CD28-independent manner.[219] Following stimulation with its ligand, 4-1BB provides costimulatory signals to both CD4+ and CD8+ T cells, with a greater effect on the expansion of CD8+ due to the upregulation of antiapoptotic genes, such as *bcl-XL* and *bfl-1*. 4-1BB signals are mediated by the activation of NF-κB, c-Jun, and p38 downstream pathways.[155] 4-1BB has also a role in activation of DCs, which induces IL-6 and IL-12 production and upregulating B7 costimulatory molecules.[220] 4-1BB plays roles in activating non-T-cells other than DCs, such as monocytes, B cells, mast cells, NK cells, and neutrophils and its engagement is associated with cellular proliferation, cytokine induction, bactericidal activity, and sustenance of T-cell effector functions.

Targeting of 4-1BB:4-1BBL pathway in cancer reveals itself as a promising approach. The adoptive transfer of *ex vivo* 4-1BB- and CD28-costimulated T cells induced antitumor immune response in some preclinical studies.[221,222] 4-1BB agonistic antibodies as antitumor therapy were broadly tested in several animal models with encouraging results. Melero et al. reported that the intraperitoneal injection of an antimurine 4-1BB mAb resulted in the eradication of established P815 mastocytoma and Ag104A sarcoma in mice.[223] Driessens et al. reviewed of subsequent studies that demonstrated the efficacy of anti-4-1BB- or 4-1BBL-expressing tumor cells vaccines in inducing specific antitumor T-cell response, suppression of tumor growth and regression of pre-established tumors in different animal models. Therapeutic effects of agonistic anti-4-1BB mAb are due to enhanced NK and CD8+ T-cell activation and IFN-γ production.[218] The current direction toward which 4-1BB-directed anticancer immunotherapy is moving is the use of anti-4-1BB mAbs in combination with other therapeutic approaches, such as antitumor necrosis factor-related apoptosis inducing ligand (TRAIL), CD40 mAbs, intratumoral delivery of IL-12 gene, DC vaccines, CTLA-4 blockade, anti-CD4 therapy, chemotherapy, and radiotherapy.[224] To date, one agonistic anti-4-1BB-humanized mAb BMS-663513 has been developed and the functional effects were demonstrated on human and monkey T cells and peripheral blood mononuclear cells, where IFN-production was enhanced compared to controls (Table 5.8). BMS-663513 is under evaluation in several phase I and II trials in patients with solid tumors and showed clinical activity. A phase II randomized study in melanoma patients with stage IV disease was stopped due to the occurrence of hepatitis.[206,225]

OX40:OX40L Costimulatory Pathway

OX40 is an inducible costimulatory receptor expressed on activated CD4+ and CD8+ T cells, but also on activated Tregs, NKT cells, NK cells, and neutrophils. OX40L expression is induced on professional APCs, as well as on T cells, with the aim of amplifying T-cell responsiveness during T-cell/T-cell interactions. In addition to APCs, other cell types can induce OX40L expression, such as Langerhans cells, mast cells, NK cells, endothelial cells, and smooth muscle cells. Based on experimental evidences from OX40 deficient mice, it has been reported that this receptor promotes effector T-cell proliferation and survival, cytokines production, as well as the generation, and the maintenance of memory T cells. Moreover, OX40 inhibits Treg functions and counteracts the generation of inducible Tregs.[226] OX40 seems to act as a late positive costimulatory receptor, which goes on after CD28 signal, in a sequential manner.[227] The prosurvival activity of OX40 is in part due to its ability to upregulate antiapoptotic genes of the Bcl-2 family. In fact, OX40 engagement by OX40L activates both PI3K/Akt and NF-κB downstream pathways.[228]

OX40 represents a promising candidate for cancer immunotherapy. As reviewed by Croft et al., different approaches have been evaluated, such as agonistic OX40 mAbs or OX40L-Ig fusion protein, tumor cells, and DCs transfection with OX40L, and agonist RNA aptamer-binding OX40. Treatment with agonistic OX40 mAbs or OX40L-Ig fusion protein resulted in enhanced antitumor immunity in several cancer models, such as sarcoma, melanoma, colon carcinoma, and glioma.[226] Several studies also reported encouraging results following the use of agonistic OX40 mAbs in combination with IL-12, anti-4-1BB, GM-CSF, DC vaccine, IL-12, and CD80 costimulation and chemotherapy.[229–231] Combination therapy with agonistic OX40 mAbs and cyclophosphamide induces a profound Tregs depletion in concomitance with an increased infiltration of effector CD8+ T cells in B16 melanoma model.[232]

A phase I/II trial is ongoing to evaluate the safety and the efficacy of a murine anti-human OX40 in combination with cyclophosphamide and radiation in patients with progressive metastatic prostate cancer (see Table 5.8). To avoid immune response to the murine mAb, a humanized OX40 agonist has been developed by Agonox, a spinoff biotech company, and it will be tested in future clinical trials.[42]

Light: HVEM Costimulatory Pathway

LIGHT, along with LTα, was identified as a ligand of the aforementioned HVEM receptor and it is a member of TNF family. LIGHT expression has been reported on activated T cells, immature DCs, monocytes, and NK cells. LIGHT is not expressed on B cells, but it can be induced following activation.[233] Experimental evidences suggested that the interaction HVEM/LIGHT results in a positive costimulatory signaling, which induces T-cell proliferation and cytokines production.[177] In fact, the constitutive expression of LIGHT in T cells of transgenic mice leads to accumulation and activation of DCs and expansion of activated effector and memory T cells.[234] Moreover, the manifestation of lymphoproliferative disorders and autoimmune disease was also observed.[235] LIGHT deficient mice have been generated and showed defects in CD8 + T-cell activation and in thymic selection. LIGHT is also a critical ligand for activating NK cells to produce IFN-γ.[233] The intracellular signaling of HVEM following LIGHT binding is mediated by TRAF proteins, which in turn activate NF-κB and c-Jun/AP-1 pathways, leading to the transcription of prosurvival and proproliferative genes, as well as genes regulating cytokines secretion. LIGHT can also engage the lymphotoxin-β-receptor (LTβR) on DCs and provide a crucial signaling that results in DCs expansion, activation and IL-2 production.[177]

Thus, LIGHT can modulate the immune response both directly by signaling via HVEM on T cells and indirectly by activating DCs through LTβR. Due to its role as immunomodulator, LIGHT could be a suitable target for cancer immunotherapy. The overexpression of LIGHT in P815 myeloma cell line induces regression of established tumors in a CD28-independent manner;[236] similar results were obtained upon LIGHT overexpression in Ag104 sarcoma cell line; in fact, this forced expression caused rejection of tumor through NK-cell activation, which, in turn, triggered tumor-specific CD8+ T-cell proliferation at the tumor site.[237] In addition, the injection of LIGHT expressing adenoviral vector into primary 4T1 mammary carcinoma has been found to promote T-cell recruitment, immune surveillance of the tumor, and elimination of metastasis.[238] A recent study showed that the LIGHT/HVEM costimulation through both LIGHT-transfected cells and HVEM agonistic mAb-induced apoptosis in fresh B-CLL cells along with an increased production of IL-8.[239] Another therapeutic approach targeting LIGHT/HVEM signaling was reported by Park et al., which developed P815 tumor cell expressing a single-chain variable fragment (scFv) of an anti-HVEM agonistic monoclonal antibody on their surface. These authors showed that tumor cells expressing anti-HVEM scFv spontaneously regress in a CD4+ and CD8+ T-cell-dependent manner when inoculated in mice and stimulated tumor-specific long-term T-cell memory. Moreover, the combination of anti-HVEM scFv expressing tumor vaccines and 4-1BB costimulation caused the regression of established tumors *in vivo*.[240] Further studies are needed to clarify the true potential of targeting this pathway in cancer immunotherapy.

CD70:CD27 Costimulatory Pathway

CD27 is another costimulatory receptor belonging to the TNF family, and it is expressed on naive T and B cells and on NK cells. CD70 has been identified as CD27 ligand and its expression is restricted to APCs. The engagement of CD27 by CD70 promotes a positive costimulatory signaling, which results in T-cell proliferation and survival, maybe in concert with CD28.[227] Like other members of the TNFR family, CD27 signaling is mediated by the recruitment of TRAF proteins.[241] Targeting CD27 could represent an attractive strategy in the field of cancer immunotherapy. Earlier studies have reported that early studies reporting that the overexpression of CD70 promoted cancer elimination through the activation of T cells and NK cells. In addition, the potential of costimulatory ligand CD70 to boost DC-based vaccine capacity to evoke effective CD8+ T-cell immunity has been explored.[242] Glouchkova et al. suggested that the modulation of the CD70/CD27 pathway might represent a novel therapeutic approach for enhancing the antileukemic response in B-cell precursor acute lymphoblastic leukemia.[243]

Recently, agonistic anti-CD27 antibodies has shown to be effective as monotherapy in reducing the outgrowth of experimental lung metastases and established subcutaneous melanoma tumors *in vivo*.[244] In addition to CD70 agonists, the soluble form of CD70 has been evaluated as powerful adjuvant in a glioblastoma model.[245] The aberrant expression of CD70 in a broad range of hematological malignancies and in some solid tumors has led to the development of CD70-specific T cells, having a chimeric antigen receptor (CAR) consisting of CD27 fused to the CD3-chain. Recently, adoptively transferred CD70-specific T cells have been found to induce regression of established murine xenografts through the recognition of CD70-expressing tumor cells.[246]

GITRL:GITR Costimulatory Pathway

Glucocorticoid-induced TNFR-related protein (GITR) is a costimulatory receptor expressed on activated T cells and, constitutively, on Tregs. Its ligand GITRL is expressed at low levels on APCs, but it gets induced following TLR stimulation.[247] Several studies have reported that GITR signaling promotes the proliferation of naive T cells and cytokines production through the recruitment of TRAF proteins and the activation of downstream pathways. Moreover, one of the first described GITR functions was the ability to protect T cells from activation-induced cell death. Controversial data have been reported about the regulation of Treg functions by GITR. In fact, experimental evidences suggest both an inhibitor and a stimulatory role for GITR. The use of GITR agonistic antibody (clone DTA-1) is also effective in stimulating antitumor immunity *in vivo*.[248] The modulation of GITR pathway is an intriguing therapeutic possibility.

The treatment with GITR-expressing adenovirus vector has been shown to be able to induce T-cell response and to reduce tumor size in mice inoculated with B16 tumor cells.[249] Nishikawa et al. reported that triggering GITR through GITRL-expressing plasmid resulted in the inhibition of tumor growth in a CMS5 sarcoma model. The protection of CD8 + T cell against Treg-mediated suppression was also observed by the authors.[250] Recently, Zhou et al. suggested that the antitumor effect of anti-GITR antibody was dependent on its ability to positive costimulates T cells rather than to suppress Treg functions, but the question is still debated.[251] Last year, a clinical study of an agonist anti-GITR antibody (TRX518) in melanoma was started but the trial was put on hold because of a major business setback of the company that makes the antibody (see Table 5.8).

CD30L:CD30 Costimulatory Pathway

CD30 receptor is an inducible costimulatory receptor expressed on activated and memory T cells following TCR/CD28 or IL-4 stimulation. The ligand of

CD30 is CD30L, which is expressed on activated T cells, as well as on macrophages, DCs, and B cells. CD30L/CD30 signaling seems to be involved in Th1 and Th2 cell responses and plays a critical role in Th17 differentiation.[252] Due to the expression of CD30 on all malignant HRS cells, this receptor represents an important target for the immunotherapy of hematological malignancies. SGN-35 (brentuximab vedotin) is an anti-CD30 antibody that has been modified by the addition of a dipeptide linker to permit attachment of microtubule polymerization monomethylauristatin E (MMAE)[210] (also Table 5.8). SGN-35 has been evaluated in phase I dose escalation study in 45 patients with relapsed or refractory CD30-positive hematologic malignancies and the maximum-tolerated dose was determined to be 1.8 mg/kg.[207] In a pivotal phase II study of SGN-35, 102 patients with relapsed or refractory Hodgkin lymphoma were treated with 1.8 mg/kg dose of SGN-35 every three weeks. A reduction in tumor volume was observed in 95% of patients and the ORR was 75%.[208] The efficacy of SGN-35 has been also evaluated in a phase II single-arm study in 58 patients with ALCL. The authors reported that the ORR was 86%.[209] A multicenter randomized phase III trial of SGN-35 (AETHERA) in posttransplant classical Hodgkin lymphoma patients at high risk for recurrence was started in April 2010.

In the light of these impressive result, the FDA approved SGN-35 for the treatment of Hodgkin lymphoma in August 2011. The high efficacy of this antibody-drug conjugate could be due to the fact that cytotoxic effect of MMAE targets not only CD30-expressing HRS cells, but also the immune-suppressive Tregs present in the tumor microenvironment because of a bystander effect; moreover, SGN-35 delivers itself an additional apoptotic signal, mainly in ALCL cells.[210]

COSTIMULATION IMMUNOTHERAPY AND TUMOR TOLERANCE

Developing tumors are typically recognized and eliminated by a protective mechanism of immunosurveillance, failure of which results in the prevalence of tumor tolerance over immunity.[253,254] The goal of tumor immunotherapy is to break such tolerance and initiate a robust, prolonged tumor-specific immune response without the harsh toxicities that traditional cancer therapies impart. High-profile accomplishments in the field have recently been made, including FDA-approval of the first cellular vaccine for cancer,[255] and demonstration that a small minority of patients with metastatic melanoma can be, for all intents and purposes, cured upon antibody mediated blockade of the T-cell inhibitory molecule CTLA-4.[126] Median overall survival in both trials, however, was only increased by 4 months. While these milestones should be celebrated as proof-of-concept that T-cell-based immunotherapy of cancer is feasible and relatively effective (compared to standard of care treatment), there is clearly room for improvement.

Blocking negative costimulatory molecules to boost antitumor T-cell responses in cancer patients is an attractive new strategy in cancer immunotherapy. Antibodies that block CTLA-4 on T cells have proven effective in treating melanoma patients.[35] The efficacy of CTLA-4 antibodies at least suggests that tumor-specific T cells can be activated in patients bearing tumors. When tumors escape immune surveillance and progress to become a solid cell mass, immune tolerance mechanisms are established in the tumor microenvironment that strongly inhibit infiltrating T-lymphocyte function.[253] For example, prostaglandin E2 secreted by monocytes and TAMs inhibits the proliferation of T cells and promotes T helper (Th)2 responses, which downregulate the antitumor Th1 response.[256]

Moreover, prostaglandin E2 promotes the secretion of IL-10 by macrophages, DCs, and tumors, which maintains the immunosuppressive environment in the tumor. Macrophages from tumor stroma also produce the immunosuppressive cytokine TGF-β, which inhibits the antitumor activities of infiltrating CTLs, NK cells, neutrophils, and macrophages. In addition, transforming growth factor-β induces the production of IL-10 by the tumor cells and downregulates the expression of the activating receptor NKG2D—an important regulator of antitumor immune surveillance—on CD8+ T cells and NK cells.[192,257] B7-H4 is the newest addition to the B7 family that has been shown to negatively regulate T-cell activation. The expression of B7-H4 in multiple nonlymphoid tissues suggests that it might mediate tolerance at the tissue level. In addition, human breast and ovarian cancers have been found to express B7-H4.[258,259] The cytokines IL-6 and IL-10 present in the ascites were shown to induce expression of B7-H4 on normal blood monocytes. However, tumor ascites had no direct effect on intracellular or cell surface expression of B7-H4 in the tumor cells. The authors also found that the cytokines IL-4 and GM-CSF suppressed IL-10-induced B7-H4 expression. Thus, the downregulation of B7-H4 may contribute to the potent adjuvant effects of GM-CSF in cancer immunotherapy. Expression of B7-H4 by TAMs inhibited the *in vitro* proliferation and effector function of CD8+ T cells specific for the tumor antigen Her-2/neu. Using morpholino antisense oligonucleotides, the authors showed that the immunosuppression was mediated specifically by B7-H4 and not other immunosuppressive effectors known to be expressed by macrophages, such as PDL-1, arginase, or inducible nitric oxide synthase.[256] The B7-H4-dependent immunosuppression by macrophages at the tumor site was then confirmed in a mouse ovarian tumor model. Macrophages treated with oligonucleotides to block B7-H4 expression reduced the growth of tumors implanted in lymphocyte-deficient mice that received T cells specific for tumor antigens. This further indicates that B7-H4 is the critical immunosuppressive molecule expressed by TAMs. A possible scenario that might explain these findings is that ovarian cancer cells secrete IL-6 and IL-10 to induce the expression of B7-H4 on infiltrating macrophages, which would then inhibit the proliferation of and cytokine production by infiltrating T cells via B7-H4. This suggests that blockade of B7-H4 enhances the activity of tumor-infiltrating T cells, shifting the balance of immunity and immune evasion in favor of tumor destruction.[192]

The above experimental evidence reveals the crucial roles of negative costimulators in preventing tissue and tumor attack by infiltrating T cells.[256,260] Enhancing the function of these molecules may be of benefit in the treatment of autoimmune diseases, whereas inhibition of their function might be an effective therapeutic strategy to boost antitumor immunity. Tumor immunity and autoimmunity are alike to some extent. Tumor reactivity and autoreactivity exist in our TCR repertoire but are restricted by many inhibitory mechanisms such as peripheral tolerance and the action of regulatory T cells. The studies discussed in this chapter, along with others, suggest that further checkpoints exist in tissues and tumors that are mediated by negative costimulatory molecules such as PD-L1 and B7-H4. These studies also suggest that cytokines (pro-or anti-inflammatory) are crucial regulators of the expression of these inhibitory molecules. A lot still needs to be learned about negative costimulation in tissues and tumors and its role in regulating T-cell activity. For instance, is positive costimulation in tissues or tumors required for the function of self- or tumor reactive T cells? And what are the differences in the function and regulation of the various negative costimulators? From our experience in studying costimulation in the context of the regulation of naive T-cell activation, we may expect to observe combinations of various positive and negative costimulatory factors that regulate T-cell activities in tissues and tumors. Thus, it may eventually be possible to design effective immunotherapies that specifically perturb autoimmune responses without impinging on immunity to infection or that break tumor tolerance without provoking autoimmune diseases.

MODULATION OF B7 PATHWAY TO AUGMENT CANCER IMMUNOTHERAPY

The B7 system is one of the most important secondary signaling mechanisms and is essential in maintaining the delicate balance between immune potency and suppression of autoimmunity. Potential therapeutic applications include immune-boosting adjuvants to conventional anticancer therapy, HSCT, antitumor vaccines, bioengineered T cells, as well as attenuation of GVHD. The B7 family is only one aspect of a complex signaling network that comprises other IGSF members, the TNFRSF, chemokines, cytokines, and adhesion molecules. However, based on a substantial evidence base and a growing therapeutic armory, the B7 family requires particular attention, as summarized in Table 5.3. The standardized approach to nomenclature is the cluster of differentiation (CD), which has not yet been applied to all members of the family. While many researchers are more familiar with their original names, which are still widely used in the literature, for the purposes of this review, the CD designation is used where ever possible.

Allogenic HSCT

Failure of allogeneic HSCT may in part be mediated by suppressive B7 signaling. Anti-CTLA-4 mAb therapy has been applied successfully in phase 2 clinical trials to treat relapsed CHL, myeloma, and leukemias after allogeneic HSCT without the anticipated exacerbation of GVHD seen in murine transplantation experiments.[19,261] Use of PD-L1/PD-1 axis blockade to enhance allogeneic T-cell responses has not yet reached clinical trial, although there is promising preclinical data in a murine AML model using TCR-engineered AML antigen-specific allogeneic T cells.[20] Late transfer of these cells led to poorer antitumor responses accompanied by PD-1 overexpression. Responses were restored by treatment with anti-PD-L1 mAb. PD-1 blockade, however, accelerated GVHD lethality.[262]

Tumor Vaccination Strategies

B7 molecules may play an essential role in cancer vaccination strategies. Mouse model immunization strategies using highly immunogenic cancer cell lines showed early success, particularly with chemokine costimulatory approaches.[263] Tumor lysate-pulsed DCs have been incorporated into some vaccination strategies,[264] showing modest success in patients with advanced lymphoma.[265] Idiotype-specific tumor vaccines have been produced for myeloma[266] and NHL[267] while immunogenic tumor-specific antigens have been identified in CLL and acute leukemia.[268,269] However, vaccination has yet to make any real impact on cancer therapy.

Combining vaccination strategies with immunosuppressive B7 pathway blockade may improve these disappointing outcomes. CTLA-4 mAb-enhanced melanoma rejection has been demonstrated in a clinical trial,[36,37,129] but studies in NHL have been disappointing, with minimal responses achieved in vaccinated patients treated with ipilimumab. Encouraging *in vitro* evidence suggests that a similar strategy could be applied to PD-1/PD-L1 axis blockade, although this has yet to be incorporated into any clinical trial. One group showed PD-L1/PD-L2 siRNA silencing improved DC-induced leukemia-specific T-cell responses,[26] while another demonstrated enhanced T-cell responses after PD-1 antibody treatment in a myeloma/DC fusion vaccination strategy.[25]

BIOENGINEERING OF T CELLS FOR CANCER IMMUNOTHERAPY

In contrast to the active immunization strategies outlined in the previous paragraph, an alternative strategy is to expand and reinfuse autologous bioengineered T cells. Autologous TILs extracted from melanoma biopsies, expanded and reinfused into immunosuppressed recipients, have shown some therapeutic success but failed to translate to other malignancies. Attempts to augment autologous T-cell specificity for tumor antigens led to TCR bioengineering approaches, first against Epstein–Barr virus (EBV)-driven lymphoproliferative tumors and subsequently other tumor-specific antigens, while clinical responses are reported, reactive clones tend to rapidly lose efficacy or die off altogether.[270–274] Subsequent developments used tumor antigen-inoculated transgenic mice whose T cells express human MHC, which expanded tumor-specific T-cell clones and hence derived TCR genes for transfection into patient-derived T cells.[275] Newer techniques incorporate novel receptor constructs into autologous T cells using CAR. Here, a rearranged, antigen-specific immunoglobulin variable region gene is combined with intracellular domains of the TCR gene, thus bypassing MHC-restricted antigen recognition. CARs have the advantage of being amenable to further augmentation with costimulatory motifs, of which CD28 and CD80 have demonstrated efficacy.[23,24] CARs incorporating costimulatory modifications have reached phase 1 clinical trials in NHL using an anti-CD19-CD28-TCRζ chain construct, and CLL, using an anti-CD19-CD137 construct[276] (a TNFRSF member). Promising results have been observed, even in refractory patients.[277] Further optimization is needed and B7 family members will play a central role in this.

ICOS and B7-H2 Costimulatory Pathway in Cancer

Angioimmunoblastic T-cell lymphoma cells express ICOS, PD-1, and CXCR5, consistent with being the malignant counterpart of T follicular helper cells (TFH) lymphocytes.[278] ICOS expression has also been described as a potential survival mechanism in nucleophosmin-anaplastic lymphoma kinase (NPM-ALK) fusion ALCL cells.[279] Although induced ICOS-L expression enhances cytotoxic T-cell-mediated tumor rejection,[136–138] there is sparse and conflicting evidence for its expression in solid tumors, while expression in myeloma and acute leukemia is widely heterogeneous. Despite these sometimes contradictory findings, the ICOS/ICOS-L axis may yet have an indirect role in enhancement of tumor immunity. ICOS is inducible on NK cells, which demonstrate cytotoxicity against ICOS-L-transfected murine leukemia cell lines.[280] Cytokine-induced killer cells demonstrate MHC-independent cytotoxicity and antitumor activity, enhanced after ICOS transfection.[281] Optimal immunostimulatory therapy using CTLA-4 mAbs may be dependent on an intact ICOS/ICOS-L pathway, with CTLA-4 blockade increasing tumor-specific IFN-γ-secreting T cells in cancer patients.[16,139]

Therapeutic Modulation of ICOS/ICOS-L

ICOS is overexpressed during acute allogeneic solid organ rejection and tolerance is improved with pathway blockade[21] which suggests that this pathway may have importance in GVHD. Murine acute GVHD is reduced if donor *Icos*$^{-co}$ mice or ICOS-blocking antibodies are used, with less gut and liver GVHD and improved survival[22,282] despite intact *Icos*$^{-co}$ donor cell cytotoxic function, cytokine-secretion, and tissue trafficking, while *Icos*$^{-/-}$ recipient mice better tolerate allogeneic HSCT with more rapid and complete donor chimerism.[22] However, a further study demonstrated more severe GVHD arising from allogeneic CD8 + *Icos*$^{-/-}$ cell transplantation compared with wild type, a contradiction perhaps explained by the differing mouse genetic backgrounds and variable use of Treg-depleting anti-CD25 mAbs.[283] ICOS appears central to GVHD modulation, although because of these controversies, a therapeutic application has yet to emerge.

COMBINATION OF COSTIMULATORY ANTIBODY–LIGAND FUSION PROTEINS FOR TARGETED CANCER IMMUNOTHERAPY

Combinatory strategies are becoming of increasing interest in cancer immunotherapy. Costimulation by individual members of the immunoglobulin-like (Ig) and TNF superfamily have already shown promising antitumor potential, thus prompting the exploration of their synergistic abilities in combinatorial approaches. Interfering with the costimulatory/inhibitory ligand-receptor network that regulates the immune response has become a promising approach in cancer immunotherapy. Thus, antagonistic antibodies directed against inhibitory receptors of the Ig superfamily (e.g., CTLA-4, PD-1) and agonistic antibodies directed against costimulatory receptors of the TNFR superfamily (e.g., 4-1BB, OX40, GITR, CD127, CD40) are being evaluated in clinical trials.[284,285] In addition, it is becoming apparent that strongest antitumor effects might be achieved by combinatorial treatments.[286,287] In preclinical models, synergistic actions have been described for the combined activation of different costimulatory receptors (e.g., 4-1BB with OX40 or CD40)[229,288,289] as well as for combined activation and blockade of costimulatory and coinhibitory receptors, respectively (e.g., anti-4-1BB mAb with either anti-CTLA-4 or anti-PD-1).[290–292] The evaluation of indicated combinations is complicated since the expression pattern of these receptors and corresponding ligands orchestrating the immune response is cell-type specific, time-dependent, and cell context-related.[10] Thus, seeking maximal antitumor potential of costimulatory/inhibitory reagents in combinatorial settings constitutes a major challenge in the field.

For immunotherapeutic approaches, costimulation has been provided either by agonistic antibodies for particular receptors or respective ligands.[293,294] Studies with ligands involved mainly multimeric recombinant proteins composed of the extracellular domain of the ligand fused to antibody Fc or multimerization domains (e.g., surfactant protein D (SP-D), modified core streptavidin (SA), and tenascin (TNC)).[295–298] Although effective costimulatory activity was achieved, undirected costimulation bears the risk of unexpected AE and autoimmunity (e.g., liver toxicity observed after anti-4-1BB mAb treatment in preclinical and clinical studies).[172] Thus, targeted approaches are being developed, creating tumor-specific antibody-fusion proteins with costimulatory ligands in order to direct, confine and improve the immune response at the tumor site.[295] Enhanced antitumor effects could be shown by target-directed costimulation with B7.1 or 4-1BBL in diverse tumor mouse models. Furthermore, combination therapies with regulatory T-cell (Treg) depletion and a bispecific antibody resulted in improved therapeutic effects.[299–301]

Previously a combinatorial approach of two costimulatory antibody–ligand fusion proteins, that target B7.2 and 4-1BBL to the tumor cell via two independent antigens, has been reported. In this model system, T cells were retargeted by a bispecific antibody, and stimulation was enhanced by target mediated costimulation of B7.2 and 4-1BBL.[302] Here we report further combinations of antibody–ligand fusion proteins with a focus on the combination of B7.1 and 4-1BBL with the costimulatory members OX40L, LIGHT and GITRL of the TNF superfamily, and we will analyze cytokine release, proliferation, and the cytotoxic potential of T cells. Because encouraging results were obtained by the combination of B7.1 and 4-1BBL, we adapted the model system for a time-shift setting, where the benefit of costimulation-assisted restimulation was shown. Finally, the antitumor potential of this combinatorial setting was confirmed *in vivo* in a lung metastasis mouse model. A targeted strategy with antibody-fusion proteins composed of a tumor-directed antibody and the extracellular domain of the costimulatory ligand B7.1, 4-1BBL, OX40L, GITRL, or LIGHT, respectively, was carried out.[303] Costimulatory activity was assessed in an experimental setting where initial T-cell activation was induced by a bispecific antibody (tumor-related antigen 9 CD3). Advantage of combined targeted costimulation was shown for either B7.1 or 4-1BBL with OX40L, GITRL, LIGHT, and 4-1BBL in terms of T-cell proliferation and IFN-c release. Since encouraging results were obtained by the combination of B7.1 and 4-1BBL, a model system for a time-shift setting was adapted. There was enhanced proliferation and granzyme B expression as well as reduced PD-1 expression on the T-cell population, which demonstrated the benefit of costimulation-assisted restimulation. Finally, the antitumor potential of this combinatorial setting was confirmed *in vivo* in a lung metastasis mouse model.[303] Thus, combinatorial approaches with costimulatory antibody–ligand fusion proteins seem a promising strategy to be further investigated for cancer immunotherapy.

Thus, for comprehensive costimulatory ligand combination assessment, spatiotemporal considerations need to be taken into account. The data from the time-shift setting system indicate that costimulation by B7.1-Db and scFv-4-1BBL is most effective when applied during scDb-mediated restimulation. In this system, costimulation showed not only the ability to further raise the proliferation and cytotoxic potential of T cells in support of repeated CD3-induced T-cell stimulation, it also showed to counteract the scDb driven enhancement of T cells expressing the inhibitory receptors PD-1, commonly associated with immune restrain. PD-1 is expressed on antigen-experienced T cells in the periphery to limit their activity during inflammatory response and autoimmunity.[304] Upregulation of its ligand PD-L1 in tumors has been identified as a mechanism of immune evasion. The importance of this checkpoint receptor in the context of cancer immunotherapy is reflected by the fact that several antagonistic antibodies are in clinical trials.[38]

It was shown in a B16 lung metastasis tumor mouse model that the application of the costimulatory antibody-fusion proteins could enhance the antitumor effect of the bispecific antibody *in vivo,* which provides evidence for the benefit of such a combinatorial approach. This suggests that even powerful tumor-directed polyclonal T-cell activation can benefit from additional costimulation.[303] On the other hand, metastases reduction, although to a much lesser extent was observed for the treatment with the costimulatory fusion proteins only, which indicates also an enhancement of the endogenous tumor-specific immune response in this rather poorly immunogenic model. Thus, the potential to enforce a broad spectrum of cancer immunotherapeutic strategies could be expected. However, extensive *in vivo* studies will be required to understand in detail the underlying immunological mechanisms. By now, the antitumor potential of individual costimulation has been widely acknowledged. Nevertheless, it has also become apparent that it might take combinatorial approaches to fully exploit this strategy. As we could corroborate in this study, the evaluation of configurations and spatiotemporal considerations are crucial. Thus, addressing these issues by establishing experimental settings with costimulatory antibody–ligand fusion proteins constitutes a valuable contribution to the field.

SUMMARY AND CONCLUSION

Improving the knowledge of T costimulatory and coinhibitory pathways over the past decade had shed light on the central roles that these costimulatory molecules play in the generation of an effective immune response. Many tumors escape from immune surveillance through the downregulation of positive costimulatory molecules and the upregulation of coinhibitory signals. Blockade of coinhibitory pathway on the one hand and the stimulation of the positive signals on the other hand have been found to enhance antitumoral immunity, both alone and in combination with traditional therapy in preclinical and clinical trials. So engaging costimulatory pathways, as well as blocking coinhibitory pathways, has therapeutic potential for treatment of cancer. But for tumor immunotherapy, there are multiple barriers to the antitumor response, and coinhibitory pathways participate in shielding tumors from immune eradication. The differential expression of coinhibitory molecules (such as B7-H4) on certain cancers provides an opportunity for selective immunotherapeutic intervention. Interference with multiple coinhibitory pathways may be needed for optimal therapeutic benefit. Despite the expression of antigens by tumor cells, spontaneous immune-mediated rejection of cancer seems to be a rare event. TCR engagement by peptide/MHCs constitutes the main signal for the activation of naive T cells but is not sufficient to initiate a productive generation and maintenance of effector cells. Full activation of T cells requires additional signals driven by costimulatory molecules present on activated APCs but rarely on tumors. Following the discovery of B7-1 (CD80), several other costimulatory molecules have been shown to contribute to T-cell activation and have relevance for improving antitumor immunity. Moreover, increasing understanding of coinhibitory receptors has highlighted key additional pathways that can dominantly inhibit antitumor T-cell function. Improving positive costimulation, and interfering with negative regulation, continues to represent an attractive immunotherapeutic approach for the treatment of cancer. The pathways with the highest potential for clinical application and translation to the clinic, are clinical trials aimed at boosting positive costimulation and antitumor immunity with agonistic CD40, 4-1BB, or OX40 antibodies, and clinical trials that block the coinhibitory receptors CTLA-4 and PD-1. However, challenges are posed by the development of inflammation or autoimmunity following immune intervention.

As established by clinical and experimental results, it is quite evident that anti-CD80 antibody treatment is effective against relapsed and refractory follicular lymphoma. Future studies in other CD80-positive hematological malignancies (e.g., diffuse large B-cell NHL, CLL, Hodgkin's lymphoma, and MM) should also be taken under consideration. Thus, anti-CD80 antibody immunotherapy may have a potent role in the treatment of CD80-bearing cancer cells because their binding can modulate the key molecules in the signaling pathway and enhance antitumor response. Considering the importance of CD80 signaling in the regulation of immune responses against cancer, the manipulation of this signaling pathway to increase immunity against cancer represents a potential therapeutic approach. Understanding the mechanisms by which tumor cells escape immune surveillance will help us to establish new and effective approaches to vaccination and immunotherapy. One of the most important immune evasion mechanism employed by tumor cells is the downregulation of the CD80 costimulatory molecule. The success of novel cancer therapies depends on the identification of functional targets that play an essential role in tumor growth and metastasis, survival, and evasion from immunosurveillance. Anti-CD80 therapy can be used to target tumors expressing CD80. The clinical success of anti-CD80 antibody for the treatment of refractory follicular lymphoma has stimulated great interest in the promise of antibody therapeutics for cancer. The qualities of galiximab, like long half-life and high specificity and safety compared with other cancer therapeutics together with its ability to bind to and modulate key players in signaling pathways that drive malignant transformation and enhance antitumor immune functions, makes it a highly desirable therapeutic agent.

Most tumors do not regress but continue to grow in spite of the presence of spontaneous or antigen induced immune responses, due to downregulation of costimulatory molecules like CD80. The existence of systemic immune responses may not by itself be sufficient to deal with the complex nature of tumor—host interactions because factors such as insufficient costimulation to induce T-cell response may further contribute to the lack of effective immunity. It is now well established that T cells are rendered anergic due to the lack of costimulatory molecule(s) expression by tumor cells. Tumor cells are able to induce antigen-specific tolerance or anergy on the basis of MHC-I-restricted antigen presentation without the expression of costimulatory molecules. This unresponsiveness, however, can be reversed when tumor cells are genetically modified to express costimulatory molecules. A plethora of studies suggest that the insertion of genes encoding CD80 into tumors generally increases their immunogenicity and can be used as vaccine. Recently, fusagene vectors were developed to encode multiple gene products like CD80 with cytokines or MHC molecules as fusion proteins from a single cistron to increase the immunogenicity of target tumor cells. The vectors generated could be used in immunotherapy for the treatment of MM, leukemias, and other cancers, as they have been shown to stimulate allogeneic mixed lymphocyte proliferation and augment increases in CTL and NK cell responses and IFN-γ release. Considering the importance of costimulation in the regulation of immune responses against relapsed cancer, the manipulation of this pathway to increase immunity represents a potential therapeutic approach. Furthermore, signaling by either anti-CD80 antibodies or through CD28-bearing T cells regresses the growth, augments the expression of proapoptotic molecules, and induces apoptosis of CD80 + lymphomas. Therefore, immunotherapy utilizing anti-CD80 antibodies is a promising future treatment especially in the case of relapse and refractory lymphomas.

Our understanding of the B7 family has expanded enormously since the costimulatory pathways were first described. Contemporary models of immune regulatory networks reflect this complexity. The promise of immune-mediated enhancement of autologous and allogeneic responses through pharmacologic manipulation of this pathway shows substantial promise. Ongoing studies investigating the role of the most recently described members of the family: B7-H3, B7-H4, B7-H6, butyrophilin, and Skint will likely reveal further potentially modifiable pathways as therapeutic targets for intervention. Whereas manipulation of the B7 family members and their ligands in suppressing GVHD and augmenting GVL after allogeneic HSCT has shown benefit in murine studies, and promising results in limited phase 2 clinical studies, this remains an area for clinical trial development. The contribution of ICOS/ICOS-L to GVHD appears to be fundamental; however, based on our current understanding of this pathway, the complexities of the interactions make predictions of clinical responses difficult to predict. After decades of study, strategies incorporating B7 family members, such as CTLA-4 and PD-1 pathway-inhibiting molecules and CAR-T cells, have finally demonstrated clear clinical benefit, fulfilling the early promise of the importance of this family in malignancies. Further studies are necessary to evaluate the safety and the efficacy of these approaches before using them in the clinical practice for human use.

REFERENCES

1. Mir MA, Agrewala JN. Influence of CD80 and CD86 costimulation in the modulation of the activation of APCs. *Curr Immunol Rev* 2007;**3**(3):160–9.
2. Suvas S, Singh V, et al. Distinct role of CD80 and CD86 in the regulation of the activation of B cell and B cell lymphoma. *J Biol Chem* 2002;**277**:7766–75.
3. Yee KW, O'Brien SM. Emerging drugs for chronic lymphocytic leukaemia. *Expert Opin Emerg Drugs* 2006;**11**:167–89.
4. Puccetti P, Grohmann U. IDO and regulatory T cells: a role for reverse signaling and non-canonical NF-κ B activation. *Nat Rev Immunol* 2007;**7**:817–23.
5. Orabona C, Belladonna ML, Vacca C, et al. Cutting edge: silencing suppressor of cytokine signaling 3 expression in dendritic cells turns CD28-Ig from immune adjuvant to suppressant. *J Immunol* 2005;**174**:6582–6.
6. Kinnear G, Jones ND, Wood KJ. Costimulation blockade: current perspectives and implications for therapy. *Transplantation* 2013;**27**:527–35.
7. Inman BA, Frigola X, Dong H, Kwon ED. Costimulation, coinhibition and cancer. *Curr Cancer Drug Targets* 2007;**7**(1):15–30.
8. Greaves P, Gribben JG. The role of B7 family molecules in hematologic malignancy. *Blood* 2013;**121**(5):734–44.
9. Mir MA, Agrewala JN. Signaling through CD80: an approach for treating lymphomas. *Expert Opin Ther Targets* 2008;**12**:969–79.
10. Mir MA, Albaradie RS, Agrewala JN. Reverse costimulation through anti-B7-1 and anti-B7-2 in the survival of Mycobacterium tuberculosis in antigen presenting cells. *IJBPAS* 2013;**2**(5):1024–43.
11. Mir MA, Agrewala JN. Influence of CD80 and CD86 costimulation in the modulation of the activation of APCs. *Curr Immunol Rev* 2007;**3**(3):160–9.
12. Driessens G, Kline J, Gajewski TF. Costimulatory and coinhibitory receptors in anti-tumor immunity. *Immunol Rev* 2009;**229**:126–44.

13. Chen L, Ashe S, Brady WA, et al. Costimulation of antitumor immunity by the B7 counter receptor for the T lymphocyte molecules CD28 and CTLA-4. *Cell* 1992;**71**:1093–102.
14. Iwai Y, Ishida M, Tanaka Y, Okazaki T, Honjo T, Minato N. Involvement of PD-L1 on tumor cells in the escape from host immune system and tumor immunotherapy by PD-L1 blockade. *Proc Natl Acad Sci USA* 2002;**99**(19):12293–7.
15. Nomi T, Sho M, Akahori T, et al. Clinical significance and therapeutic potential of the programmed death-1 ligand/programmed death-1 pathway in human pancreatic cancer. *Clin Cancer Res* 2007;**13**(7):2151–7.
16. Fu T, He Q, Sharma P. The ICOS/ICOSL pathway is required for optimal antitumor responses mediated by anti-CTLA-4 therapy. *Cancer Res* 2011;**71**(16):5445–54.
17. Latchman Y, Wood CR, Chernova T, et al. PD-L2 is a second ligand for PD-1 and inhibits T cell activation. *Nat Immunol* 2001;**2**(3):261–8.
18. Dong H, Strome SE, Salomao DR, et al. Tumor-associated B7-H1 promotes T-cell apoptosis: a potential mechanism of immune evasion. *Nat Med* 2002;**8**(8):793–800.
19. Blazar BR, Taylor PA, Panoskaltsis-Mortari A, Sharpe AH, Vallera DA. Opposing roles of CD28: B7 and CTLA-4: B7 pathways in regulating in vivo alloresponses in murine recipients of MHC disparate T cells. *J Immunol* 1999;**162**(11):6368–77.
20. Koestner W, Hapke M, Herbst J, et al. PD-L1 blockade effectively restores strong graft-versus-leukemia effects without graft-versus-host disease after delayed adoptive transfer of T-cell receptor gene-engineered allogeneic CD8 + T cells. *Blood* 2011;**117**(3):1030–41.
21. Ozkaynak E, Gao W, Shemmeri N, et al. Importance of ICOS-B7RP-1 costimulation in acute and chronic allograft rejection. *Nat Immunol* 2001;**2**(7):591–6.
22. Taylor PA, Panoskaltsis-Mortari A, Freeman GJ, et al. Targeting of inducible costimulator (ICOS) expressed on alloreactive T cells down-regulates graft-versus-host disease (GVHD) and facilitates engraftment of allogeneic bone marrow (BM). *Blood* 2005;**105**(8):3372–80.
23. Maher J, Brentjens RJ, Gunset G, Riviere I, Sadelain M. Human T-lymphocyte cytotoxicity and proliferation directed by a single chimeric TCRzeta/CD28 receptor. *Nat Biotech* 2002;**20**(1):70–5.
24. Stephan MT, Ponomarev V, Brentjens RJ, et al. T-cell-encoded CD80 and 4-1BBL induce auto- and transcostimulation, resulting in potent tumor rejection. *Nat Med* 2007;**13**(12):1440–9.
25. Rosenblatt J, Glotzbecker B, Mills H, et al. PD-1 blockade by CT-011, anti-PD-1 antibody, enhances ex vivo tcell responses to autologous dendritic cell/myeloma fusion vaccine. *J Immunother* 2011;**34**(5):409–18.
26. Hobo W, Maas F, Adisty N, et al. siRNA silencing of PD-L1 and PD-L2 on dendritic cells augments expansion and function of minor histocompatibility antigen-specific CD8 + T cells. *Blood* 2010;**116**(22):4501–11.
27. Zippelius A, Batard P, Rubio-Godoy V, et al. Effector function of human tumor-specific CD8 T c ells in melanoma lesions: a state of local functional tolerance. *Cancer Res* 2004;**64**(8):2865–73.
28. Antonia SJ, Seigne J, Diaz J, et al. Phase I trial of a B7-1 (CD80) gene modified autologous tumor cell vaccine in combination with systemic interleukin-2 in patients with metastatic renal cell carcinoma. *J Urol* 2002;**167**:1995–2000.
29. Raez LE, Cassileth PA, Schlesselman JJ, et al. Allogeneic vaccination with a B7.1 HLA-A gene-modified adenocarcinoma cell line in patients with advanced non-small-cell lung cancer. *J Clin Oncol* 2004;**22**(14):2800–7.

30. Fishman M, Hunter TB, Soliman H, et al. Phase II trial of B7-1 (CD-86) transduced, cultured autologous tumor cell vaccine plus subcutaneous interleukin-2 for treatment of stage IV renal cell carcinoma. *J Immunother* 2008;**31**(1):72–80.
31. Kaufman HL, Cohen S, Cheung K, et al. Local delivery of vaccinia virus expressing multiple costimulatory molecules for the treatment of established tumors. *Hum Gene Ther* 2006;**17**(2):239–44.
32. DiPaola RS, Plante M, Kaufman H, et al. A phase I trial of pox PSA vaccines (PROSTVAC®-VF) with B7-1, ICAM-1, and LFA-3 co-stimulatory molecules (TRICOM) in patients with prostate cancer. *J Transl Med* 2006;**4**:191–2.
33. Kaufman HL, Kim-Schulze S, Manson K, et al. Poxvirus based vaccine therapy for patients with advanced pancreatic cancer. *J Transl Med* 2007;**5**:191–2.
34. Maker AV, Yang JC, Sherry RM, et al. Intrapatient dose escalation of anti-CTLA-4 antibody in patients with metastatic melanoma. *J Immunother* 2006;**29**(4):455–63.
35. Phan GQ, Yang JC, Sherry RM, Hwu P, Topalia SL, et al. Cancer regression and autoimmunity induced by cytotoxic T lymphocyte-associated antigen 4 blockade in patients with metastatic melanoma. *Proc Natl Acad Sci USA* 2003;**100**:8372–7.
36. Ribas A, Camacho LH, Lopez-Berestein G, et al. Antitumor activity in melanoma and anti-self responses in a phase I trial with the anti-cytotoxic T lymphocyte-associated antigen 4 monoclonal antibody CP-675,206. *J Clin Oncol* 2005;**23**:8968–77.
37. Ribas A, Antonia S, Sosman J. Results of a phase II clinical trial of 2 doses and schedules of CP-675206, an anti- CTLA4 monoclonal antibody, in patient (pts) with advanced melanoma. *J Clin Oncol* 2007;**25**:191,210,228.
38. Rini BI, Stein M, Shannon P, et al. Phase 1 dose-escalation trial of tremelimumab plus sunitinib in patients with metastatic renal cell carcinoma. *Cancer* 2011;**117**(4):758–67.
39. Chung KY, Gore I, Fong L, et al. Phase II study of the anti-cytotoxic T-lymphocyte-associated antigen 4 monoclonal antibody, tremelimumab, in patients with refractory metastatic colorectal cancer. *J Clin Oncol* 2010;**28**(21):3485–90.
40. Berger R, Rotem-Yehudar R, Slama G, et al. Phase I safety and pharmacokinetic study of CT-011, a humanized antibody interacting with PD-1, in patients with advanced hematologic malignancies. *Clin Cancer Res* 2008;**14**(10):3044–51.
41. Brahmer JR, Topalian S, Wollner I, et al. Safety and activity of MDX-1106 (ONO-4538), an anti-PD-1 monoclonal antibody, in patients with selected refractory or relapsed malignancies. *J Clin Oncol* 2008;**26**:3006.
42. Garber JK. Beyond ipilimumab: new approaches target the immunological synapse. *J Natl Cancer Inst* 2011;**103**(14):1079–82.
43. Kantoff PW, Schuetz TJ, Blumenstein BA, et al. Overall survival analysis of a phase II randomized controlled trial of a Poxviral-based PSA-targeted immunotherapy in metastatic castration-resistant prostate cancer. *J Clin Oncol* 2010;**28**(7):1099–105.
44. Li G, Wu X, Zhang F, et al. Triple expression of B7-1, B7-2 and 4-1BBL enhanced antitumor immune response against mouse H22 hepatocellular carcinoma. *J Cancer Res Clin Oncol* 2011;**137**:695–703.
45. Pan D, Wei X, Liu M, et al. Adenovirus mediated transfer of p53, GM-CSF and B7-1 suppresses growth and enhances immunogenicity of glioma cells. *Neurol Res* 2010;**32**(5):502–9.
46. Song J, Lei FT, Xiong X, Haque R. Intracellular signals of T cell costimulation. *Cell Mol Immunol* 2008;**5**(4):239–47.
47. Hurwitz AA, Foster BA, Kwon ED, et al. Combination immunotherapy of primary prostate cancer in a transgenic mouse model using CTLA-4 blockade. *Cancer Res* 2000;**60**(9):2444–8.

48. Gregor PD, Wolchok JD, Ferrone CR, et al. CTLA-4 blockade in combination with xenogeneic DNA vaccines enhances T-cell responses, tumor immunity and autoimmunity to self antigens in animal and cellular model systems. *Vaccine* 2004;**22**(13–14):1700–8.
49. Sutmuller RPM, Van Duivenvoorde LM, Van Elsas A, et al. Synergism of cytotoxic T lymphocyte-associated antigen 4 blockade and depletion of CD25 + regulatory T cells in antitumor therapy reveals alternative pathways for suppression of autoreactive cytotoxic T lymphocyte responses. *J Exp Med* 2001;**194**(6):823–32.
50. Davila E, Kennedy R, Cells E. Generation of antitumor immunity by cytotoxic T lymphocyte epitope peptide vaccination, CpG-oligodeoxynucleotide adjuvant, and CTLA-4 blockade. *Cancer Res* 2003;**63**(12):3281–8.
51. Demaria S, Kawashima N, Yang AM, et al. Immune mediated inhibition of metastases after treatment with local radiation and CTLA-4 blockade in a mouse model of breast cancer. *Clin Cancer Res* 2005;**11**(2):728–34.
52. Mokyr MB, Kalinichenko T, Gorelik L, Bluestone JA. Realization of the therapeutic potential of CTLA-4 blockade in low-dose chemotherapy-treated tumor-bearing mice. *Cancer Res* 1998;**58**(23):5301–4.
53. Shahinian A, Pfeffer K, et al. Differential T cell costimulatory requirements in CD28-deficient mice. *Science* 1993;**261**:609–12.
54. Snapper CM, Paul WE. Interferon-gamma and B cell stimulatory factor-1 reciprocally regulate Ig isotype production. *Science* 1987;**236**:944–7.
55. Freeman GJ, Boussiotis VA, et al. B7-1 and B7-2 do not deliver identical costimulatory signals, since B7-2 but not B7-1 preferentially costimulates the initial production of IL-4. *Immunity* 1995;**2**:523–32.
56. Sethna MP, van Parijs L, et al. A negative regulatory function of B7 revealed in B7-1 transgenic mice. *Immunity* 1994;**1**:415–21.
57. Ikemizu S, Gilbert RJ, et al. Structure and dimerization of a soluble form of B7-1. *Immunity* 2000;**12**:51–60.
58. Bajorath J, Peach RJ, Linsley PS. Immunoglobulin fold characteristics of B7-1 (CD80) and B7-2 (CD86). *Protein Sci* 1994;**3**:2148–50.
59. Leonard JP, Friedberg JW, et al. A phase I/II study of galiximab (an anti-CD80 monoclonal antibody) in combination with rituximab for relapsed or refractory, follicular lymphoma. *Ann Oncol* 2007;**18**:1216–23.
60. Gordon LI, Cheson BD, et al. Genentech, Inc. Phase I results from a multicenter trial of galiximab (anti-CD80 antibody, IDEC-114) in combination with rituximab for the treatment of follicular lymphoma. *Blood* 2003;**102**:307b.
61. Budd CR. Activation-induced cell death. *Curr Opin Immunol* 2001;**13**(3):356–62.
62. Gottschalk AR, Boise LH, et al. Identification of immunosuppressant-induced apoptosis in a murine B-cell line and its prevention by bcl-x but not bcl-2. *Proc Natl Acad Sci USA* 1994;**91**(15):7350–4.
63. Lee H, Choi J-K, Li M, Kaye K, Kieff E, Jung JU. Role of cellular tumor necrosis factor receptor-associated factors in NF-κB Activation and lymphocyte transformation by herpes virus Saimiri STP. *J Virol* 1999;**73**(5):3913–19.
64. Zheng P, Sarma S, Guo Y, Liu Y. Two mechanisms for tumor evasion of preexisting cytotoxic T-cell responses: lessons from recurrent tumors. *Cancer Res* 1999;**59**:3461–7.
65. Matulonis UA, Dosiou C, Lamont C, et al. Role of B7-1 in mediating an immune response to myeloid leukemia cells. *Blood* 1995;**85**:2507–15.

66. Wu TC, Huang AY, Jaffee EM, et al. A reassessment of the role of B7-1 expression in tumor rejection. *J Exp Med* 1995;**182**:1415–21.
67. Matsumoto K, Anasetti C. The role of T cell costimulation by CD80 in the initiation and maintenance of the immune response to human leukemia. *Leuk Lymphoma* 1999;**35**:427–35.
68. Huang AY, Bruce AT, Pardoll DM, et al. Does B7-1 expression confer antigen-presenting cell capacity to tumors in vivo?. *J Exp Med* 1996;**183**:769–76.
69. Reiser H, Freeman GJ, et al. Murine B7 antigen provides an efficient costimulatory signal for activation of murine T lymphocytes via the T-cell receptor/CD3 complex. *Proc Natl Acad Sci USA* 1992;**89**:271–5.
70. Kelly JM, Darcy PK, Markby JL, Godfrey DI, et al. Induction of tumor-specific T cell memory by NK cell-mediated tumor rejection. *Nat Immunol* 2002;**3**:83.
71. Harding FA, Allison JP. CD28-B7 interactions allow the induction of CD8 + cytotoxic T lymphocytes in the absence of exogenous help. *J Exp Med* 1993;**177**:1791–6.
72. Townsend SE, Allison JP. Tumor rejection after direct costimulation of CD8 + T cells by B7-transfected melanoma cells. *Science* 1993;**259**:368–70.
73. Tirapu I, Huarte E, Guiducci C, et al. Low surface expression of B7-1 CD80 is an immunoescape mechanism of colon carcinoma. *Cancer Res* 2006;**66**:2442–50.
74. Chambers BJ, Salcedo M, Ljunggren HG. Triggering of natural killer cells by the costimulatory molecule CD80 B7-1. *Immunity* 1996;**5**:311–17.
75. Heise CP, Shi F, Albertini MR, Mahvi DM. B7.1 expression eliminates tumor resistance to IL-12 gene therapy. *Cancer Gene Ther* 2001;**8**:118–27.
76. Baskar S, Ostrand-Rosenberg S, et al. Constitutive expression of B7 restores immunogenicity of tumor cells expressing truncated major histocompatibility complex class II molecules. *Proc Natl Acad Sci USA* 1993;**90**(12):5687–90.
77. Sakate Y, Yashiro M, Tanaka H, et al. Usefulness of inhibiting the lymph node metastasis in human gastric carcinoma by B71 gene transfection. *J Surg Res* 2004;**122**: 89–95.
78. Yu X, Abe R, Hodes RJ. The role of B7-CD28 co-stimulation in tumor rejection. *Int Immunol* 1998;**10**:791–7.
79. Bai XF, Liu J, May Jr. KF, et al. B7-CTLA4 interaction promotes cognate destruction of tumor cells by cytotoxic T lymphocytes in vivo. *Blood* 2002;**99**:2880–9.
80. Sojka DK, Donepudi M, et al. Melphalan and other anticancer modalities up-regulate B7-1 gene expression in tumor cells. *J Immunol* 2000;**164**:6230–6.
81. Lohr J, Knoechel B, Jiang S, et al. The inhibitory function of B7 costimulators in T cell responses to foreign and self-antigens. *Nat Immunol* 2003;**4**:664–9.
82. Liu J, Xia X, Torrero M, et al. The mechanism of exogenous B7.1-enhanced IL-12-mediated complete regression of tumors by a single electroporation delivery. *Int J Cancer* 2006;**119**:2113–18.
83. Putzer BM, Rodicker F, Hitt MM, et al. Improved treatment of pancreatic cancer by IL-12 and B7.1 costimulation: antitumor efficacy and immunoregulation in a nonimmunogenic tumor model. *Mol Ther* 2002;**5**:405–12.
84. Singh NP, Miller RW, Yolcu ES, et al. Primary tumor cells resected from cancer patients and decorated with a novel form of CD80 protein serve as effective antigen-presenting cells for the induction of autologous T cell immune responses ex vivo. *Hum Gene Ther* 2006;**17**:334–46.

85. Si SY, Hu PZ, Huang YY, et al. Tumor cells with B7.1 and transmembrane anchored staphylococcal enterotoxin A generate effective antitumor immunity. *Biochem Biophys Res Commun* 2006;**347**:208–14.
86. Van Ginderachter JA, Geldhof AB, et al. B7-1, IFN γ and anti-CTLA-4 co-operate to prevent T-cell tolerization during immunotherapy against a murine T-lymphoma. *Int J Cancer* 2000;**87**:539–47.
87. Baskar S, Glimcher L, et al. Major histocompatibility complex class II + B7-1 + tumor cells are potent vaccines for stimulating tumor rejection in tumor-bearing mice. *J Exp Med* 1995;**181**:619–29.
88. Chan L, Hardwick N, Darling D, et al. IL-2/B7.1 CD80 fusagene transduction of AML blasts by a self-inactivating lentiviral vector stimulates T cell responses in vitro: a strategy to generate whole cell vaccines for AML. *Mol Ther* 2005;**11**:120–31.
89. Wen XY, Mandelbaum S, Li ZH, et al. Tricistronic viral vectors co-expressing interleukin-12 (IL-12) and CD80 (B7-1) for the immunotherapy of cancer: preclinical studies in myeloma. *Cancer Gene Ther* 2001;**8**:361–70.
90. Carlring J, Shaif-Muthana M, Sisley K, et al. Apoptotic cell death in conjunction with CD80 costimulation confers uveal melanoma cells with the ability to induce immune responses. *Immunology* 2003;**109**:41–8.
91. Waterhouse P, Penninger JM, et al. Lymphoproliferative disorders with early lethality in mice deficient in Ctla-4. *Science* 1995;**270**:985–8.
92. Ruiz-Ruiz C, Munoz-Pinedo C, Lopez-Rivas A. Interferon-γ treatment elevates caspase-8 expression and sensitizes human breast tumor cells to a death receptor-induced mitochondria-operated apoptotic program. *Cancer Res* 2000;**60**:5673–80.
93. Bogner C, Sandherr M, Perker M, et al. Cyclin E but not bcl-2, bax or mcl-1 is differentially expressed in ZAP 70-positive and ZAP 70-negative B-CLL cells. *Ann Hematol* 2006;**85**:458–62.
94. Logue EC, Sha WC. CD28-B7 bidirectional signaling: a two-way street to activation. *Nat Immunol* 2004;**5**:1103–5.
95. Orabona C, Grohmann U, et al. CD28 induces immunostimulatory signals in dendritic cells via CD80 and CD86. *Nat Immunol* 2004;**5**:1134–42.
96. Harris M. Monoclonal antibodies as therapeutic agents for cancer [review]. *Lancet Oncol* 2004;**5**(5):292–302.
97. Keating MJ. Management of chronic lymphocytic leukemia: a changing field. *Rev Clin Exp Hematol* 2002;**6**(4):350–65.
98. Hurwitz H, Fehrenbacher L, Cartwright T, et al. Bevacizumab a monoclonal antibody to vascular-endothelial growth factor prolongs survival in first-line colorectal cancer: results of a phase III trial of bevacizumab in combination with bolus IFL (irinotecan, 5 fluorouracil, leucovorin) as first-line therapy in subjects with metastatic colorectal cancer. *Proc Am Soc Clin Oncol* 2003;**22**:202.
99. Plosker GL, Figgitt DP. Rituximab: a review of its use in non-Hodgkin's lymphoma and chronic lymphocytic leukaemia [review]. *Drugs* 2003;**63**:803–43.
100. Demidem A, Lam T, Alas S, et al. Chimeric anti-CD20 (IDEC-C2B8) monoclonal antibody sensitizes a B cell lymphoma cell line to cell killing by cytotoxic drugs. *Cancer Biother Radiopharm* 1997;**12**:177–85.
101. Davis M. Ethics in phase II trials of cancer therapies. *Perspectives Prof* 2000;**20**(1):E1.
102. Kennett RG. Monoclonal antibodies. Hybrid myelomas—a revolution in serology and immunogenetics. *Am J Hum Genet* 1979;**31**(5):539–47.

103. Morrison SL, Johnson MJ, Herzenberg LA, Oi VT. Chimeric human antibody molecules: mouse antigen-binding domains with human constant region domains. *Proc Natl Acad Sci USA* 1984;**81**(21):6851–5.
104. Czuczman MS, Thall A, et al. Phase I/II study of galiximab, an anti-CD80 antibody, for relapsed or refractory follicular lymphoma. *J Clin Oncol* 2005;**23**:4390–8.
105. Hariharan HK, Murphy T, et al. Combining galiximab with the chemotherapeutic agents fludarabine or doxorubicin improves efficacy in animal models of lymphoma. ASCO Annual Meeting Proceedings. *J Clin Oncol* 2007;**3**:3040.
106. Gottlieb AB, Kang S, Linden KG, et al. Evaluation of safety and clinical activity of multiple doses of the anti-CD80 monoclonal antibody, galiximab, in patients with moderate to severe plaque psoriasis. *Clin Immunol* 2004;**111**:28–37.
107. Wang S, Chen L. Co-signaling molecules of the B7-CD28 family in positive and negative regulation of T lymphocyte responses. *Microbes Infect* 2004;**6**:759–66.
108. Leget GA, Czuczman MS. Use of rituximab, the new FDA-approved antibody. *Curr Opin Oncol* 1998;**10**(6):548–51.
109. Hiddemann W, Cheson BD. How we manage follicular lymphoma. *Leukemia* 2014;**28**(7):1388–95.
110. Forstpointner R, Unterhalt M, et al. Maintenance therapy with rituximab leads to a significant prolongation of response duration after salvage therapy with a combination of rituximab, fludarabine, cyclophosphamide, and mitoxantrone (R-FCM) in patients with recurring and refractory follicular and mantle cell lymphomas: results of a prospective randomized study of the German Low Grade Lymphoma Study Group (GLSG). *Blood* 2006;**108**(13):4003–8.
111. Colombat P, Brousse N, Salles G, Morschhauser F, et al. Rituximab induction immunotherapy for first-line low-tumor-burden follicular lymphoma: survival analyses with 7-year follow-up. *Ann Oncol* 2012;**23**(9):2380–5.
112. Liu Q, Fayad L, Cabanillas F, Hagemeister FB, Ayers GD, et al. Improvement of overall and failure-free survival in stage IV follicular lymphoma: 25 years of treatment experience at The University of Texas M.D. Anderson Cancer Center. *J Clin Oncol* 2006;**24**(10):1582–9.
113. Marcus NJ. Pain in cancer patients unrelated to the cancer or treatment. *Cancer Invest* 2005;**23**(1):84–93.
114. Young RC. Initial therapy for early ovarian carcinoma. *Cancer* 1987;**60**(Suppl. 8):2042–9.
115. Bhat S, Czuczman MS. Galiximab: a review. *Expert Opin Biol Ther* 2010;**10**(3):451–8.
116. Vinjamaram S, Czuczman MS, Hernandez-Ilizaliturri FJ. The use of galiximab in non-Hodgkin lymphoma. *Clin Lymphoma Myeloma* 2008;**8**(5):277–82.
117. Czuczman MS, Leonard JP, Jung S, Johnson JL, et al. Phase II trial of galiximab (anti-CD80 monoclonal antibody) plus rituximab (CALGB 50402): follicular Lymphoma International Prognostic Index (FLIPI) score is predictive of upfront immunotherapy responsiveness. *Ann Oncol* 2012;**23**(9):2356–62.
118. Yuan J, Adamow M, Ginsberg BA, et al. Integrated NYESO-1 antibody and CD8 + T-cell responses correlate with clinical benefit in advanced melanoma patients treated with ipilimumab. *Proc Natl Acad Sci USA* 2011;**108**(40):16723–8.
119. Korman AJ, Peggs KS, Allison JP. Checkpoint blockade in cancer immunotherapy. *Adv Immunol* 2006;**90**:297–339.
120. Weber J, Thompson JA, Hamid O, et al. A randomized, double-blind, placebo-controlled, phase II study comparing the tolerability and efficacy of ipilimumab administered with or without prophylactic budesonide in patients with unresectable stage III or IV melanoma. *Clin Cancer Res* 2009;**15**(17):5591–8.

121. Hamid O, Chin K, Li J, et al. Dose effect of ipilimumab in patients with advanced melanoma: results from a phase II, randomized, dose-ranging study. *J Clin Oncol* 2008;**26**:489s.
122. Day SJO, Maio M, Chiarion-Sileni V, et al. Efficacy and safety of ipilimumab monotherapy in patients with pretreated advanced melanoma: a multicenter single-arm phase II study. *Ann Oncol* 2010;**21**(8):1712–17.
123. Wolchok JD, Neyns B, Linette G, et al. Ipilimumab monotherapy in patients with pretreated advanced melanoma: a randomised, double-blind, multicentre, phase 2, dose-ranging study. *Lancet Oncol* 2010;**11**(2)):155–64.
124. Hersh EM, O'Day SJ, Powderly J, et al. A phase II multicenter study of ipilimumab with or without dacarbazine in chemotherapy-naïve patients with advanced melanoma. *Invest New Drugs* 2011;**29**(3):489–98.
125. Robert C, Thomas L, Bondarenko I, et al. Ipilimumab plus dacarbazine for previously untreated metastatic melanoma. *N Engl J Med* 2011;**364**(26):2517–26.
126. Hodi FS, O'Day SJ, McDermott DF, et al. Improved survival with ipilimumab in patients with metastatic melanoma. *N Engl J Med* 2010;**363**:711–23.
127. Yang JC, Hughes M, Kammula U, et al. Ipilimumab (anti-CTLA4 antibody) causes regression of metastatic renal cell cancer associated with enteritis and hypophysitis. *J Immunother* 2007;**30**(8):825–30.
128. Lynch TJ, Bondarenko IN, Luft A, et al. Phase II trial of ipilimumab (IPI) and paclitaxel/carboplatin (P/C) in firstline stage IIIb/IV non small cell lung cancer (NSCLC). *J Clin Oncol* 2010;**102**:1388–97.
129. Ribas A, Bozon VA, Lopez-Berestein G, et al. Phase 1 trial of monthly doses of the human anti-CTLA4monoclonal antibody CP-675,206 in patients with advanced melanoma. *J Clin Oncol* 2005;**23**(16S):7524.
130. Kirkwood JM, Lorigan P, Hersey P, Hauschild A, Robert C, McDermott D, et al. Phase II trial of tremelimumab (CP-675,206) in patients with advanced refractory or relapsed melanoma. *Clin Cancer Res* 2010;**16**(3):1042–8.
131. Ascierto PA, Marincola FM, Ribas A. Anti-CTLA4 monoclonal antibodies: the past and the future in clinical application. *J Transl Med* 2011;**9**:196.
132. Ying H, Yang L, Qiao G, et al. Cutting edge: CTLA-4-B7 interaction suppresses Th17 cell differentiation. *J Immunol* 2010;**185**:1375–8.
133. McHugh RS, Whitters MJ, Piccirillo CA, et al. CD4 + CD25 + immunoregulatory T cells: gene expression analysis reveals a functional role for the glucocorticoid induced TNF receptor. *Immunity* 2002;**16**(2):311–23.
134. Swallow MM, Wallin JJ, Sha WC. B7h, a novel costimulatory homolog of B7.1 and B7.2, is induced by TNFα. *Immunity* 1999;**11**(4):423–32.
135. Simpson TR, Quezada SA, Allison JP. Regulation of CD4 T cell activation and effector function by inducible costimulator (ICOS). *Curr Opin Immunol* 2010;**22**:326–32.
136. Liu X, Bai XF, Wen J, et al. B7H costimulates clonal expansion of, and cognate destruction of tumor cells by, CD8 + T lymphocytes in vivo. *J Exp Med* 2001;**194**(9):1339–48.
137. Wallin JJ, Liang L, Bakardjiev A, Sha WC. Enhancement of CD8 + T cell responses by ICOS/B7h costimulation. *J Immunol* 2001;**167**(1):132–9.
138. Zuberek K, Ling V, Wu P, et al. Comparable in vivo efficacy of CD28/B7, ICOS/GL50, and ICOS/GL50B costimulatory pathways in murine tumor models: IFNγ-dependent enhancement of CTL priming, effector functions, and tumor specific memory CTL. *Cell Immunol* 2003;**225**(1):53–63.

139. Liakou CI, Kamat A, Tang DN, et al. CTLA-4 blockade increases IFNγ-producing CD4 + ICOS hi cells to shift the ratio of effector to regulatory T cells in cancer patients. *Proc Natl Acad Sci USA* 2008;**105**(39)):14987–92.
140. Vonderheide RH, Lorusso PM, Khalil M, et al. Tremelimumab in combination with exemestane in patients with advanced breast cancer and treatment-associated modulation of inducible costimulator expression on patient T cells. *Clin Cancer Res* 2010;**16**(13):3485–94.
141. Lee H, Kim JH, Yang SY, et al. Peripheral blood gene expression of B7 and CD28 family members associated with tumor progression and microscopic lymphovascular invasion in colon cancer patients. *J Cancer Res Clin Oncol* 2010;**136**(9):1445–52.
142. Bogunovic D, O'Neill DW, Belitskaya-Levy I, et al. Immune profile and mitotic index of metastatic melanoma lesions enhance clinical staging in predicting patient survival. *Proc Nat Acad Sci USA* 2009;**106**(48):20429–34.
143. Strauss L, Bergmann C, Szczepanski MJ, Lang S, Kirkwood JM, Whiteside TL. Expression of ICOS on human melanoma-infiltrating CD4 + CD25 highFoxp3 + T regulatory cells: implications and impact on tumor-mediated immune suppression. *J Immunol* 2008;**180**(5):2967–80.
144. Martin-Orozco N, Li Y, Wang Y, et al. Melanoma cells express ICOS ligand to promote the activation and expansion of T-regulatory cells. *Cancer Res* 2010;**70**(23):9581–90.
145. Riley JL. PD-1 signaling in primary T cells. *Immunol Rev* 2009;**229**(1):114–25.
146. Butte MJ, Keir ME, Phamduy TB, Sharpe AH, Freeman GJ. Programmed death-1 ligand 1 interacts specifically with the B7-1 costimulatory molecule to inhibit T-cell responses. *Immunity* 2007;**27**(1):111–22.
147. Carreras J, Lopez-Guillermo A, Roncador G, et al. High numbers of tumor-infiltrating programmed cell death 1-positive regulatory lymphocytes are associated with improved overall survival in follicular lymphoma. *J Clin Oncol* 2009;**27**(9):1470–6.
148. Steidl C, Shah SP, Woolcock BW, et al. MHC class II transactivator CIITA is a recurrent gene fusion partner in lymphoid cancers. *Nature* 2011;**471**(7338):377–81.
149. Green MR, Monti S, Rodig SJ, et al. Integrative analysis reveals selective 9p24.1amplification, increased PD-1 ligand expression, and further induction via JAK2 in nodular sclerosing odgkin lymphoma and primary mediastinal large B-cell lymphoma. *Blood* 2010;**116**(17):3268–77.
150. Liu J, Hamrouni A, Wolowiec D, et al. Plasma cells from multiple myeloma patients express B7-H1 (PD-L1) and increase expression after stimulation with IFN-{gamma} and TLR ligands via a MyD88-,TRAF6-, and MEK-dependent pathway. *Blood* 2007;**110**(1):296–304.
151. Hallett WHD, Jing W, Drobyski WR, Johnson BD. Immunosuppressive effects of multiple myeloma are overcome by PD-L1 blockade. *Biol Blood Marrow Transplant* 2011;**17**(8):1133–45.
152. Benson Jr. DM, Bakan CE, Mishra A, et al. The PD-1/PD-L1 axis modulates the natural killer cell versus multiple myeloma effect: a therapeutic target for CT-011, a novel monoclonal anti-PD-1 antibody. *Blood* 2010;**116**(13):2286–94.
153. Blank C, Brown I, Peterson AC, et al. PD-L1/B7H-1 inhibits the effector phase of tumor rejection by Tcell receptor (TCR) transgenic CD8 + T cells. *Cancer Res* 2004;**64**(3):1140–5.
154. Saudemont A, Buffenoir G, Denys A, et al. Gene transfer of CD154 and IL12 cDNA induces an antileukemic immunity in a murine model of acute leukemia. *Leukemia* 2002;**16**(9):1637–44.

155. Saudemont A, Quesnel B. In a model of tumor dormancy, long-term persistent leukemic cells have increased B7-H1 and B7.1 expression and resist CTL-mediated lysis. *Blood* 2004;**104**(7):2124–33.
156. Tamura H, Dan K, Tamada K, et al. Expression of functional B7-H2 and B7.2 costimulatory molecules and their prognostic implications in de novo acute myeloid leukemia. *Clin Cancer Res* 2005;**11**(16):5708–17.
157. Berthon C, Driss V, Liu J, et al. In acute myeloid leukemia, B7-H1 (PD-L1) protection of blasts from cytotoxic T cells is induced by TLR ligands and interferon-gamma and can be reversed using MEK inhibitors. *Cancer Immunol Immunother* 2010;**59**(12):1839–49.
158. Ramsay AG, Clear AJ, Fatah R, Gribben JG. Multiple inhibitory ligands induce impaired T-cell immunologic synapse function in chronic lymphocytic leukemia that can be blocked with lenalidomide: establishing a reversible immune evasion mechanism in human cancer. *Blood* 2012;**120**(7):1412–21.
159. Aue G, Njuguna N, Tian X, et al. Lenalidomide-induced upregulation of CD80 on tumor cells correlates with T-cell activation, the rapid onset of a cytokine release syndrome and leukemic cell clearance in chronic lymphocytic leukemia. *Haematologica* 2009;**94** (9):1266–73.
160. Kozako T, Yoshimitsu M, Fujiwara H, et al. PD-1/PD-L1 expression in human T-cell leukemia virus type 1 carriers and adult T-cell leukemia/lymphoma patients. *Leukemia* 2009;**23**(2):375–82.
161. Thompson RH, Dong H, Kwon ED. Implications of B7-H1 expression in clear cell carcinoma of the kidney for prognostication and therapy. *Clin Cancer Res* 2007;**13** (2):709s–15s.
162. Zang X, Allison JP. The B7 family and cancer therapy: costimulation and coinhibition. *Clin Cancer Res* 2007;**13**(18):5271–9.
163. Thompson RH, Gillett MD, Cheville JC, et al. Costimulatory B7-H1 in renal cell carcinoma patients: indicator of tumor aggressiveness and potential therapeutic target. *Proc Natl Acad Sci USA* 2004;**101**(49):17174–9.
164. Ghebeh H, Mohammed S, Al-Omair A, et al. The B7-H1 (PD-L1) T lymphocyte-inhibitory molecule is expressed in breast cancer patients with infiltrating ductal carcinoma: correlation with important high-risk prognostic factors. *Neoplasia* 2006;**8** (3):190–8.
165. Nakanishi J, Wada Y, Matsumoto K, Azuma M, Kikuchi K, Ueda S. Overexpression of B7-H1 (PD-L1) significantly associates with tumor grade and postoperative prognosis in human urothelial cancers. *Cancer Immunol Immunother* 2007;**56**(8)):1173–82.
166. Li B, Vanroey M, Wang C, Chen THT, Korman A, Jooss K. Anti-programmed death-1 synergizes with granulocyte macrophage colony-stimulating factor-secreting tumor cell immunotherapy providing therapeutic benefit to mice with established tumors. *Clin Cancer Res* 2009;**15**(5):1623–34.
167. Durgan K, Ali M, Warner P, Latchman YE. Targeting NKT cells and PD-L1 pathway results in augmented antitumor responses in a melanoma model. *Cancer Immunol Immunother* 2011;**60**(4):547–58.
168. Mangsbo SM, Sandin LC, Anger K, Korman AJ, et al. Enhanced tumor eradication by combining CTLA-4 or PD-1 blockade with CpG therapy. *J Immunother* 2010;**33** (3):225–35.
169. Curiel TJ, Wei S, Dong H, et al. Blockade of B7-H1 improves myeloid dendritic cell-mediated antitumor immunity. *Nat Med* 2003;**9**(5):562–7.

170. Martin-Orozco N, Dong C. Inhibitory costimulation and anti-tumor immunity. *Semin Cancer Biol* 2007;**17**(4):288–98.
171. Mkrtichyan M, Najjar YG, Raulfs EC, et al. Anti-PD-1 synergizes with cyclophosphamide to induce potent antitumor vaccine effects through novel mechanisms. *Eur J Immunol* 2011;**41**(10):2977–86.
172. Ascierto PA, Simeone E, Sznol M, Fu YX, Melero I. Clinical experiences with anti-CD137 and anti-PD1 therapeutic antibodies. *Semin Oncol* 2010;**37**(5):508–16.
173. Brahmer JR, Tykodi SS, Chow LQ, et al. Safety and activity of anti-PD-L1 antibody in patients with advanced cancer. *N Engl J Med* 2012;**366**(26):2455–65.
174. Topalian SL, Hodi FS, Brahmer JR, et al. Safety, activity, and immune correlates of anti-PD-1 antibody in cancer. *N Engl J Med* 2012;**366**(26):2443–54.
175. Patnaik A, Kang SP, Tolcher AW, et al. Phase I study of MK-3475 (anti-PD-1 monoclonal antibody) in patients with advanced solid tumors. *J Clin Oncol* 2012;**30**(Suppl.):215.
176. Del Rio ML, Lucas CL, Buhler L, Rayat G, Rodriguez-Barbosa JI. HVEM/LIGHT/BTLA/CD160 cosignaling pathways as targets for immune regulation. *J Leukoc Biol* 2010;**87**(2):223–35.
177. Murphy TL, Murphy KM. Slow down and survive: enigmatic immunoregulation by BTLA and HVEM. *Annu Rev Immunol* 2010;**28**:389–411.
178. Vendel AC, Calemine-Fenaux J, Izrael-Tomasevic A, Chauhan V, et al. B and T lymphocyte attenuator regulates B cell receptor signaling by targeting Syk and BLNK. *J Immunol* 2009;**182**(3):1509–17.
179. Hidi HM, Thibult ML, Chetaille B, et al. High expression of the inhibitory receptor BTLA in T-follicular helper cells and in B-cell small lymphocytic lymphoma/chronic lymphocytic leukemia. *Am J Clin Pathol* 2009;**132**(4):589–96.
180. Han L, Wang W, Fang Y, et al. Soluble B and T lymphocyte attenuator possesses antitumor effects and facilitates heat shock protein 70 vaccine-triggered antitumor immunity against amurine TC-1 cervical cancer model in vivo. *J Immunol* 2009;**183**(12):7842–50.
181. Derré L, Rivals JP, Jandus C, et al. BTLA mediates inhibition of human tumor-specific CD8 + T cells that can be partially reversed by vaccination. *J Clin Invest* 2010;**120**(1):157–67.
182. Maeda M, Carpenito C, Russell RC, et al. Murine CD160, Ig-like receptor on NK Cells and NKT cells, recognizes classical and nonclassical MHC class I and regulates NK cell activation. *J Immunol* 2005;**175**(7):4426–32.
183. Cai G, Anumanthan A, Brown JA, Greenfield EA, Zhu B, Freeman GJ. CD160 inhibits activation of human CD4 + T cells through interaction with herpes virus entry mediator. *Nat Immunol* 2008;**9**(2):176–85.
184. Liu FT, Giustiniani J, Farren T, et al. CD160 signaling mediates PI3K-dependent survival and growth signals in chronic lymphocytic leukemia. *Blood* 2010;**115**(15):3079–88.
185. Farren TW, Giustiniani J, Liu F-T, et al. Differential and tumor-specific expression of CD160 in B-cell malignancies. *Blood* 2011;**118**(8):2174–83.
186. Chabot S, Jabrane-Ferrat N, Bigot K, et al. A novel antiangiogenic and vascular normalization therapy targeted against human CD160 receptor. *J Exp Med* 2011;**208**(5):973–86.
187. Kleeff J, Loos M, Hedderich DM, Friess H. B7-H3 and its role in antitumor immunity. *Clin Dev Immunol* 2010;**17**(10):3100–11 [article 683875].
188. Sica GL, Choi IH, Zhu G, et al. B7-H4, a molecule of theB7 family, negatively regulates T cell immunity. *Immunity* 2003;**18**(6):849–61.
189. Zang X, Loke P, Kim J, Murphy K, Waitz R, Allison JP. B7x: a widely expressed B7 family member that inhibits T cell activation. *Proc Nat Acad Sci USA* 2003;**100**(18):10388–92.

190. He C, Qiao H, Jiang H, Sun X. The inhibitory role of b7-h4 in antitumor immunity: association with cancer progression and survival. *Clin Dev Immunol* 2011;**378**:79–83 [article ID 695834, 8 pages].
191. Quandt D, Fiedler E, Boettcher D, Marsch W Ch, Seliger B. B7-H4 expression in human melanoma: its association with patients' survival and antitumor immune response. *Clin Cancer Res* 2011;**17**(10):3100–11.
192. Kryczek I, Zou L, Rodriguez P, et al. B7-H4 expression identifies a novel suppressive macrophage population in human ovarian carcinoma. *J Exp Med* 2006;**203**(4):871–81.
193. Qian Y, Shen L, Xu C, et al. Development of a novel monoclonal antibody to B7-H4: characterization and biological activity. *Eur J Med Res* 2011;**16**(7):295–302.
194. Banchereau J, Dubois B, Fayette J, et al. Functional CD40 antigen on B cells, dendritic cells and fibroblasts. *Adv Exp Med Biol* 1995;**378**:79–83.
195. Elgueta R, Benson MJ, De Vries VC, Wasiuk A, Guo Y, Noelle RJ. Molecular mechanism and function of CD40/CD40L engagement in the immune system. *Immunol Rev* 2009;**229**(1):152–72.
196. Quezada SA, Jarvinen LZ, Lind EF, Noelle RJ. CD40/CD154 interactions at the interface of tolerance and immunity. *Annu Rev Immunol* 2004;**22**:307–28.
197. Kikuchi T, Worgall S, Singh R, Moore MAS, Crystal RG. Dendritic cells genetically modified to express CD40 ligand and pulsed with antigen can initiate antigen specific humoral immunity independent of CD4 + T cells. *Nat Med* 2000;**6**(10):1154–9.
198. Ahonen CL, Wasiuk A, Fuse S, et al. Enhanced efficacy and reduced toxicity of multifactorial adjuvants compared with unitary adjuvants as cancer vaccines. *Blood* 2008;**111**(6):3116–25.
199. Nowak AK, Robinson BWS, Lake RA. Synergy between chemotherapy and immunotherapy in the treatment of established murine solid tumors. *Cancer Res* 2003;**63**(15):4490–6.
200. Honeychurch J, Glennie MJ, Johnson PWM, Illidge TM. Anti-CD40 monoclonal antibody therapy in combination with irradiation results in a CD8 T-cell dependent immunity to B-cell lymphoma. *Blood* 2003;**102**(4):1449–57.
201. Vonderheide RH, Flaherty KT, Khalil M, et al. Clinical activity and immune modulation in cancer patients treated with CP-870,893, a novel CD40 agonist monoclonal antibody. *J Clin Oncol* 2007;**25**(7):876–83.
202. Ruter J, Antonia SJ, Burris HA, Huhn RD, Vonderheide RH. Immune modulation with weekly dosing of an agonist CD40 antibody in a phase I study of patients with advanced solid tumors. *Cancer Biol Ther* 2010;**10**(10):983–93.
203. Advani R, Forero-Torres A, Furman RR, et al. Phase I study of the humanized anti-CD40 monoclonal antibody dacetuzumab in refractory or recurrent non-Hodgkin's lymphoma. *J Clin Oncol* 2009;**27**(26):4371–7.
204. Hussein M, Berenson JR, Niesvizky R, et al. A phase I multidose study of dacetuzumab (SGN-40; humanized anti-CD40 monoclonal antibody) in patients with multiple myeloma. *Haematologica* 2010;**95**(5):845–8.
205. Furman RR, Forero-Torres A, Shustov A, Drachman JG. A phase I study of dacetuzumab (SGN-40, a humanized anti-CD40 monoclonal antibody) in patients with chronic lymphocytic leukemia. *Leuk Lymphoma* 2010;**51**(2):228–35.
206. Sznol M, Hodi FS, Margolin K, et al. Phase I study of BMS-663513, a fully human anti-CD137 agonist monoclonal antibody, in patients (pts) with advanced cancer (CA). *J Clin Oncol* 2008;**26**:3007.
207. Younes A, Bartlett NL, Leonard JP, et al. Brentuximab vedotin (SGN-35) for relapsed CD30-positive lymphomas. *N Engl J Med* 2010;**363**(19):1812–21.

208. Chen RW, Gopal AK, Smith SE, et al. Results from a pivotal phase II study of Bretuximab vedutin (SGN-35) in patients with relapsed or refractory Hodgkin Lymphoma (HL). *J Clin Oncol* 2011;**29**(Suppl. 15):225.
209. Barlett NL, Grove LE, Kennedy D, Sievers EL, Forero-Torres A. Objective responses with Bretuximab vedutin (SGN-35) retreatment in CD30-positive hemalogic malignancies: a case series. *J Clin Oncol* 2010;**28**(Suppl. 15):225.
210. Katz J, Janik JE, Younes A. Brentuximab vedotin (SGN-35). *Clin Cancer Res* 2011;**17**(20):6428–36.
211. Gladue RP, Paradis T, Cole SH, et al. The CD40 agonist antibody CP-870,893 enhances dendritic cell and B-cell activity and promotes anti-tumor efficacy in SCID-hu mice. *Cancer Immunol Immunother* 2011;**60**(7):1009–17.
212. Carpenter EL, Mick R, Rüter J, Vonderheide RH. Activation of human B cells by the agonist CD40 antibody CP-870,893 and augmentation with simultaneous toll-like receptor 9 stimulation. *J Transl Med* 2009;**7**:93,219.
213. Lewis TS, McCormick RS, Emmerton K, et al. Distinct apoptotic signaling characteristics of the anti-CD40 monoclonal antibody dacetuzumab and rituximab produce enhanced antitumor activity in non-Hodgkin lymphoma. *Clin Cancer Res* 2011;**17**(14):4672–81.
214. Tai YT, Catley LP, Mitsiades CS, et al. Mechanisms by which SGN-40, a humanized anti-CD40 antibody, induces cytotoxicity in human multiple myeloma cells: clinical implications. *Cancer Res* 2004;**64**(8):2846–52.
215. Lapalombella R, Gowda A, Joshi T, et al. The humanized CD40 antibody SGN-40 demonstrates pre-clinical activity that is enhanced by lenalidomide in chronic lymphocytic leukaemia. *Br J Haematol* 2009;**144**(6):848–55.
216. Luqman M, Klabunde S, Lin K, et al. The antileukemia activity of a human anti-CD40 antagonist antibody, HCD122, on human chronic lymphocytic leukemia cells. *Blood* 2008;**112**(3):711–20.
217. Vinay DS, Kwon BS. 4-1BB signaling beyond T cells. *Cell Mol Immunol* 2011;**8**(4):281–4.
218. Vinay DS, Kwon BS. Immunotherapy targeting 4-1BB and its ligand. *Int J Hematol* 2006;**83**(1):23–8.
219. Saoulli K, Lee SY, Cannons JL, et al. CD28-independent, TRAF2-dependent costimulation of resting T cells by 4-1BB ligand. *J Exp Med* 1998;**187**(11):1849–62.
220. Cheuk ATC, Mufti GJ, Guinn BA. Role of 4-1BB: 4-1BB ligand in cancer immunotherapy. *Cancer Gene Ther* 2004;**11**(3):215–26.
221. Strome SE, Martin B, Flies D, et al. Enhanced therapeutic potential of adoptive immunotherapy by in vitro CD28/4-1BB costimulation of tumor-reactive T cells against a poorly immunogenic, major histocompatibility complex class I negative A9P melanoma. *J Immunother* 2000;**23**(4):430–7.
222. Li Q, Carr A, Ito F, Teitz-Tennenbaum S, Chang AE. Polarization effects of 4-1BB during CD28 costimulation in generating tumor-reactive T cells for cancer immunotherapy. *Cancer Res* 2003;**63**(10)):2546–52.
223. Melero I, Shuford WW, Newby SA, et al. Monoclonal antibodies against the 4-1BB T-cell activation molecule eradicate established tumors. *Nat Med* 1997;**3**(6):682–5.
224. Lee H, Park H-J, Sohn H-J, Kim JM, Kim SJ. Combinatorial therapy for liver metastatic colon cancer: dendritic cell vaccine and low-dose agonistic anti-4-1BB antibody co-stimulatory signal. *J Surg Res* 2011;**169**(1):e43–50.
225. Molckovsky A, Siu LL. First-in-class, first-in-human phase I results of targeted agents: highlights of the 2008 American society of clinical oncology meeting. *J Hematol Oncol* 2008;**1**:221.

226. Croft M, So T, Duan W, Soroosh P. The significance of OX40 and OX40L to T-cell biology and immune disease. *Immunol Rev* 2009;**229**(1):173–91.
227. Croft M. Costimulation of T cells by OX40, 4-1BB, and CD27. *Cytokine Growth Factor Rev* 2003;**14**(3–4):265–73.
228. Song J, So T, Croft M. Activation of NF-κB1 by OX40 contributes to antigen-driven T cell expansion and survival. *J Immunol* 2008;**180**(11):7240–8.
229. Pan PY, Zang Y, Weber K, Meseck ML, Chen SH. OX40 ligation enhances primary and memory cytotoxic T lymphocyte responses in an immunotherapy for hepatic colon metastases. *Mol Ther* 2002;**6**(4):528–36.
230. Ali SA, Ahmad M, Lynam J, et al. Anti-tumour therapeutic efficacy of OX40L in murine tumour model. *Vaccine* 2004;**22**(27–28):3585–94.
231. Cuadros C, Dominguez AL, Lollini PL, et al. Vaccination with dendritic cells pulsed with apoptotic tumors in combination with Anti-OX40 and Anti-4-1BB monoclonal antibodies induces T cell-mediated protective immunity in Her-2/neu transgenic mice. *Int J Cancer* 2005;**116**(6):934–43.
232. Hirschhorn-Cymerman D, Rizzuto GA, Merghoub T, et al. OX40 engagement and chemotherapy combination provides potent antitumor immunity with concomitant regulatory T cell apoptosis. *J Exp Med* 2009;**206**(5):1103–16.
233. Cai G, Freeman GJ. The CD160, BTLA, LIGHT/HVEM pathway: a bidirectional switch regulating T-cell activation. *Immunol Rev* 2009;**229**(1):244–58.
234. Shaikh RB, Santee S, Granger SW, et al. Constitutive expression of LIGHT on T cells leads to lymphocyte activation, inflammation, and tissue destruction. *J Immunol* 2001;**167** (11):6330–7.
235. Wang J, Lo JC, Foster A, et al. The regulation of T cell homeostasis and autoimmunity by T cell-derived LIGHT. *J Clin Invest* 2001;**108**(12):1771–80.
236. Tamada K, Shimozaki K, Chapoval AI, et al. Modulation of T-cell-mediated immunity in tumor and graft-versus-host disease models through the LIGHT co-stimulatory pathway. *Nat Med* 2000;**6**(3):283–9.
237. Yu P, Lee Y, Liu W, et al. Priming of naive T cells inside tumors leads to eradication of established tumors. *Nat Immunol* 2004;**5**(2):141–9.
238. Yu P, Lee Y, Wang Y, et al. Targeting the primary tumor to generate CTL for the effective eradication of spontaneous metastases. *J Immunol* 2007;**179**(3):1960–8.
239. Pasero C, Barbarat B, Just-Landi S, et al. A role for HVEM, but not lymphotoxin-β receptor, in LIGHT-induced tumor cell death and chemokine production. *Eur J Immunol* 2009;**39**(9):2502–14.
240. Park JJ, Anand S, Zhao Y, et al. Expression of anti-HVEM single-chain antibody on tumor cells induces tumor-specific immunity with long-term memory. *Cancer Immunol Immunother* 2012;**61**(2):203–14.
241. Ward RC, Kaufman HL. Targeting costimulatory pathways for tumor immunotherapy. *Int Rev Immunol* 2007;**26**(3–4):161–96.
242. Keller AM, Xiao Y, Peperzak V, Naik SH, Borst J. Costimulatory ligand CD70 allows induction of CD8 + Tcell immunity by immature dendritic cells in a vaccination setting. *Blood* 2009;**113**(21):5167–75.
243. Glouchkova L, Ackermann B, Zibert A, et al. The CD70/CD27 pathway is critical for stimulation of an effective cytotoxic T cell response against B cell precursor acute lymphoblastic leukemia. *J Immunol* 2009;**182**(1):718–25.
244. Roberts DJ, Franklin NA, Kingeter LM, et al. Control of established melanoma by CD27 stimulation is associated with enhanced effector function and persistence, and reduced

PD-1 expression of tumor infiltrating CD8+ T cells. *J Immunother* 2010;**33**(8):769–79.

245. Miller J, Eisele G, Tabatabai G, et al. Soluble CD70: a novel immunotherapeutic agent for experimental glioblastoma: laboratory investigation. *J Neurosurg* 2010;**113**(2):280–5.
246. Shaffer DR, Savoldo B, Yi Z, et al. T cells redirected against CD70 for the immunotherapy of CD70-positive malignancies. *Blood* 2011;**117**(16)):4304–14.
247. Watts TH. TNF/TNFR family members in costimulation of T cell responses. *Annu Rev Immunol* 2005;**23**:23–68.
248. Placke T, Kopp HG, Salih HR. Glucocorticoid induced TNFR-related (GITR) protein and its ligand in antitumor immunity: functional role and therapeutic modulation. *Clin Dev Immunol* 2010:224. [article ID 239083: 10 pages].
249. Calmels B, Paul S, Futin N, Ledoux C, Stoeckel F, Acres B. Bypassing tumor-associated immune suppression with recombinant adenovirus constructs expressing membrane bound or secreted GITR-L. *Cancer Gene Ther* 2005;**12**(2):198–205.
250. Nishikawa H, Kato T, Hirayama M, et al. Regulatory T cell resistant CD8+ T cells induced by glucocorticoid-induced tumor necrosis factor receptor signaling. *Cancer Res* 2008;**68**(14):5948–54.
251. Zhou P, L'Italien L, Hodges D, Schebye XM. Pivotal roles of CD4+ effector T cells in mediating agonistic anti-GITR mAb-induced-immune activation and tumor immunity in CT26 tumors. *J Immunol* 2007;**179**(11):7365–75.
252. Sun X, Yamada H, Shibata K, et al. CD30 ligand/CD30 plays a critical role in Th17 differentiation in mice. *J Immunol* 2010;**185**(4):2222–30.
253. Dunn GP, Old LJ, Schreiber RD. The immunobiology of cancer immunosurveillance and immunoediting. *Immunity* 2004;**21**:137–48.
254. Gajewski TF, Meng Y, Blank C, et al. Immune resistance orchestrated by the tumor microenvironment. *Immunol Rev* 2006;**213**:131–45.
255. Kantoff PW, Higano CS, Shore ND, et al. Sipuleucel-T immunotherapy for castrationresistant prostate cancer. *N Engl J Med* 2010;**363**:411–22.
256. Ben-Baruch A. Inflammation-associated immune suppression in cancer: the roles played by cytokines, chemokines and additional mediators. *Semin Cancer Biol* 2006;**16**:38–52.
257. Cheng L, Jiang J, Gao R, Wei S, Nan F, Li S, et al. B7-H4 expression promotes tumorigenesis in ovarian cancer. *Int J Gynecol Cancer* 2009;**19**(9):1481–6.
258. Tringler B, Liu W, Corral L, Torkko KC, Enomoto T, et al. B7-H4 overexpression in ovarian tumors. *Gynecol Oncol* 2006;**100**:44–52.
259. Tringler B, Zhuo S, Pilkington G, Torkko KC. B7-H4 is highly expressed in ductal and lobular breast cancer. *Clin Cancer Res* 2005;**11**:1842–8.
260. Keir ME, Liang SC, Guleria I, Latchman YE, Qipo A, et al. Tissue expression of PD-L1 mediates peripheral T cell tolerance. *J Exp Med* 2006;**203**:883–95.
261. Bashey A, Medina B, Corringham S, et al. CTLA4 blockade with ipilimumab to treat relapse of malignancy after allogeneic hematopoietic cell transplantation. *Blood* 2009;**113**(7):1581–8.
262. Blazar BR, Carreno BM, Panoskaltsis-Mortari A, et al. Blockade of programmed death-1 engagement accelerates graft-versus-host disease lethality by an IFN-gamma-dependent mechanism. *J Immunol* 2003;**171**(3):1272–7.
263. Dranoff G, Jaffee E, Lazenby A, et al. Vaccination with irradiated tumor cells engineered to secrete murine granulocyte-macrophage colony-stimulating factor stimulates potent, specific, and long-lasting antitumor immunity. *Proc Natl Acad Sci USA* 1993;**90**(8):3539–43.

264. Inaba K, Metlay JP, Crowley MT, Steinman RM. Dendritic cells pulsed with protein antigens in vitro can prime antigen-specific, MHC-restricted T cells in situ. *J Exp Med* 1990;**172**(2):631–40.
265. Hsu FJ, Benike C, Fagnoni F, et al. Vaccination of patients with B-cell lymphoma using autologous antigen-pulsed dendritic cells. *Nat Med* 1996;**2**(1):52–8.
266. Osterborg A, Yi Q, Henriksson L, et al. Idiotype immunization combined with granulocyte macrophage colony-stimulating factor in myeloma patients induced type I, major histocompatibility complex restricted, CD8- and CD4-specific T-cell responses. *Blood* 1998;**91**(7):2459–66.
267. Navarrete MA, Heining-Mikesch K, Schuler F, et al. Upfront immunization with autologous recombinant idiotype Fab fragment without prior cytoreduction in indolent B-cell lymphoma. *Blood* 2011;**117**(5):1483–91.
268. Krackhardt AM, Witzens M, Harig S, et al. Identification of tumor-associated antigens in chronic lymphocytic leukemia by SEREX. *Blood* 2002;**100**(6):2123–31.
269. Oka Y, Tsuboi A, Taguchi T, et al. Induction of WT1 (WilmsÆ tumor gene)-specific cytotoxic T lymphocytes by WT1 peptide vaccine and the resultant cancer regression. *Proc Natl Acad Sci USA* 2004;**101**(38):13885–90.
270. Rooney CM, Smith CA, Ng CY, et al. Use of gene-modified virus-specific T lymphocytes to control Epstein-Barr-virus-related lymphoproliferation. *Lancet* 1995;**345**(8941):9–13.
271. Kawakami Y, Eliyahu S, Delgado CH, et al. Cloning of the gene coding for a shared human melanoma antigen recognized by autologous T cells infiltrating into tumor. *Proc Natl Acad Sci USA* 1994;**91**(9):3515–19.
272. Clay TM, Custer MC, Sachs J, Hwu P, Rosenberg SA, Nishimura MI. Efficient transfer of a tumor antigen-reactive TCR to human peripheral blood lymphocytes confers antitumor reactivity. *J Immunol* 1999;**163**(1):507–13.
273. Stanislawski T, Voss RH, Lotz C, et al. Circumventing tolerance to a human MDM2-derived tumor antigen by TCR gene transfer. *Nat Immunol* 2001;**2**(10):962–70.
274. Morgan RA, Dudley ME, Wunderlich JR, et al. Cancer regression in patients after transfer of genetically engineered lymphocytes. *Science* 2006;**314**(5796):126–9.
275. Johnson LA, Morgan RA, Dudley ME, et al. Gene therapy with human and mouse T-cell receptors mediates cancer regression and targets normal tissues expressing cognate antigen. *Blood* 2009;**114**(3):535–46.
276. Kochenderfer JN, Dudley ME, Feldman SA, et al. B-cell depletion and remissions of malignancy along with cytokine-associated toxicity in a clinical trial of anti-CD19 chimeric-antigen-receptor-transduced T cells. *Blood* 2012;**119**(12):2709–20.
277. Porter DL, Levine BL, Kalos M, Bagg A, June CH. Chimeric antigen receptor-modified T cells in chronic lymphoid leukemia. *N Engl J Med* 2011;**365**(8):725–33.
278. Marafioti T, Paterson JC, Ballabio E, et al. The inducible T-cell co-stimulator molecule is expressed on subsets of T cells and is a new marker of lymphomas of T follicular helper cell-derivation. *Haematologica* 2010;**95**(3):432–9.
279. Zhang Q, Wang H, Kantekure K, et al. Oncogenic tyrosine kinase NPM-ALK induces expression of the growth-promoting receptor ICOS. *Blood* 2011;**118**(11):3062–71.
280. Ogasawara K, Yoshinaga SK, Lanier LL. Inducible costimulator costimulates cytotoxic activity and IFN-gamma production in activated murine NK cells. *J Immunol* 2002;**169**(7):3676–85.
281. He M, Wang Y, Shi WJ, et al. Immunomodulation of inducible co-stimulator (ICOS) in human cytokine-induced killer cells against cholangiocarcinoma through ICOS/ICOS ligand interaction. *J Dig Dis* 2011;**12**(5):393–400.

282. Hubbard VM, Eng JM, Ramirez-Montagut T, et al. Absence of inducible costimulator on alloreactive T cells reduces graft versus host disease and induces Th2 deviation. *Blood* 2005;**106**(9):3285–92.
283. Yu XZ, Liang Y, Nurieva RI, Guo F, Anasetti C, Dong C. Opposing effects of ICOS on graft-versus host disease mediated by CD4 and CD8 T cells. *J Immunol* 2006;**176**(12):7394–401.
284. Pardoll D, Drake C. Immunotherapy earns its spot in the ranks of cancer therapy. *J Exp Med* 2012;**209**(2):201–9.
285. Schaer DA, Murphy JT, Wolchok JD. Modulation of GITR for cancer immunotherapy. *Curr Opin Immunol* 2012;**24**(2):217–24.
286. Melero I, Martinez-Forero I, Dubrot J, Suarez N, Palazón A, Chen L. Palettes of vaccines and immunostimulatory monoclonal antibodies for combination. *Clin Cancer Res* 2009;**15**(5):1507–9.
287. Takeda K, Kojima Y, Uno T, Hayakawa Y, Teng MW, Yoshizawa H, et al. Combination therapy of established tumors by antibodies targeting immune activating and suppressing molecules. *J Immunol* 2010;**184**(10):5493–501.
288. Serghides L, Bukczynski J, Wen T, Wang C, Routy JP, et al. Evaluation of OX40 ligand as a costimulator of human antiviral memory CD8 T cell responses: comparison with B7.1 and 4–1BBL. *J Immunol* 2005;**175**(10):6368–77.
289. Uno T, Takeda K, Kojima Y, Yoshizawa H, Akiba H, et al. Eradication of established tumors in mice by a combination antibody-based therapy. *Nat Med* 2006;**12**(6):693–8.
290. Kocak E, Lute K, Chang X, May Jr. KF, Exten KR, Zhang H, et al. Combination therapy with anti-CTL antigen-4 and anti-4-1BB antibodies enhances cancer immunity and reduces autoimmunity. *Cancer Res* 2006;**66**(14):7276–84.
291. Curran MA, Kim M, Montalvo W, Al-Shamkhani A, Allison JP. Combination CTLA-4 blockade and 4-1BB activation enhances tumor rejection by increasing T-cell infiltration, proliferation, and cytokine production. *PLoS One* 2011;**6**(4):e19499.
292. Hirano F, Kaneko K, Tamura H, Dong H, Wang S, Ichikawa M, et al. Blockade of B7–H1 and PD-1 by monoclonal antibodies potentiates cancer therapeutic immunity. *Cancer Res* 2005;**65**(3):1089–96.
293. Melero I, Hervas-Stubbs S, Glennie M, Pardoll DM, Chen L. Immunostimulatory monoclonal antibodies for cancer therapy. *Nat Rev Cancer* 2007;**7**(2):95–106.
294. Murphy KA, Lechner MG, Popescu FE, Bedi J, et al. An in vivo immunotherapy screen of costimulatory molecules identifies Fc-OX40L as a potent reagent for the treatment of established murine gliomas. *Clin Cancer Res* 2012;**18**(17):4657–68.
295. Lechner MG, Russell SM, Bass RS, Epstein AL. Chemokines, costimulatory molecules and fusion proteins for the immunotherapy of solid tumors. *Immunotherapy* 2011;**3**(11):1317–40.
296. Kanagavelu SK, Snarsky V, Termini JM, Gupta S, Barzee S, et al. Soluble multi-trimeric TNF superfamily ligand adjuvants enhance immune responses to a HIV-1 Gag DNA vaccine. *Vaccine* 2012;**30**(4):691–702.
297. Sharma RK, Schabowsky RH, Srivastava AK, Elpek KG, et al. 4-1BB ligand as an effective multifunctional immunomodulator and antigen delivery vehicle for the development of therapeutic cancer vaccines. *Cancer Res* 2010;**70**(10):3945–54.
298. Wyzgol A, Müller N, Fick A, Munkel S, Grigoleit GU, et al. Trimer stabilization, oligomerization, and antibody-mediated cell surface immobilization improve the activity of

soluble trimers of CD27L, CD40L, 41BBL, and glucocorticoid-induced TNF receptor ligand. *J Immunol* 2009;**183**(3):1851–61.

299. Zhang N, Sadun RE, Arias RS, Flanagan ML, Sachsman SM, et al. Targeted and untargeted CD137L fusion proteins for the immunotherapy of experimental solid tumors. *Clin Cancer Res* 2007;**13**(9):2758–67.
300. Liu A, Hu P, Khawli LA, Epstein AL. B7.1/NHS76: a new costimulator fusion protein for the immunotherapy of solid tumors. *J Immunother* 2006;**29**(4):425–35.
301. Liu R, Jiang W, Yang M, Guo H, Zhang Y, Wang J, et al. Efficient inhibition of human B-cell lymphoma in SCID mice by synergistic antitumor effect of human 4-1BB ligand/anti-CD20 fusion proteins and anti-CD3/anti-CD20 diabodies. *J Immunother* 2010;**33**(5):500–9.
302. Hornig N, Kermer V, Frey K, Diebolder P, Kontermann RE, Müller D. Combination of a bispecific antibody and costimulatory antibody-ligand fusion proteins for targeted cancer immunotherapy. *J Immunother* 2012;**35**(5):418–29.
303. Hornig N, Reinhardt K, Kermer V, Kontermann RE, Müller D. Evaluating combinations of costimulatory antibody–ligand fusion proteins for targeted cancer immunotherapy. *Cancer Immunol Immunother* 2013;**62**:1369–80.
304. Fife BT, Bluestone JA. Control of peripheral T-cell tolerance and autoimmunity via the CTLA-4 and PD-1 pathways. *Immunol Rev* 2008;**224**:166–82.

Chapter 6

T-Cell Costimulation and Its Applications in Diseases

INTRODUCTION TO T-CELL COSTIMULATION

T cells are dependent on antigen presenting cells (APCs) for at least two distinct stimuli for their optimum activation and effector function. The first signal is provided by the engagement of clonotypic T-cell receptor (TCR) with major histocompatibility complex (MHC)–peptide complex on APCs. The second signal is non-MHC-restricted and delivered by costimulatory molecules. The best-defined costimulatory molecules are the CD80 and Cd86 on APCs and their ligands CD28/CTLA-4 on T cells. The significance of costimulatory molecules in T-cell activation gained considerable impetus following the observation that occupancy of TCR alone is generally inadequate for exerting complete T-cell activation. Thus an encounter with an antigen can lead to two quite distinct outcomes in T cells: proliferation and differentiation into effector cells; or inactivation or death. Which outcome occurs is determined by the appropriate delivery of costimulatory signals.[1–4]

Activation of T lymphocytes is a critical component of the immunological response to foreign protein molecules. TCR recognition of peptide-loaded MHC molecules provides antigen specificity and initiates the required steps for T-cell activation, although additional signals are needed for complete T-cell activation. A two-signal model for lymphocyte activation was first proposed as a mechanism for self:nonself discrimination in B cells by Bretscher and Cohn in 1970[5] and was subsequently expanded to incorporate CD8 T-cell activation by Lafferty et al.[6] in 1975. They showed that engagement of the TCR by peptide-loaded MHC in the absence of other signals is insufficient to activate the T cell, and in fact may render it unresponsive to further antigenic stimulation, a condition termed anergy.[7,8] They further showed that provision of additional, non-MHC-restricted signals provided by professional APC, resulted in the T cell becoming fully activated leading to clonal expansion and development of effector function. Thus, the two-signal

Developing Costimulatory Molecules for Immunotherapy of Diseases.
DOI: http://dx.doi.org/10.1016/B978-0-12-802585-7.00006-6

model, where signal one is defined as the binding of peptide/MHC complexes and signal two refers to the additional, costimulatory signal(s), provided a potential mechanism for peripheral tolerance.[9,10] The most studied and well characterized costimulatory receptor/ligand complex is the CD28/B7 interaction.[11,12]

COSTIMULATION MEDIATED BY CD28 COSTIMULATORY PATHWAY IN T CELLS

CD28 was first identified by antibodies recognizing a 44 kDa protein on the surface of human T cells as type 1 transmembrane protein. In humans, CD28 is expressed on approximately 80% of CD4+ T cells and 50% of CD8+ T cells and has been detected on plasma cells, neutrophils, and eosinophils.[13,14] In contrast to humans, in mouse 100% of both CD4 and CD8 T cells express CD28.[15] CD28 is the founding member of the immunoglobulin (Ig) family of costimulatory receptors that now includes the receptors: cytotoxic T lymphocyte-associated antigen 4 (CTLA-4, CD152), inducible costimulator (ICOS), programmed death receptor 1 (PD-1), and B & T lymphocyte attenuator (BTLA).

CD28 signaling causes the initial activation of naive CD4 T cells by increasing the sensitivity of the T cell to antigen receptor engagement, and as a result proliferation is induced at otherwise submitogenic concentrations of antigen.[16,17] Cytokine production is greatly increased, most significantly IL-2. CD28 costimulation results in a 50-fold increase in IL-2 secretion by both transcriptional and posttranscriptional regulation of expression.[18] In addition, cell survival is enhanced by CD28 costimulation, in part by inducing expression of anti-apoptotic proteins including Bcl-X_L.[19,20] Thus, by a variety of mechanisms, CD28-mediated costimulation greatly enhances the T cells effector response to antigen.

Whether CD28 can activate signaling independent of TCR engagement or function only in a TCR dependent manner has been controversial. The ability of certain "superagonistic" anti-CD28 antibodies to independently activate T cells suggests that in some circumstances CD28 can function in the absence of a TCR derived signal.[21] Importantly, the existence of both TCR dependent and independent pathways is not mutually exclusive, and it is likely that both are operative and important.

CD28 COSTIMULATION ENHANCES T-CELL SURVIVAL

A major consequence of CD28 signaling is protection from cell death. The two dominant pathways of apoptosis in T cells are (1) receptor mediated (i.e., tumor necrosis factor (TNF) family) or (2) mitochondrial-associated proteins (i.e., the Bcl family) both of which are modulated via CD28 signaling.[11] CD28 costimulation prevents activation induced cell death (AICD) by inhibiting the expression of CD95L expression (*cis*-mediated death) on the

T cell and by decreasing the formation of the death-inducing signaling complex (DISC). CD28 stimulation increases the protein expression of c-FLIPs, which compete with procaspase 8 for binding to the death domains of CD95 and FADD, and thereby preventing the conversion of procaspase 8 to active caspase 8 and the induction of cell death.[22] CD28-deficient cells are more sensitive to Fas-mediated cell death. CD28 stimulation also induces the upregulation of anti-apoptotic factors including Bcl-X_L. The overexpression of Bcl-X_L in CD28-deficient mice restores cellular survival but not proliferation; thereby, separating these two CD28-dependent functions.[19,23]

CD28 T-CELL COSTIMULATION IN DISEASES

Perhaps surprisingly, mutations in CD28 have not been identified as the genetic basis for any human disease. However, mouse models of disease have been shown to depend on CD28 function. The use of CD28- and B7-deficient cells has implicated this pathway in the generation of a TH2 response required for the destruction of islet cells (autoimmune diabetes in the NOD mouse model)[1] and in the activation of newly recruited T cells responsible for epitope spreading (relapsing EAE in the EAE mouse model).[24] CD28 has been shown to be required in a model of allergic airway inflammation.[25,26] In the absence of CD28 or in the CD28-AYAA knockin mice, antibody production and germinal center formation is markedly reduced.[27] Thus, in a number of model systems, CD28 plays a critical role.

So, an understanding of costimulation and the mechanism by which it regulates immune responses provides new avenues for the development of therapeutics. As CD28 decreases the threshold required to activate naive T cells, as well as increasing the survival of activated T cells, one can envision development of drugs that either potentiate or downregulate an immune response. Although global inhibition of CD28 function would be anticipated to profoundly inhibit T-cell function, more specific targeting of specific regions of the extracellular or intracellular regions of CD28 via antibodies, small molecule mimetics or siRNAs could potentially alter some aspects of CD28 effects whereas leaving others intact.

CD28 COSTIMULATION IN PRIMARY T-CELL RESPONSES

The importance of CD8 + T cells in the resolution of viral infection is widely accepted. Activation of naive CD8 + T cells during virus infection occurs in local draining lymph nodes, where dendritic cells (DCs) present viral antigens to CD8 + T cells.[28,29] During naive CD8 + T cell–DC interactions, costimulatory signals delivered by molecules such as CD28 (signal two) determine whether CD8 + T cells will become activated and expand, or they will be suboptimally activated. Studies examining primary infection of mice with viruses such as VSV, MHV-68, and influenza type A virus, indicated that CD28 was required for primary expansion of antiviral CD8+ T cells.[30–33] In one of the earliest CTLA-4-Ig blocking studies, using influenza virus, Lumsden et al. identified that the loss of CD28 signaling negatively impacted both CD4+ and CD8+ T cells.[34] In this study, there was a significant decrease in the production of antiviral antibodies, decreased expansion of virus-specific CTLs, and a loss of IFN-γ and cytotoxic function by those cells which did expand. Ultimately these CTLA-4-Ig blocked mice resolved the infection, yet it was delayed in comparison to controls. In a complimentary study by Bertram et al., influenza virus-infected CD28 −/− mice exhibited substantially decreased expansion of virus-specific CD8+ T cells at the peak of the primary response whether virus was delivered intraperitoneally or intranasally.[32] Halstead et al. also showed that both dominant and subdominant primary CD8+ T-cell responses against influenza virus are greatly reduced in CD28 knockout mice.[33] In contrast, studies using lymphochoriomeningitis virus (LCMV) infection of mice, initially showed that an efficient primary CD8+ T-cell response could be generated in the absence of CD28 costimulation. CD28 knockout mice (CD28 −/−) were infected with LCMV, and despite the absence of CD28 signaling, virus CD8+ T cells expanded and viral burden was eliminated at levels comparable to wild-type controls. Similar CD8+ T-cell expansion was observed against all measured epitopes of LCMV, including subdominant epitopes.[35,36] The reason for this discrepancy in the lack of requirement for a CD28-mediated signal in LCMV infection became apparent from studies that showed that if sufficiently high levels of TCR stimulation were obtained, the need for costimulation could be overcome.[37] Viola and Lanzavecchia elegantly showed in *in vitro* studies, that independent of the nature of the TCR stimuli, TCR stimulation must exceed a minimum threshold in order to achieve complete activation of a T-cell clone. However, in the presence of CD28 costimulation, that threshold is significantly lowered.[38] Kundig et al. utilized LCMV infection and showed that the disparity in requirement for CD28 in primary LCMV infection versus VSV infection was due to differences in TCR signal duration.[37] Indeed, of all the viruses examined, LCMV is the only virus whose natural host is the mouse and therefore it replicates much more rapidly and extensively than any of the other viruses examined. As a result, antigen presentation persists for a longer period of time and at higher levels, providing a strong and sustained TCR signal which overcomes the need for CD28 costimulation.[37]

When viral infection is cleared the effector T-cell population undergoes a steady contraction until a small stable memory pool is formed. Memory cells respond faster and more effectively in the event of secondary insult to the host.[39] One of the major contributing factors to the rapidity of memory T-cell responses is their potentially higher affinity for antigen that leads to a lower threshold of activation.[40,41] Given that the strength of TCR signaling and predetermined threshold of activation can affect the need for costimulation, it is reasonable to question whether or not memory T cells have a requirement for CD28 costimulation during re-activation.

CD28-B7 Costimulation and Its Effect on CD8 + Memory T-Cell Responses

Costimulation signals have been recognized as critical for optimal T-cell responses and result from important interaction between receptors on the surface of T cells and their ligands on APCs. CD28 receptor costimulatory family has been found to be a major player in providing costimulation to CD8+ T cells. Recent studies using viral infection models have highlighted the importance of CD28 costimulation signals during memory responses against viruses. PD-1 another member of the CD28 family may contribute to functional defects of helpless memory CD8+ T cells. The delivery of costimulatory molecules such as CD28, 4-1BB, and OX40 can help boost the generation and function of virus-specific memory CD8+ T cells. Taken together this suggests that the use of costimulatory molecules as adjuvants along with viral antigens in vaccines may facilitate the generation of effective antigen-specific memory CD8+ T-cell responses. Understanding the costimulatory requirements of memory CD8+ T cells therefore may lead to improved vaccines that target antiviral CD8+ T-cell memory.

After pathogen clearance effector T cells undergo contraction and a memory T-cell pool is formed. These memory cells respond faster and more effectively in the event of secondary insult to the host because of their higher precursor frequency and higher affinity for antigen that leads to a lower threshold of activation. As the requirement for costimulation affects the strength of TCR signaling and the threshold of activation it is important to determine whether or not memory T cells have a requirement for CD28 costimulation during re-activation. Early studies relied on *in vitro* experiments to address this. More recently however, the availability of new reagents and of genetically modified mice have allowed the direct assessment *in vivo* of the requirement of CD28 signaling by memory CD8 + T cells. During antiviral CD8+ T-cell responses costimulatory signals from the CD28 family affect different phases of the immune response. It has now become apparent that different members of this family play important roles in the initiation phase, the generation and maintenance of memory, quality of memory, and the secondary response.

Memory CD8+ T-cell immune responses have been considered for a number of years not to require costimulation based on several studies that used *in vitro* systems of restimulation or CD28-deficient mice.[42,43] It has been demonstrated recently that CD28 plays a critical role in the secondary CD8+ T-cell response,[44,45] thus challenging the notion that costimulation is not required by memory CD8+ T cells. To circumvent the problem of generating virus-specific memory cells in CD28-deficient mice that have an impaired primary response, memory CD8+ T cells, were generated in wild-type mice by *in vivo* viral infections. Following the development of intact primary T-cell responses, and the generation of memory CD8+ T cells, the requirement of the memory population for CD28 costimulation during a secondary response was examined by blocking CD28 binding to its ligands with either CTLA-4-Ig, anti-B7 or anti-CD28 monoclonal antibodies or transfer of memory cells to CD80/CD86 double deficient mice (B7.1 and B7.2 knockouts).[44,45]

Interestingly, virus-specific memory CD8+ T cells that were generated in the absence of CD28 costimulation expanded approximately 9 times, whereas virus-specific memory CD8+ T cells that were generated in C57Bl/6 mice expanded more than 40 times. These findings were further substantiated when virus-specific memory CD8+ T cells were generated in C57Bl/6 mice and transferred into CD80/CD86-deficient mice or wild-type control mice, challenged, and analyzed five days later for expansion of the virus-specific memory population. The importance of CD28 signaling during secondary responses was further supported with vaccinia virus infections where the lack of CD28 signaling impaired the responses of memory virus-specific CD8+ T cells.[45]

Thus the CD28 requirement of memory CD8+ T cells for expansion has been shown in multiple viral infections such as influenza type A virus, HSV, vaccinia virus, and murine gamma herpes virus and is required for rapid pathogen clearance. The reduced expansion of virus-specific memory CD8+ T cells in the absence of costimulation challenges the paradigm that memory immune responses occur independently of costimulatory signals. CD28 signaling during primary response may be affecting the quality of memory CD8+ T cells generated while the expansion of memory T cells clearly requires CD28 costimulation signals for optimal secondary responses and normal pathogen clearance.[44,45] This CD28 requirement by memory cells is not restricted to CD8+ T cells, CD4+ T cells have also been shown to require *in vivo* CD28 costimulation.[46] This information has important implications in designing efficient vaccination strategies against pathogens and tumors that can downregulate costimulatory signals.

The Future Prospectus

The need for potent CD8+ T-cell eliciting vaccines remains largely unfulfilled. Discovery of adjuvants and strategies that enhance the generation, maintenance, and quality of memory CD8+ T cells is important for the development of effective vaccines against viruses, intracellular pathogens, and tumors. Costimulatory molecules from the CD28 and the TNFR family augment the immune response during viral infections and contribute to different phases of CD8+ T-cell responses as seen in Figure 6.1A–C. It appears that the CD28 and CD27 are required to initiate a primary CD8+ T-cell response.[47]

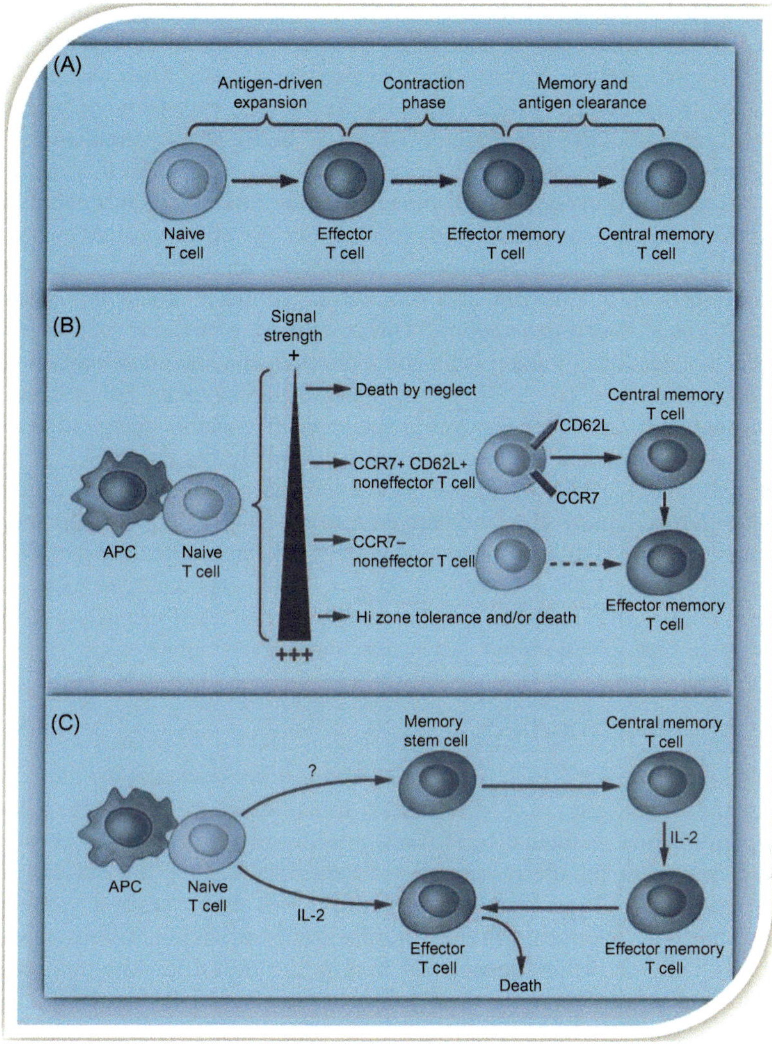

FIGURE 6.1 (A–C) Models of CD8+ T-cell differentiation to distinct memory cell subsets. (A) In the linear differentiation model, an autonomous antigen-triggered differentiation process consisting of conversion from naive to effector to TEM cell occurs, followed by the appearance of TCM cells after antigen clearance through a process of dedifferentiation.[117] (B) The signal strength model proposes that naive T cells progress through hierarchical thresholds for proliferation and differentiation as the strength and duration of the interaction with APCs is increased. T cells receiving the weakest signals do not survive, whereas high-intensity signaling causes the development of terminally differentiated effector T cells that cannot survive into the memory phase. The TCM cells, being the least differentiated of the antigen-stimulated T cells, retain the developmental options of naive T cells, including their capacity for marked clonal expansion.[118,119] (C) The memory stem cell model proposes that the cells within the TCM cell compartment are self-renewing and serve as a source of effector T cells.[197,198]

For secondary responses of memory CD8+ T cells, costimulatory molecules such as CD28, 4-1BB, OX40, and CD27 all seem to play a role in shaping the memory responses either by providing pro-survival signals or by enhancing the quality of the memory CD8 + T cells. Secondary expansion of memory CD8 + T cells requires professional APC66,[48] and CD28 costimulation.[44,45] TNFR family members as costimulatory molecules could also be used as adjuvants. Indeed DNA and adenovirus-based vaccines have shown that expression of 4-1BBL, OX40L, and CD70 leads to increased T-cell expansion, enhanced CTL activity, and antibody response.[49,50] Agonistic antibodies to TNF family members such as 4-1BB can also provide an adjuvant effect and enhance memory CD8 + T-cell generation.[51] Direct delivery of ligands such as using 4-1BBL to "decorate" tumor cells may provide costimulatory signals that enhance antitumor CTL.[52–54] An alternative strategy may be the use of oligonucleotide-based ligands known as aptamers, an example being multivalent 4-1BBL aptamers that act as agonists that can directly trigger CD8 + T cells and inhibit tumors in mice.[55] Chronic viral infections are characterized by accumulation of functionally impaired antigen-specific CD8 + T cells, and studies have shown that 4-1BBL in combination with CD80 can induce the expansion of the antigen-specific CD8 + T cells from this impaired pool.[56] Therefore such strategies may prove valuable for the design of effective vaccines not only against acute viral infections but also against chronic viral infections.

CONCLUDING REMARKS

Animal models of viral infections have shown that costimulatory molecules of both the CD28 and the TNFR family, as indicated in Table 6.1, help in the generation and maintenance of virus-specific memory CD8+ T cells, but are also important for the re-activation of memory CD8+ T cells and secondary responses. These costimulatory molecules may act in a redundant fashion, but they may also provide an opportunity to augment virus-specific memory CD8+ T-cell responses and may prove useful in designing effective vaccines against chronic viral infections such as HBV and HIV.[57] A number of questions still remain about the function of costimulatory molecules in memory antiviral CD8+ T-cell responses (see "Unanswered Questions" below). The function of CD28 and TNFR family members has been studied for RNA and DNA viruses, and studies have been done to delineate their functions at the acute and chronic stages of disease. However the redundancy in the function of these molecules questions whether there is a hierarchy in the expression and function of the costimulatory molecules. Although agonistic antibodies may enhance responses when CD28 signaling is absent.[58] This does not necessarily suggest a switch in costimulation requirements. It may however suggest that the lack of critical costimulatory molecules may be overcome by targeting alternative receptors with monoclonal antibodies or aptamers.

TABLE 6.1 Chimeric Antigen Receptor (CAR) T Cells Using CD28 Costimulatory Molecules in Clinical Trials

Cancer	CAR Target	CAR Endodomains	Number of Patients	Clinical Outcomes
Lymphoma	CD19	CD28 and CD3-ζ	1	PR
Lymphoma	CD19	CD28 and CD3-ζ	4	3 PR, 1 died of influenza
CLL	CD19	CD28 and CD3-ζ	4	1 CR, 2 PR, 1 SD
CLL	CD19	CD28 and CD3-ζ	4	1 CR, 1 PR, 2 PD
Lymphoma	CD19	CD28 and CD3-ζ	6	1 PR, 5 SD
CLL	CD19	CD28 and CD3-ζ	8	1 PR, 2 SD, 3 NR, 1 PD, 1 died of sepsis-like disease (symptoms preceded T-cell transfer)
ALL	CD19	CD28 and CD3-ζ	1	CR
ALL	CD19	CD28 and CD3-ζ	5	5 CR
ALL	CD19	CD28 and CD3-ζ	16	10 CR, 4 CRi, 2 NR
CLL	CD19	4-1BB and CD3-ζ	1	CR
CLL	CD19	4-1BB and CD3-ζ	3	2 CR, 1 PR
ALL	CD19	4-1BB and CD3-ζ	2	2 CR

CLL, chronic lymphocytic leukemia; ALL, acute lymphocytic leukemia; PR, partial response; CR, complete response; SD, stable disease; PD, progressive disease; NR, no objective response; CRi, complete response with incomplete count recovery; NED, no evidence of disease.

The recent discovery of the important role of costimulatory molecules such as CD28 during re-activation of memory CD8 + T cells would raise the danger that therapeutic blocking of costimulation in transplantation and autoimmunity may impair the host's ability to respond to viral infection. On the other hand, some viral infections manipulate costimulation to evade the immune response. A number of viruses such as measles and HIV down-regulate B7 family members so as to hamper CTL responses.[59–61] This would suggest that successfully priming CTL vaccines may not be very effective against such viruses. A strategy against such pathogens and tumors may be to "add back" costimulatory ligands to reverse the impairment of CTL responses, or to generate memory, if possible, which is less dependent on CD28 costimulation. One of the hallmarks of chronic viral infections is the occurrence of systemic inflammation; the effect of different pro-inflammatory cytokines on the expression of costimulatory receptors and their ligands during different phases of viral infections is still poorly understood.

The expression of TNFR or CD28 costimulatory molecules or their corresponding ligands on the APCs is necessary for an effective antiviral CD8 + T-cell response, especially for vaccinations against viral infections. The important interplay between different costimulatory molecules for the generation, maintenance, and functionality of memory CD8 + T cells, indicates that the design of preventive vaccines will require we further understand the important contributions of costimulation to effective antiviral memory CD8 + T-cell responses.

UNANSWERED QUESTIONS

- Can one cell provide multiple costimulatory signals?
- Do different APC provide different costimulatory signals?
- What is the importance of redundant signaling?
- Do central and effector memory CD8 + T cells differ in their requirement for costimulation?
- Does persistent viral load alter expression of costimulatory molecules on APC?
- What is the effect of costimulation on tertiary memory?
- Does chronic infection change costimulation requirements of CD8 + T cells?
- Can costimulatory ligand combination enhance adjuvant activity?

PROMOTING T-CELL FUNCTION BY MODULATING COSTIMULATION OR CO-INHIBITION

The development of an antitumor T-cell mediated immune response is a multistep process in which tumor-associated antigens (TAAs) expressed by the tumor cells are processed and presented by professional APCs to circulating T cells, which become activated. The quality and potency of this T-cell response will depend on the nature of the antigen presented, the functionality of the APC itself, and the cytokines and costimulatory interactions that occur in the T-cell/APC microenvironment.[62] Once activated, TAA-specific effector T cells can migrate to the tumor site and target malignant cells expressing the cognate antigen epitope displayed in the context of a MHC molecule.

Optimally effective cancer immunotherapy may require combinatorial approaches. Synergistic combinations could include means of activating T cells, such as vaccination or the transfer of *ex-vivo* activated and expanded tumor-reactive T cells, coupled with means of sustaining T-cell activation, such as agonistic antibodies to costimulatory receptors or blocking antibodies to co-inhibitory receptors. As many clinical-grade reagents are now available, potential combinations are abundant. Currently, there are over 20 registered clinical trials to study the combination of ipilimumab with vaccines, radiation, chemotherapy, hormonal therapy, cytokines, anti-PD-1, and targeted therapy agents in patients with a broad range of cancers.

Immune activation is tightly regulated by co-receptors expressed on T cells (Figure 6.1A–C). Costimulatory receptors include CD28 and ICOS (inducible T-cell co-stimulator) of the Ig superfamily, as well as 4-1BB, OX40, CD27, CD30, CD40, GITR (glucocorticoid inducible TNF receptor-related protein), and HVEM (herpes-virus entry mediator) of the TNFR superfamily.[63,64] These costimulatory signals are counterbalanced by co-inhibitory members of the Ig superfamily including CTLA-4, PD-1, BTLA (B and T lymphocyte attenuator), lymphocyte activation gene-3 (LAG-3), TIM3 (T-cell immunoglobulin and mucin domain-containing protein 3), and VISTA (V-domain immunoglobulin suppressor of T-cell activation) on T cells.[65–69] The idea of blocking the immune co-inhibitors as a therapeutic anticancer strategy was suggested by James Allison over a decade ago.[70] Anti-CTLA-4 was used as a prototype but antibodies that either stimulate costimulatory TCRs or block other inhibitory immune-checkpoint molecules have been examined more recently.

TURNING ON THE STIMULATORS: ANTIBODIES TO 4-1BB (CD137), OX40 (134), GITR, AND CD40

Animal models and clinical trials have focused on targeting the 4-1BB, OX40, GITR, and CD40 members of the TNFR superfamily. 4-1BB is expressed on activated T cells, activated NK cells, DCs, and endothelial cells.[62] 4-1BB enhances T-cell function by promoting T-cell survival and memory generation,[71] activating APCs and endothelial cells, reducing T regulatory cell (Treg) suppressive capacity, and enhancing effector T-cell resistance to Treg suppression.[72,73] Agonistic anti-4-1BB monoclonal antibodies alone or in combination with vaccination can enable rejection of syngeneic tumors in preclinical models.[74–77] Phase I and II clinical trials with a fully humanized monoclonal anti-4-1BB antibody in patients with melanoma and renal cell carcinoma (RCC) showed only very mild antitumor activity,[78] suggesting that anti-4-1BB antibody may require combinations with other agents in order to demonstrate relevant antitumor activity.

OX40, expressed on activated CD4+ and CD8 + T cells, functions as a late costimulatory receptor.[62,79] Ligation of OX40 enhances immune responses by prolonging CD4+ and CD8 + T-cell survival and memory generation, which prevents T-cell tolerance that impairs the suppressor function of Treg and suppresses the generation of inducible Treg. An agonistic anti-OX40 antibody increases antitumor activity in a number of animal models.[80–83] Other reports indicate that anti-OX40 antibodies can work in combination with anti-4-1BB or vaccination to augment antitumor immune responses.[84,85]

GITR is also expressed after T-cell activation, is constitutively expressed at high levels on Tregs, and can be further induced after Treg activation.[48,86] GITR enhances proliferation and function of CD4+ and CD8 + T cells, inhibits Treg function, and elicits effector T-cell resistance to Treg-mediated suppression.[87,88] GITR may increase intratumor effector T cells to Tregs ratio and anti-GITR antibodies elicit antitumor responses in a number of animal models.[89,90] In addition, anti-GITR antibodies can be combined with vaccination, chemotherapy, or anti-CTLA-4 antibody to augment antitumor activity.[91]

CD40 is mainly expressed on APCs and endothelial cells, and its binding to its ligand (CD40L/CD154) on activated T cells results in persistent T-cell activation as well as expansion and activation of APCs. An agonistic anti-CD40 antibody has been shown to cause regression of pancreatic cancer in both human and mice via activation of macrophages, suggesting a T-cell independent antitumor mechanism.[92] CD40 is also expressed on many types of tumor cells and its ligation may promote tumor cell apoptosis and growth arrest. An initial phase I clinical trial using an agonistic anti-CD40 antibody in patients with advanced solid tumors demonstrated modest antitumor activity.[93] Overall, agonistic antibodies against immune co-stimulators have demonstrated modest antitumor activities in early phases of clinical trials. The combination of agonistic antibodies with other treatment modalities may be needed to achieve optimal antitumor activity.

TURNING OFF THE BRAKES: ANTIBODIES AGAINST CTLA-4 (CD152), PD-1 (CD279), AND PD-L1

CTLA-4 is expressed by activated CD4+ and CD8 + T cells. Upon T-cell activation, CTLA-4 is rapidly mobilized from intracellular vesicles to the immune synapse where it outcompetes co-stimulator CD28 for binding to its ligands B7-1 and B7-2 and, as a result, ablates T-cell activation (Figure 6.2B). In addition, CTLA-4 mediates cell cycle arrest and is essential for Treg suppression.[63] In human studies, anti-CTLA-4 enhances frequency of CD4+ and CD8+ T cells as well as the antibody response to tumor antigens.[94,95] In animal models, blocking monoclonal antibody against CTLA-4

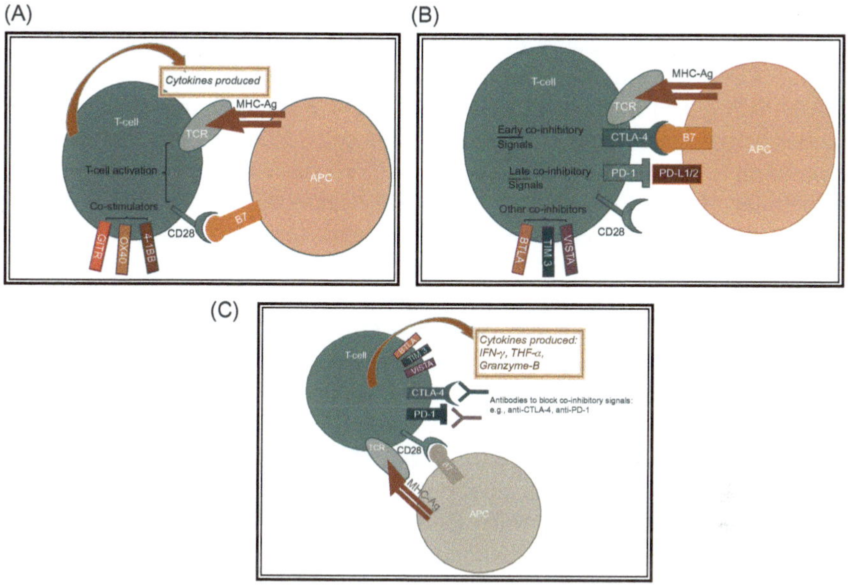

FIGURE 6.2 **Modulation of T-cell activation and current strategies promoting effector T-cell functions.** (A) Augmenting T-cell activation by positive costimulation. Antigenic presentation triggers T-cell activation and occurs when a peptide bound to MHC molecule on an APC interacts with T-cell receptor (TCR) on the surface of a T cell. In order to achieve optimal activation, additional costimulatory signals are required and primarily involve interaction between CD28 on T cells and B7 on APCs. Other T-cell positive co-stimulators include 4-1BB, OX40, and GITR. (B) Limiting T cell activation by negative costimulation. After T cell activation, cytotoxic T lymphocyte-associated protein 4 (CTLA-4) is mobilized to the cell surface and binds to B7 with greater affinity than CD28 and therefore prevents signaling through CD28. Later inhibitory signals can be provided by co-inhibitors such as programmed cell death-1 (PD-1), which binds to PD-1 ligand 1 (PD-L1). Other co-inhibitors of T cell activation include VISTA, TIM3, and BTLA. (C) Sustaining T-cell activation through blockade of negative costimulatory molecules. Blocking antibodies against CTLA-4 or PD-1 are currently employed to neutralize co-inhibitory receptors and prevent dampening of the T-cell response. Blockade of these inhibitory immune checkpoints results in enhanced and sustained activation of tumor-specific T cells that produce cytokines including TNF-α, interferon-γ (IFN-γ), and granzyme-B.

promotes antitumor activity.[63,96,97] Phase I and II clinical trials indicate that an anti-CTLA-4 antibody, ipilimumab, has significant antitumor activity in patients with advanced melanoma.[98,99] A phase III randomized controlled trial in patients with metastatic melanoma showed that ipilimumab improved median overall survival by 3.7 months,[100] leading to FDA approval of ipilimumab for the treatment of patients with metastatic melanoma. A second randomized phase III clinical trial recently showed that addition of ipilimumab to standard dacarbazine chemotherapy improved overall survival by 2.1 months in patients with metastatic melanoma.[101]

PD-1 is expressed by activated CD4+ and CD8+ T cells, NK T cells, and APCs. It has two ligands, PD-L1 and PD-L2, with distinct expression profiles.[102] PD-L1, the main target for PD-1, is expressed broadly on T cells, B cells, APCs, and nonhematopoietic cells. PD-L2 is largely restricted to activated macrophages, myeloid DCs, and mast cells. PD-1 −/− mice develop autoimmunity with high titers of autoantibodies, consistent with PD-1's role as an inhibitor of T and B cells.[103,104] Anti-PD-1 antibodies reduce tumor metastasis and growth in animal models,[105,106] whereas forced expression of PD-L1 in murine tumor cell lines enhances *in vivo* tumor growth.[107] In a phase I trial in 39 patients with refractory metastatic melanoma, colorectal cancer, prostate cancer, nonsmall-cell lung cancer (NSCLC), or RCC, anti-PD-1 antibody (MDX-1106) resulted in complete or partial response in three patients and less significant tumor regression in two other patients.[108] A recent phase I clinical trial with an anti-PD-1 antibody (BMS-936558) showed promising antitumor activity in patients with advanced NSCLC, RCC, and melanoma.[109] Another phase I trial with anti-PD-L1 antibody showed mild to modest antitumor activity in patients with advanced NSCLC, melanoma, and RCC.[110] Blocking antibodies against other T-cell co-inhibitors including LAG-3 and TIM3 are still at early stages of development as potential anticancer agents.[65,69]

ADOPTIVE T-CELL TRANSFER

The adoptive transfer of T cells is a promising approach to treat cancers. Primary human T cells can be modified using viral and non-viral vectors to promote the specific targeting of cancer cells via the introduction of exogenous TCRs or chimeric antigen receptors (CARs). This gene transfer displays the potential to increase the specificity and potency of the anticancer response while decreasing the systemic adverse effects that arise from conventional treatments that target both cancerous and healthy cells.

The transfusion of T cells, also called adoptive T-cell therapy, is an effective treatment for viral infections and has induced regression of cancer in early stage clinical trials. Adoptive T-cell therapy for cancer is a form of transfusion therapy consisting of the infusion of various mature T-cell subsets with the goal of eliminating a tumor and preventing its recurrence. However, recent advances in cellular immunology and tumor biology are guiding new approaches to adoptive T-cell therapy. For example, use of engineered T cells is being tested as a strategy to improve the functions of effector and memory T cells, and manipulation of the host to overcome immunotoxic effects in the tumor microenvironment has led to promising results in early stage clinical trials.[111–113]

Allogeneic and autologous sources of T cells derived from several anatomic sites have been tested. Indeed, in the 1970s, Chester Southam and colleagues demonstrated that subcutaneous growth of human tumor autografts to patients bearing advanced cancers was inhibited by the co-transfer of autologous leukocytes in about half of the patients.[114] This finding suggested that lymphocytes with a specific inhibitory effect on the implantation and growth of cancer cells were present in many patients and could be mined as potential candidates for adoptive immunotherapy. The primary advantage of using CD8 + T cells for adoptive therapy, as opposed to other cytolytic cells, such as NK cells, is their ability to specifically target tumor cells through the recognition of differentially expressed tumor proteins presented on the cell surface. Using T cells for adoptive therapy is also attractive due to the long clonal life span of T cells,[115,116] which allows both therapeutic and immunoprophylactic scenarios to be envisioned. In addition, T cells are well suited for genetic manipulation, which has enabled the evaluation of genetically enhanced or retargeted T cells in pilot clinical trials for cancer as well as other diseases.

Adoptive T-cell therapy depends on the ability to optimally select or genetically engineer cells with targeted antigen specificity and then induce the cells to proliferate while preserving their effector function and engraftment and homing abilities. T-cell populations are heterogeneous and comprise memory cells, effector cells, and Tregs exist in several distinct stages of differentiation. Naive CD4+ and CD8+ T cells undergo unique developmental programs after antigen activation, which results in the generation of effector memory and long-lived central memory T cells, TEM cells, and TCM cells, respectively. Three models by which memory CD8+ T cells can be generated have been proposed (Figure 6.1A–C). Models of CD8+ T-cell differentiation to distinct memory cell subsets. **(A) Linear differentiation model,** an autonomous antigen-triggered differentiation process consisting of conversion from naive to effector to TEM cell occurs, followed by the appearance of TCM cells after antigen clearance through a process of dedifferentiation.[117] **(B) The signal strength model** proposes that naive T cells progress through hierarchical thresholds for proliferation and differentiation as the strength and duration of the interaction with APCs is increased.[118,119] T cells receiving the weakest signals do not survive, whereas high-intensity signaling causes the development of terminally differentiated effector T cells that cannot survive into the memory phase. The TCM cells, being the least differentiated of the antigen-stimulated T cells, retain the developmental options of naive T cells, including their capacity for marked clonal expansion. **(C) The memory stem cell model** proposes that the cells within the TCM cell compartment are self-renewing and serve as a source of effector T cells.

IMPROVING SIGNALING CAPACITIES—SECOND- AND THIRD-GENERATION CARs

T cells play a major role in antitumor immunity. CD8+ CTLs efficiently destroy tumor cells, whereas CD4+ T cells improve the antigen-presenting

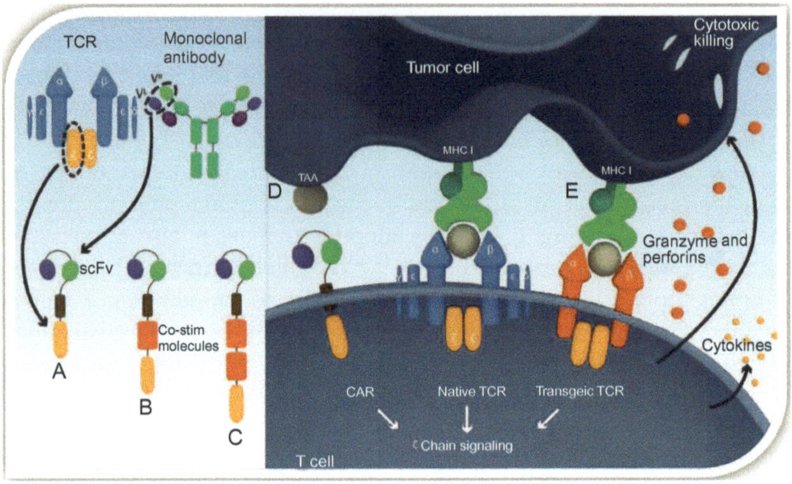

FIGURE 6.3 **Genetic engineering and adoptive transfer of patient T cells.** Lymphocytes are isolated from the peripheral blood of a cancer patient and transduced with a vector encoding either a new antigen-specific TCR or CAR. The engineered T cells are then expanded *ex vivo* before being adoptively transferred back to the patient. Important factors to consider during optimization of a clinical protocol are indicated.

capacity of DCs and support the stimulation of tumor-reactive CTLs. Following these findings. T-cell-based immunotherapeutic strategies for the treatment of tumor patients were developed. CD4+ and CD8+ T lymphocytes are powerful components of adaptive immunity, which essentially contribute to the elimination of tumors. Due to their cytotoxic capacity, T cells emerged as attractive candidates for specific immunotherapy of cancer. A promising approach is the genetic modification (see Figure 6.3) of T cells with CARs. The development of an antitumor T-cell mediated immune response is a multistep process in which TAAs expressed by the tumor cells are processed and presented by professional APCs to circulating T cells, which become activated. The quality and potency of this T-cell response will depend on the nature of the antigen presented, the functionality of the APC itself, and the cytokines and costimulatory interactions that occur in the T-cell/APC microenvironment. Once activated, TAA-specific effector T cells can migrate to the tumor site and target malignant cells expressing the cognate antigen epitope displayed in the context of a MHC molecule.[120]

T-cell proliferation and survival require antigenic stimulation by APCs expressing costimulatory molecules. Many tumor cells lack expression of costimulatory molecules, such as CD80 and CD86, and substantially reduce the opportunity of T cells to successfully encounter the antigen in a suitably costimulatory environment.[121,122] One way to circumvent this problem is to use CARs or transgenic αβTCRs to retarget virus-specific CTLs, rather than "random" T cells. Such virus-specific CTLs should receive optimal activation and costimulation following engagement of their native (virus-specific) αβTCRs with viral latent antigens expressed by professional APCs, thus enabling superior antitumor activity mediated by their tumor-reactive transgenic receptor. This hypothesis has been tested in a clinical trial performed at our institution, in which we compared the longevity of polyclonal activated T cells and polyclonal EBV-specific CTLs each expressing a CAR targeting the GD2 antigen, which is expressed on neuroblastoma.[123,124] The EBV-specific CTLs remained detectable substantially longer (>18 months) than their activated T-cell counterparts (<1 month), suggesting the beneficial effects of costimulation of EBV-specific CTLs provided by APCs expressing EBV-latent antigens.[124] An alternative means for providing T-cell costimulation is to force the expression of costimulatory ligands, such as CD80 and 4-1BBL, for the costimulatory receptors they already possess.[125] Post-infusion, these molecules will ensure there is "autocostimulation" and a bystander "transcostimulation," which substitutes for the lack of appropriate costimulation from the tumor cells. Preclinical studies have shown that incorporation of these molecules in CAR-modified T cells enhances their ability to produce effector cytokines (IFNγ, IL-2, TNFα) and, in an *in vivo* mouse model, promotes tumor rejection in mice with large tumor burden.[125]

A CAR, sometimes referred to as a T-body, chimeric immune receptor, or chimeric artificial receptor, is a transmembrane molecule, which is composed of an extracellular binding domain derived from a single chain antibody fragment (scFv), for recognition of a TAA and intracellular signaling domains for T-cell activation. Hence, upon CAR binding to a TAA on the cell surface of a target cell, the CAR T-cell, will induce apoptosis in the target cell using the same mechanisms as ordinary T cells [Figure 6.2B]. In contrast to a TCR, which recognizes a peptide fragment of an antigen presented by an HLA molecule on the surface of target cells, a CAR molecule recognizes an intact cell surface antigen, thus tumor cell recognition is HLA independent so there is no restriction in terms of patient selection.[126]

CARs are antibody-based extracellular receptor structures anchored into the cell membrane of T cells with a cytoplasmic domain which mediates signal transduction. Eshhar and colleagues introduced the concept of CARs as early as 1989. Several groups have since confirmed the ability to redirect T cells using receptors encompassing different scFvs fused to the CD3 zeta or Fc receptor gamma (FcRc) signaling domains. CARs are molecules combining antibody-based specificity for tumor-associated surface antigens with TCR-activating intracellular domains with specific antitumor cellular immune activity.[47,127] These CARs allow a T cell to achieve MHC-independent primary activation through single chain variable fragment (scFv) antigen-specific extracellular regions fused to intracellular domains that provide T-cell activation and costimulatory signals. Most investigators have achieved efficient CAR gene transfer of human tumor and HIV antigens into human T cells via retrovirus or HIV-derived lentivirus, and some of these cell therapy products have advanced to phase I/II trials.[124,128–130] Adoptive transfer of CTLs has shown great promise in both viral infections and cancers. Results from recent clinical trials indicate improved clinical results with CARs introduced with retroviral vectors.[129,130] Second- and third-generation CARs also provide appropriate costimulatory signals via CD28 and/or CD137 (4-1BB) intracellular activation motifs, which augment cytokine secretion and antitumor activity in a variety of solid-tumor and leukemia models.[131,132] After many years of disappointing results with CAR T-cell therapy, improved culture systems and cell engineering technologies are leading to CAR T cells with more potent antitumor effects.[133]

First-generation CARs consist of a binding moiety specifically recognizing a tumor cell surface antigen and a lymphocyte activating signaling chain. The CAR-mediated recognition induces cytokine production and tumor-directed cytotoxicity of T cells. Second- and third-generation CARs include signal sequences from various costimulatory molecules resulting in enhanced T-cell persistence and sustained antitumor reaction. Clinical trials revealed that the adoptive transfer of T cells engineered with first-generation CARs represents a feasible concept for the induction of clinical responses in some tumor patients. However, further improvement is required, which may be achieved by second- or third-generation CAR-engrafted T cells.

FIRST-GENERATION CARs

CARs are generated by fusing two distinct functional fragments. The most widely used combination is the antigen binding specific fragment composed of the single chain (scFv) obtained from the variable domains of the heavy and light chains of a monoclonal antibody, and the signaling domain derived from the CD3 chain[127] (Figure 6.4). These simple molecules are currently defined as first-generation CARs, and when expressed by CD8 and CD4 T-cell subsets, they provide specific binding to antigens expressed on the cell surface of tumor cells and simultaneous activation of the cytotoxic machinery (granzyme-B and perforin) of T cells through the CD3 zeta chain signaling immunoreceptor tyrosine-based activation motif (ITAM). Due to the antibody-mediated antigen recognition, the cytotoxic function of CAR-redirected T cells does not depend on the canonical antigen processing and MHC-restricted presentation typical of native TCRs. The first-generation CAR molecules, with only an scFv against a cell surface antigen expressed on tumor cells and the cytoplasmic CD3 zeta chain signaling domain, were found to have limited clinical activity for the treatment of ovarian cancer,[129] lymphoma,[130] renal cancer,[55] and neuroblastoma.[134] In a study first-generation CAR T cells demonstrated transient cell division and suboptimal cytokine production and failed to produce prolonged T-cell expansion and

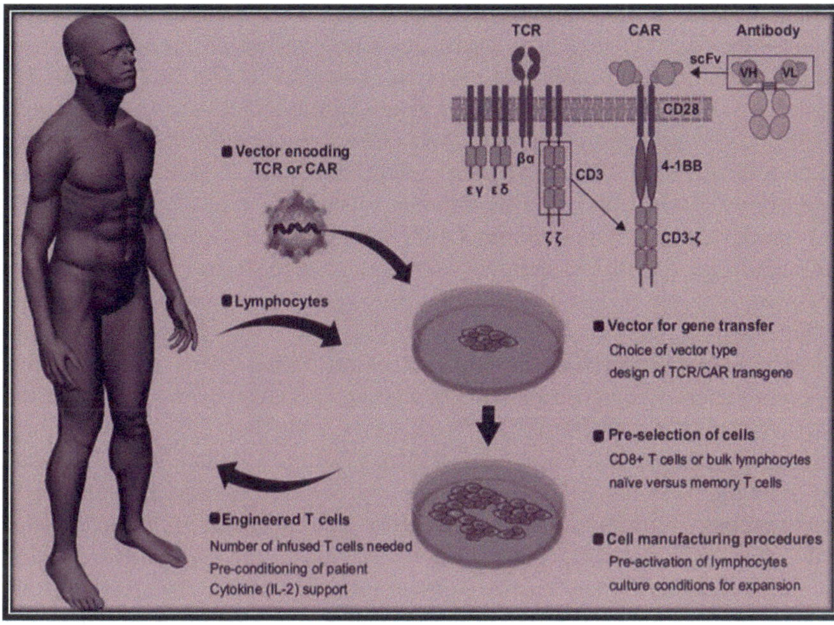

FIGURE 6.4 **Redirecting T-cell specificity.** T-cell specificity can be redirected by the expression of chimeric antigen receptors (CARs) or transgenic α- and β-TCR chains. (A) CARs are composed of two distinct fragments. The first is obtained by linking the variable heavy and light regions of a monoclonal antibody of known specificity into a single chain (scFv) and the second is the signaling region of the native TCR ζ-chain. (B) Second-generation CARs incorporate costimulatory molecules such as CD28 and 4-1BB. (C) Third-generation CARs include two or more costimulatory molecules. (D) CARs are activated after the scFv portion binds to an extracellular antigen thus the antigen recognition is MHC-independent. (E) Transgenic TCRs recognize specific peptides presented in the context of MHC class I molecules.

sustained antitumor effects. This may not be surprising given that the signal through the TCR-CD3 zeta chain alone is insufficient for priming resting T cells.[47] Although first-generation CARs could initiate a cytotoxic antitumor response in grafted T cells, it soon became obvious that signals from ITAM-bearing receptors alone can only induce transient cell division and suboptimal cytokine secretion but cannot provide prolonged polyclonal expansion and sustained antitumor reaction *in vivo*. According to the prevailing two-signaling model for lymphocyte activation, full activation and proliferation of T cells require a costimulatory signal through CD28-B7 interaction in addition to signaling through the TCR/CD3 complex.

SECOND-GENERATION CARs

However, several preclinical models showed that first-generation CARs do not fully activate modified T cells upon engagement with the antigen, as these molecules lack costimulatory properties. To overcome this obstacle, second-generation CARs have been generated in which intracytoplasmic domains, derived from costimulatory molecules such as CD2837, or CD134/OX40 or CD137/4-1BB, are incorporated within CARs to fully activate T cells.[135–137] Second-generation CARs were constructed to provide signaling both through the CD3 zeta chain and, primarily, the CD28 costimulatory molecule by placing the signaling domains in series as a single gene multidomain product. Constructs with the CD28 signaling domain proximal and the zeta chain distal to the membrane were found to be better expressed than constructs with the opposite orientation and were capable of mediating up to 20 times more interleukin (IL)-2 production upon stimulation with solid-phase antigen compared with first-generation CARs.[138,139] Subsequently, CAR constructs with costimulatory signaling domains from CD28, ICOS, OX40 (CD134), or 4-1BB (CD137) in series with the CD3 zeta signaling region were evaluated using resting human primary T cells.[140] It was found that second-generation CARs, providing any of these B7 or tumor necrosis factor receptor (TNFR) family costimulatory signals in series with CD3 zeta, confer self-sufficient antigendriven clonal expansion and enhanced effector function in resting human T cells. Furthermore, addition of the CD28 signaling domain to CARs has been shown to enhance CAR T-cell resistance to regulatory T cells.[141]

It has been reported that CAR T cells with a 4-1BB signaling domain have improved *in vivo* persistence, tumor localization, and antitumor activity compared with CAR T cells with the CD28 signaling domain.[142,143] Furthermore, a CAR with the CD27 signaling domain together with the CD3 zeta domain was recently evaluated. The greatest impact of CD27 was noted *in vivo*, where transferred CAR T cells with CD27 demonstrated heightened persistence after infusion, which facilitated improved regression of human cancer in a xenogeneic allograft model.[144] However, side-by-side comparisons of otherwise identical CAR T cells with either CD28, ICOS, OX40, 4-1BB, or CD27 signaling domains, in clinical trials under equivalent conditions, need to be performed before a general conclusion can be drawn as to which costimulatory domain is the most appropriate for CAR constructs.

THIRD-GENERATION CARs

Third-generation CARs have also been constructed containing CD3 zeta, CD28, and the OX40 or the 4-1BB signaling domain.[135,145] Third-generation CARs, in which two costimulatory molecules (CD28 and 4-1BB or CD28 and OX40) are encoded in tandem, have also been generated, and preclinical experiments suggest that these molecules may be even more potent than second-generation CARs[136,137,145] (Figure 6.4). These receptors may provide a full complement of activation, proliferation, and survival signals for enhanced antitumor activity. Despite encouraging preclinical results and some early clinical data, the use of third-generation CARs might have some disadvantages. One concern is that low avidity "off-target" binding may trigger third-generation CARs with potent activation signals that can lead to a lethal "cytokine storm." One patient treated with a third-generation CAR targeting Her2 died from adverse events due to Her2 expression in the lungs that led to excessive cytokine release and respiratory distress.[146] In addition, third-generation CARs may reduce the signal threshold to a level at which the activation of grafted T cells can occur without triggering antigens. Signal leakage may be a problem for clinical applications of these CARs. Moreover, the exact amino acid sequence and order of the intracellular signaling domains are based on empirical findings, and the optimal CAR format for T-cell activation remains unclear.

Virus-mediated gene transfer seems to be the most efficient gene delivery method, as it allows robust expression of CARs by T cells and minimizes the time of their *ex vivo*. In addition the incorporation of costimulatory endodomains (CD28 or 4-1BB) within CARs is essential in supporting their *in vivo* persistence.[147,148] Trials that include lympho-depleting chemotherapy regimens prior to the T-cell infusion may have better clinical outcomes as they reduce the tumor burden and provide an environment for the infused T cells that favors homeostatic expansion.[149] For example, impressive results were reported in three patients with aggressive, heavily pre-treated chronic lymphocytic leukemia (CLL) who received chemotherapy 1–4 days prior to the infusion of T cells transduced with a lentiviral vector encoding a CD19-specific CAR, incorporating the 4-1BB costimulatory endodomain.[147] In this trial, the infused cells showed logarithmic expansion *in vivo* and migration to the site of disease with remarkable cytotoxic effects against tumor cells (two complete and one partial remission), and persistence for more than 180 days. In contrast, CAR T-cell expansion observed *in vivo* in clinical trials using CD19-specific CARs that incorporate the CD28 signaling endodomain have produced less striking results,[45] which suggests that the "late activation" signaling pathways recruited by 4-1BB may be critical for functional, long-term expansion and engraftment of CAR-redirected T cells. However, given the diversity of the trials developed so far, systematic assessment of whether 4-1BB is responsible for the better outcome observed in one clinical trial may require a formal comparison between CAR T cells encoding CD28 and CAR T cells encoding 4-1BB infused in the same patient, in a similar way to the direct comparison of first- and second-generation (CD28 costimulation) CD19-specific CAR reported previously.[148]

Is the current design of CAR molecules ideal? Potent third-generation CARs have been generated to combine "early" (CD28) and "late" costimulatory signals (4-1BB or OX40) for complete T-cell activation.[135,137] However, combinations of these molecules raise safety concerns since they may induce T cells to produce excessive amounts of cytokines and promote severe cytokine storms as observed in a patient treated at the National Cancer

Institute.[150] One trial has been published using a CD19-specific third-generation CAR (CD28 and 4-1BB). The infusion of these cells did not produce significant side effects, but the CAR for this study was delivered in T cells by DNA electroporation, and required extensive *ex vivo* culture before infusion, which may exhaust these T cells and thus underestimate their potential toxicities.[151] Many CARs may also be immunogenic, as the scFv are usually derived from mouse hybridomas. Although CAR T cells can still be detected for months after infusion, humanized scFv may be preferable in the future to reduce the immunogenicity. Several significant issues still remain to be resolved before designing large phase II studies using CAR technology.

Although first-generation CARs could initiate a cytotoxic antitumor response in grafted T cells, it soon became obvious that signals from ITAM-bearing receptors alone can only induce transient cell division and suboptimal cytokine secretion but cannot provide prolonged polyclonal expansion and sustained antitumor reaction *in vivo*. According to the prevailing two-signaling model for lymphocyte activation, full activation and proliferation of T cells require a costimulatory signal through CD28-B7 interaction in addition to signaling through the TCR/CD3 complex.[152] Providing the costimulatory signal in trans through B7-expressing cells sustained proliferation of single ITAM-bearing CAR-expressing lymphocytes and led to enhanced antitumor response in mouse models.[153] A more straightforward strategy comprised the CD28 signaling in the CAR concept, either in two separate molecules or combined in a single CD28-ITAM receptor fusion protein.[154,155] Placement of the CD28 domain proximal to the CD3ζ chain and immediately distal to the transmembrane domain resulted in good surface expression, whereas in the opposite way the surface expression seems to be inhibited.[156] Therefore, all published second-generation CARs follow the general outline TM domain-CD28-ITAM-bearing signaling chain (Figure 6.4). Subsequently, it has been shown that the synergistic action of the two-signaling domains in one single CAR resulted in sustained proliferation of grafted lymphocytes and increased levels of IL-2, interferon (IFN)-γ, and granulocyte macrophage colony-stimulating factor (GM-CSF) secretion [73] independent of exogenous B7/CD28 costimulation. Due to CD28 costimulation the expression of anti-apoptotic proteins like B-cell lymphoma-(Bcl-) 2 is upregulated and induction of AICD is delayed.[140,157–159]

Finally, studies in mouse models supported the *in vitro* findings that T cells grafted with recombinant CD28-ITAM receptors have also higher proliferation capacities resulting in an enhanced antitumor activity.[136,159–161] A transgenic mouse model proved that even naive resting T cells can become fully activated, proliferate in antigen-induced manner, and secrete IL-2 through a chimeric receptor incorporating the costimulatory CD28 sequences in addition to an activating ITAM receptor chain.[162] One major drawback off cellular immunotherapy might be that adoptively transferred cells are rapidly impaired in their effector function by the immunosuppressive milieu, which tumor cells create in their surroundings.[163] However, engrafting T cells with second-generation CARs increases substantially the threshold of the modified cells against inhibitory effects mediated by transforming growth factor-β and against the suppressive action of Tregs.[141,164] Resistance to these cells is an important issue for immunotherapy, as tumor-infiltrating Tregs counteract against adoptively transferred tumor-specific T cells.[165] Another way of improving signaling capacities is the incorporation of Src family kinases or their adaptor molecules, which regulate the very beginning of the signaling cascade resulting from TCR triggering. The 56 kDa Lck kinase is one of the Src-homology kinases, which most likely phosphorylates CD3 ITAM motifs after TCR engagement and is noncovalently linked to either the CD4 or CD8 molecule. Incorporation of the p56Lck or its adaptor CD4 in a CAR with CD3ζ or CD28-CD3ζ signaling chains decreased signaling threshold of receptor grafted T cells.[156]

In recent years, further costimulatory molecules from the B7 family and the TNFR superfamily came into the focus of research.[166,167] Not surprisingly, a number of these molecules were also tested in the context of CARs, which led to the development of the third-generation of CARs with three different signaling moieties in the intracellular chain (Figure 6.4). Brentjens et al. generated a series of chimeric receptors bearing signaling sequences from CD28, DAP10, CD134 (OX40), and CD137 (4-1BB) in addition to the CD3ζ chain.[161] However, only the CD28-CD3ζ chain construct was able to induce significant proliferation of grafted T cells after antigen contact independently of exogenous B7 costimulation. In contrast, when cells expressing B7 molecules were used as targets, all T cells grafted with CARs having CD3ζ and costimulatory sequences proliferate better than those cells grafted with CD3ζ CAR.[161] Also in terms of IL-2 and IFN-γ secretion, T cells grafted with CD28-CD3ζ CAR always outcompeted T cells modified with receptors having other signaling combinations.[161] Similar results were obtained by another study, which also included the ICOS in the analyzed series of signaling moieties.[140] Secretion of inflammatory cytokines like TNF-α, IFN-γ, and GM-CSF was similar for T cells engrafted with CD28-CD3ζ and ICOS-CD3ζ CARs; however, IL-2 secretion and induction of proliferation was better with the CD28-CD3ζ construct.[140]

Thus, both studies have proven that for antigen-induced proliferation and high-level cytokine secretion the signal from CD28 is required and sufficient, but inclusion of further costimulatory molecules enhances proliferation capacities and apoptosis resistance in the grafted T cells.[168] It is now established that physiologically optimal activation requires CD28 engagement followed by costimulation through other T-cell signaling molecules.[169] Consequently, CARs which can simultaneously transmit multiple signals from CD28, CD3ζ, and an additional costimulatory molecule in the engrafted cell have been constructed. One of the most important "secondary" costimulatory molecules is OX40 (CD134), for which studies have shown that its signaling can further augment CD28-activated T-cell responses, enhancing proliferation, cytokine secretion, and survival.[170] Integration of OX40 in a third-generation CAR in combination with CD28 and CD3ζ chain leads to sustained *in vitro* proliferation and increased IL-2 secretion by grafted human primary T cells.[135] A number of studies pointed out the important role of the CD137/CD137L interaction for T-cell survival and AICD resistance.[125,171,172] Integration of CD137 signaling in CARs increased expression of anti-apoptotic protein Bcl-xL, induced sustained proliferation and survival of the grafted T cells, and was associated with higher effector cytokine production and antigen-specific tumor cell lysis.[132,173] In a mouse model, an established xenograft was controlled by retargeted T cells containing a CD28-CD137-CD3ζ CAR.[145] If targeted cancer cells are B7.1/B7.2 positive, chimeric CD137-CD3ζ CARs can be even more sufficient than a CD28-CD3ζ CAR.[132] Despite these encouraging results, the use of CARs with a tripartite signaling domain has to be carefully investigated, and it remains to be seen if CARs with tripartite signaling moieties reduce the signal threshold to a level where activation of grafted T cells can occur without antigen triggering.

In contrast to TCRs, CARs recognize TAAs independent of HLA. The typical CAR consists of four separate domains that are assembled from individual units: (1) the single chain variable fragment (scFv) domain, (2) the extracellular scaffold/linker, (3) the transmembrane domain, and (4) the signaling endodomain.[174] The specificity of the CAR is imparted by the scFv domain, which is directed against a TAA. Other molecules can be substituted for the scFv domain, including cytokines, pattern-recognition receptors, and cell surface molecules, to dock the CAR to the respective ligands of these molecules.[175–177] The scFv domain is attached to the transmembrane region via an extracellular scaffold. Optimal recognition of the TAA is affected by the extracellular length of the CAR. TAAs presented proximal to the plasma membrane may be more efficiently recognized by a CAR containing a longer scaffold, and conversely, TAAs presented further from the cell membrane may be more efficiently recognized by a CAR containing a shorter scaffold.[178,179] Moreover, the source of the scaffold may greatly affect the effectiveness and *in vivo* function of the CAR. CARs targeting the B-cell antigen CD19 that have been used for clinical trials contain scaffolds derived from CD28, CD8, IgG1, or IgG4. The IgG motifs found in CARs may bind to endogenous Fc receptors, leading to clearance of CAR^+ T cells expressing the IgG motifs and the nonspecific activation of NK cells. *In vivo* binding between CAR^+ T cells containing the IgG scaffolds and endogenous cells expressing Fc receptors can apparently be reduced by mutagenesis of the IgG scaffolds.[180] The transmembrane domain links the extracellular scFv domain and scaffold to the signaling endodomain. Oligomerization of the transmembrane domain may favor CAR signaling, but few studies have systematically analyzed different transmembrane domains.[181]

Signaling via the CAR molecule occurs via the addition of various endodomains to the cytoplasmic portion of the chimeric molecule. First-generation CARs signaled via immunoreceptor ITAMs from the CD3-ζ chain or FcR-γ.[127] A second costimulatory signal is included in second-generation CARs: the signaling endodomains of proteins such as CD28, 4-1BB, OX40, and ICOS.[182] CARs containing two or more costimulatory molecules in addition to CD3-ζ are commonly referred to third-generation CARs. A competitive repopulation experiment demonstrated a survival advantage for second-generation CAR$^+$ T cells infused into lymphoma patients compared to first-generation designs.[148] The ability to infuse more than one population of CAR$^+$ T cells into a given recipient is appealing to help understand the immunobiology which favors the sustained persistence and, thus, the enhanced therapeutic activity of a given CAR species. However, the expense associated with generating two infusion products from two recombinant viral vectors diminishes the enthusiasm for this otherwise appealing experimental approach.

To help reduce the barriers to combining gene therapy with T-cell therapy, our laboratory at MD Anderson Cancer Center in Houston, Texas, has employed electroporation using a commercially available Nucleofector device (Lonza Inc., Allendale, New Jersey, USA) to stably express CARs in primary human T cells for clinical trials.[183] Circulating T cells are electrotransferred with both the CAR-containing transposon and a hyperactive SB transposase, which catalyzes the cut-and-paste insertion of the transposon into the host genome. The apparent transient expression of the SB transposase in manufactured T cells helps to minimize the genotoxicity that arises via the continuous reintegration of the transposon. Transient expression of this fish-derived transposase also reduces the risk of the recipient developing an immune response to the transposase after the cells are infused. This improvement is significant, as an anti-transgene immune response could prompt the clearance and rejection of the genetically modified cells.[184] After gene transfer, the T cells are selectively propagated on activating and propagating cells (AaPCs) in the presence of stimulatory soluble cytokines for 4 weeks. The clinical-grade AaPCs are genetically modified K-562 cells that are available as a master cell bank. The AaPCs support the selective numeric expansion of CAR$^+$ T cells by expressing a TAA and the costimulatory molecules CD86, 4-1BB, and membrane-bound IL-15.[185]

Currently, to maintain patient safety, the manufacture of clinical-grade SB-modified CAR$^+$ T cells occurs over a period of 3–5 weeks to enable the loss of the DNA plasmid containing the SB transposase.[185–187] Indeed, polymerase chain reaction (PCR) is used to confirm the absence of the SB transposase prior to infusion. Redirected T-cell specificity mediated by the CAR is evaluated via a chromium release assay. Sterility is verified via visual inspection, a negative result for mycoplasma based on a PCR assay, and a negative result for endotoxin based on the limulus amoebocyte lysate test. The absence of genotoxicity is determined by the lack of growth of the genetically modified T-cell population upon removal of the AaPCs and cytokines, as well as by demonstrating a normal karyotype. The electroporated and propagated T cells are evaluated via flow cytometry for (1) viability, (2) the expression of the CAR, (3) the memory phenotype, (4) the absence of AaPCs, (5) exhaustion markers, and (6) telomere length. The presence of a polyclonal TCR repertoire is validated by flow cytometry or using bar-coded probes to confirm the lack of skewing of the numerically expanded T cells.[188]

CAR T CELLS IN CLINICAL TRIALS

CAR^+ T cells typically engineered by introducing DNA via a virus or a SB system have been successfully infused into patients with either solid or hematologic malignancy (see Table 6.1). Transfer of autologous T cells transduced with retrovirus to enforce the expression of a CD19-specific CAR containing the CD28 and CD3-ζ endodomains after a preparative chemotherapy regimen led to the prolonged eradication of CD19 + cells in a follicular lymphoma patient.[189] Later studies conducted using CD19-specific CAR + T cells in eight lymphoma and CLL patients found favorable responses in six of these patients, including 1 CR lasting more than 15 months and 5 partial responses (PRs) lasting at least 7 months. The expected adverse events associated with targeting CD19 include long-term B-cell aplasia in about half of the patients. In addition to these long-term toxicities, acute adverse events manifested as symptoms of inflammation, such as fever, fatigue, and hypotension. The loss of humoral immunity can be life-threatening, as 1 patient has died of culture-verified influenza 18 days after receiving an infusion of CAR^+ T cells.[149]

Current T-cell immunotherapy relies on harvesting T cells either from the patient, who may produce few or defective T cells due to the malignancy itself and prior treatment of the malignancy, or from an HLA-matched allogeneic donor, which includes the risk of GVHD. Due to their inherent antitumor activity and lack of HLA restriction, γδ T cells are an intriguing candidate therapy that can be pre-prepared from unrelated third-party donors and infused on demand. Artificial nucleases are another means to improve T cells for adoptive immunotherapy. Zinc-finger nucleases, transcription activator-like effector nucleases, and CRISPR/Cas9 introduce double-stranded DNA breaks at specific sites, which leads to repair by nonhomologous end joining, which may result in gene inactivation.[190–194] These technologies display potential for modulating the immune response to generate a favorable outcome in cancer immunotherapy. Artificial nucleases, such as CTLA-4 and programmed cell death-1 (PD-1), can be used to remove negative regulators of the anticancer response.[109,110,195] Furthermore, artificial nucleases could be used to remove the TCR from the αβ T cells used for immunotherapy to eliminate the HLA alloreactivity of the infused T cells to reduce the risk of GVHD and to generate an off-the-shelf T-cell product.[196]

REFERENCES

1. Lenschow DJ, Walunas TL, Bluestone JA. CD28/B7 system of T cell co-stimulation. *Annu Rev Immunol* 1996;**14**:233–58.
2. Frauwirth KA, Thompson CB. Activation and inhibition of lymphocytes by co-stimulation. *J Clin Invest* 2002;**109**:295–9.
3. Jenkins MK. The ups and downs of T cell co-stimulation. *Immunity* 1994;**1**:443–6.
4. Chambers CA. The expanding world of co-stimulation: the two-signal model revisited. *Trends Immunol* 2001;**22**:217–23.
5. Bretscher P, Cohn M. A theory of self-nonself discrimination. *Science* 1970;**169**:1042–9.
6. Lafferty KJ, Cunningham AJ. A new analysis of allogeneic interactions. *Aust J Exp Biol Med Sci* 1975;**53**:27–42.
7. Jenkins MK, Chen CA, Jung G, Mueller DL, Schwartz RH. Inhibition of antigen-specific proliferation of type 1 murine T cell clones after stimulation with immobilized anti-CD3 monoclonal antibody. *J Immunol* 1990;**144**:16–22.
8. Linsley PS, Ledbetter JA. The role of the CD28 receptor during T cell responses to antigen. *Annu Rev Immunol* 1993;**11**:191–212.
9. Bluestone JA. New perspectives of CD28-B7-mediated T cell costimulation. *Immunity* 1995;**2**:555–9.
10. June CH, Bluestone JA, Nadler LM, Thompson CB. The B7 and CD28 receptor families. *Immunol Today* 1994;**15**:321–30.
11. Rudd CE, Taylor A, Schneider H. CD28 and CTLA-4 coreceptor expression and signal transduction. *Immunol Rev* 2009;**229**:12–26.
12. Sharpe AH. Mechanisms of costimulation. *Immunol Rev* 2009;**229**:5–11.
13. Lee KP, Taylor C, Petryniak B, Turka LA, June CH, Thompson CB. The genomic organization of the CD28 gene. Implications for the regulation of CD28 mRNA expression and heterogeneity. *J Immunol* 1990;**145**:344–52.
14. Woerly G, Lacy P, Younes AB, Roger N, Loiseau S, Moqbel R, et al. Human eosinophils express and release IL-13 following CD28-dependent activation. *J Leukoc Biol* 2002;**72**:769–79.
15. Gross JA, St John T, Allison JP. The murine homologue of the T lymphocyte antigen CD28. Molecular cloning and cell surface expression. *J Immunol* 1990;**144**:3201–10.
16. Bachmann MF, McKall-Faienza K, Schmits R, Bouchard D, Beach J, Speiser DE, et al. Distinct roles for LFA-1 and CD28 during the activation of naive T cells: adhesion versus costimulation. *Immunity* 1997;**7**:549–57.
17. Bachmann MF, Sebzda E, Kündig TM, Shahinian A, Speiser DE, Mak TW, et al. T cell responses are governed by avidity and co-stimulatory thresholds. *Eur J Immunol* 1996;**26**:2017–22.
18. Fraser JD, Irving BA, Crabtree GR, Weiss A. Regulation of interleukin-2 gene enhancer activity by the T cell accessory molecule CD28. *Science* 1991;**251**:313–16.
19. Boise LH, Minn AJ, Noel PJ, June CH, Accavitti MA, Lindsten T, et al. CD28 costimulation can promote T cell survival by enhancing the expression of Bcl-x_L. *Immunity* 1995;**3**:87–98.
20. Sperling AI, Auger JA, Ehst BD, Rulifson IC, Thompson CB, Bluestone JA. CD28/B7 interactions deliver a unique signal to naive T cells that regulates cell survival but not early proliferation. *J Immunol* 1996;**157**:3909–17.
21. Luhder F, Huang Y, Dennehy KM, Guntermann C, Muller I, Winkler E, et al. Topological requirements and signaling properties of T cell-activating, anti-CD28 antibody superagonists. *J Exp Med* 2003;**197**:955–66.

22. Kirchhoff S, Muller WW, Li-Weber M, Krammer PH. Up-regulation of c-FLIPshort and reduction of activation-induced cell death in CD28-costimulated human T cells. *Eur J Immunol* 2000;**30**:2765–74.
23. Dahl AM, Klein C, Andres PG, London CA, Lodge MP, Mulligan RC, et al. Expression of Bcl-XL restores cell survival, but not proliferation and effector differentiation, in CD28-deficient T lymphocytes. *J Exp Med* 2000;**191**:2031–8.
24. Miller SD, Vanderlugt CL, Lenschow DJ, Pope JG, Karandikar NJ, Dal Canto MC, et al. Blockade of CD28/B7-1 interaction prevents epitope spreading and clinical relapses of murine EAE. *Immunity* 1995;**3**:739–45.
25. Harris N, Campbell C, Le Gros G, Ronchese F. Blockade of CD28/B7 co-stimulation by mCTLA4-Hγ1 inhibits antigen-induced lung eosinophilia but not Th2 cell development or recruitment in the lung. *Eur J Immunol* 1997;**27**:155–61.
26. Harris N, Peach R, Naemura J, Linsley PS, Le Gros G, Ronchese F. CD80 costimulation is essential for the induction of airway eosinophilia. *J Exp Med* 1997;**185**:177–82.
27. Dodson LF, Boomer JS, Deppong CM, Shah DD, Sim J, Bricker TL, et al. Targeted knock-in mice expressing mutations of CD28 reveal an essential pathway for costimulation. *MCB* 2009;**29**:3710–21.
28. Belz GT, Smith CM, Kleinert L, Reading P, Brooks A, Shortman K, et al. Distinct migrating and nonmigrating dendritic cell populations are involved in MHC class I-restricted antigen presentation after lung infection with virus. *Proc Natl Acad Sci USA* 2004;**101**:8670–5.
29. Legge KL, Braciale TJ. Accelerated migration of respiratory dendritic cells to the regional lymph nodes is limited to the early phase of pulmonary infection. *Immunity* 2003;**18**:265–77.
30. McAdam AJ, Farkash EA, Gewurz BE, Sharpe AH. B7 costimulation is critical for antibody class switching and CD8(+) cytotoxic T-lymphocyte generation in the host response to vesicular stomatitis virus. *J Virol* 2000;**74**:203–8.
31. Fuse S, Obar JJ, Bellfy S, Leung EK, Zhang W, Usherwood EJ. CD80 and CD86 control antiviral CD8 + T-cell function and immune surveillance of murine gammaherpesvirus 68. *J Virol* 2006;**80**:9159–70.
32. Bertram EM, Lau P, Watts TH. Temporal segregation of 4-1BB versus CD28-mediated costimulation: 4-1BB ligand influences T cell numbers late in the primary response and regulates the size of the T cell memory response following influenza infection. *J Immunol* 2002;**168**:3777–85.
33. Halstead ES, Mueller YM, Altman JD, Katsikis PD. In vivo stimulation of CD137 broadens primary antiviral CD8 + T cell responses. *Nat Immunol* 2002;**3**:536–41.
34. Lumsden JM, Roberts JM, Harris NL, Peach RJ, Ronchese F. Differential requirement for CD80 and CD80/CD86-dependent costimulation in the lung immune response to an influenza virus infection. *J Immunol* 2000;**164**:79–85.
35. Shahinian A, Pfeffer K, Lee KP, Kundig TM, Kishihara K, Wakeham A, et al. Differential T cell costimulatory requirements in CD28-deficient mice. *Science* 1993;**261**:609–12.
36. Suresh M, Whitmire JK, Harrington LE, Larsen CP, Pearson TC, Altman JD, et al. Role of CD28-B7 interactions in generation and maintenance of CD8 T cell memory. *J Immunol* 2001;**167**:5565–73.
37. Kundig TM, Shahinian A, Kawai K, Mittrucker HW, Sebzda E, Bachmann MF, et al. Duration of TCR stimulation determines costimulatory requirement of T cells. *Immunity* 1996;**5**:41–52.
38. Viola A, Lanzavecchia A. T cell activation determined by T cell receptor number and tunable thresholds. *Science* 1996;**273**:104–6.

39. Sprent J, Surh CD. T cell memory. *Annu Rev Immunol* 2002;**20**:551–79.
40. Busch DH, Pamer EG. T cell affinity maturation by selective expansion during infection. *J Exp Med* 1999;**189**:701–10.
41. Savage PA, Boniface JJ, Davis MM. A kinetic basis for T cell receptor repertoire selection during an immune response. *Immunity* 1999;**10**:485–92.
42. Bachmann MF, Gallimore A, Linkert S, Cerundolo V, Lanzavecchia A, Kopf M, et al. Developmental regulation of Lck targeting to the CD8 coreceptor controls signaling in naive and memory T cells. *J Exp Med* 1999;**189**:1521–30.
43. Flynn K, Mullbacher A. Memory alloreactive cytotoxic T cells do not require costimulation for activation in vitro. *Immunol Cell Biol* 1996;**74**:413–20.
44. Borowski AB, Boesteanu AC, Mueller YM, Carafides C, Topham DJ, Altman JD, et al. Memory CD8 + T cells require CD28 costimulation. *J Immunol* 2007;**179**:6494–503.
45. Fuse S, Zhang W, Usherwood EJ. Control of memory CD8 + T cell differentiation by CD80/CD86-CD28 costimulation and restoration by IL-2 during the recall response. *J Immunol* 2008;**180**:1148–57.
46. Ndejembi MP, Teijaro JR, Patke DS, Bingaman AW, Chandok MR, Azimzadeh A, et al. Control of memory CD4 T cell recall by the CD28/B7 costimulatory pathway. *J Immunol* 2006;**177**:7698–706.
47. Brocker T, Karjalainen K. Adoptive tumor immunity mediated by lymphocytes bearing modified antigen-specific receptors. *Adv Immunol* 1998;**68**:257–69.
48. Nocentini G, Giunchi L, Ronchetti S, Krausz LT, Bartoli A, Moraca R, et al. A new member of the tumor necrosis factor/nerve growth factor receptor family inhibits T cell receptor-induced apoptosis. *Proc Natl Acad Sci USA* 1997;**94**:6216–21.
49. Du X, Zheng G, Jin H, Kang Y, Wang J, Xiao C, et al. The adjuvant effects of co-stimulatory molecules on cellular and memory responses to HBsAg DNA vaccination. *J Gene Med* 2007;**9**:136–46.
50. Bukczynski J, Wen T, Ellefsen K, Gauldie J, Watts TH. Costimulatory ligand 4-1BBL (CD137L) as an efficient adjuvant for human antiviral cytotoxic T cell responses. *Proc Natl Acad Sci USA* 2004;**101**:1291–6.
51. Munks MW, Mourich DV, Mittler RS, Weinberg AD, Hill AB. 4-1BB and OX40 stimulation enhance CD8 and CD4 T-cell responses to a DNA prime, poxvirus boost vaccine. *Immunology* 2004;**112**:559–66.
52. Sharma RK, Elpek KG, Yolcu ES, Schabowsky RH, Zhao H, Bandura-Morgan L, et al. Costimulation as a platform for the development of vaccines: a peptide-based vaccine containing a novel form of 4-1BB ligand eradicates established tumors. *Cancer Res* 2009;**69**:4319–26.
53. Li Q, Ai J, Song Z, Liu J, Shan B. 4-1BB (CD137) ligand enhanced anti-tumor immune response against mouse forestomach carcinoma in vivo. *Cell Mol Immunol* 2008;**5**:379–84.
54. Kober J, Leitner J, Klauser C, Woitek R, Majdic O, Stockl J, et al. The capacity of the TNF family members 4-1BBL, OX40L, CD70, GITRL, CD30L and LIGHT to costimulate human T cells. *Eur J Immunol* 2008;**38**:2678–88.
55. Lamers CH, Sleijfer S, Vulto AG, et al. Treatment of metastatic renal cell carcinoma with autologous T-lymphocytes genetically retargeted against carbonic anhydrase IX: first clinical experience. *J Clin Oncol* 2006;**24**:e20–2.
56. McNamara JO, Kolonias D, Pastor F, Mittler RS, Chen L, Giangrande PH, et al. Multivalent 4-1BB binding aptamers costimulate CD8 + T cells and inhibit tumor growth in mice. *J Clin Invest* 2008;**118**:376–86.

57. Wang C, Wen T, Routy JP, Bernard NF, Sekaly RP, Watts TH. 4-1BBL induces TNF receptor-associated factor 1-dependent Bim modulation in human T cells and is a critical component in the costimulation-dependent rescue of functionally impaired HIV-specific CD8 T cells. *J Immunol* 2007;**179**:8252–63.
58. Van Gool SW, de Boer M, Ceuppens JL. CD28 ligation by monoclonal antibodies or B7/BB1 provides an accessory signal for the cyclosporin A-resistant generation of cytotoxic T cell activity. *J Immunol* 1993;**150**:3254–63.
59. Servet-Delprat C, Vidalain PO, Bausinger H, Manie S, Le Deist F, Azocar O, et al. Measles virus induces abnormal differentiation of CD40 ligand-activated human dendritic cells. *J Immunol* 2000;**164**:1753–60.
60. Chaudhry A, Das SR, Hussain A, Mayor S, George A, Bal V, et al. The Nef protein of HIV-1 induces loss of cell surface costimulatory molecules CD80 and CD86 in APCs. *J Immunol* 2005;**175**:4566–74.
61. Majumder B, Janket ML, Schafer EA, Schaubert K, Huang XL, Kan-Mitchell J, et al. Human immunodeficiency virus type 1 Vpr impairs dendritic cell maturation and T-cell activation: implications for viral immune escape. *J Virol* 2005;**79**:7990–8003.
62. Watts TH. TNF/TNFR family members in costimulation of T cell responses. *Annu Rev Immunol* 2005;**23**:23–68.
63. Peggs KS, Quezada SA, Allison JP. Cancer immunotherapy: co-stimulatory agonists and co-inhibitory antagonists. *Clin Exp Immunol* 2009;**157**:9–19.
64. Fonsatti E, Maio M, Altomonte M, Hersey P. Biology and clinical applications of CD40 in cancer treatment. *Semin Oncol* 2010;**37**:517–23.
65. Ngiow SF, von Scheidt B, Akiba H, Yagita H, Teng MW, Smyth MJ. Anti-TIM3 antibody promotes T cell IFN-gamma-mediated antitumor immunity and suppresses established tumors. *Cancer Res* 2011;**71**:3540–51.
66. Wang L, Rubinstein R, Lines JL, Wasiuk A, Ahonen C, Guo Y, et al. VISTA, a novel mouse Ig superfamily ligand that negatively regulates T cell responses. *J Exp Med* 2011;**208**:577–92.
67. Sedy JR, Gavrieli M, Potter KG, Hurchla MA, Lindsley RC, Hildner K, et al. B and T lymphocyte attenuator regulates T cell activation through interaction with herpesvirus entry mediator. *Nat Immunol* 2005;**6**:90–8.
68. Goldberg MV, Drake CG. LAG-3 in cancer immunotherapy. *Curr Top Microbiol Immunol* 2011;**344**:269–78.
69. Sierro S, Romero P, Speiser DE. The CD4-like molecule LAG-3, biology and therapeutic applications. *Expert Opin Ther Targets* 2011;**15**:91–101.
70. Leach DR, Krummel MF, Allison JP. Enhancement of antitumor immunity by CTLA-4 blockade. *Science* 1996;**271**:1734–6.
71. Myers L, Lee SW, Rossi RJ, Lefrancois L, Kwon BS, Mittler RS, et al. Combined CD137 (4-1BB) and adjuvant therapy generates a developing pool of peptide-specific CD8 memory T cells. *Int Immunol* 2006;**18**:325–33.
72. Morris GP, Chen L, Kong YC. CD137 signaling interferes with activation and function of CD4+ CD25 + regulatory T cells in induced tolerance to experimental autoimmune thyroiditis. *Cell Immunol* 2003;**226**:20–9.
73. Robertson SJ, Messer RJ, Carmody AB, Mittler RS, Burlak C, Hasenkrug KJ. CD137 costimulation of CD8 + T cells confers resistance to suppression by virus-induced regulatory T cells. *J Immunol* 2008;**180**:5267–74.

74. Melero I, Shuford WW, Newby SA, Aruffo A, Ledbetter JA, Hellström KE, et al. Monoclonal antibodies against the 4-1BB T-cell activation molecule eradicate established tumors. *Nat Med* 1997;**3**:682–5.
75. Miller RE, Jones J, Le T, Whitmore J, Boiani N, Gliniak B, et al. 4-1BB-specific monoclonal antibody promotes the generation of tumor-specific immune responses by direct activation of CD8 T cells in a CD40-dependent manner. *J Immunol* 2002;**169**:1792–800.
76. Wilcox RA, Flies DB, Zhu G, Johnson AJ, Tamada K, Chapoval AI, et al. Provision of antigen and CD137 signaling breaks immunological ignorance, promoting regression of poorly immunogenic tumors. *J Clin Invest* 2002;**109**:651–9.
77. Ito F, Li Q, Shreiner AB, Okuyama R, Jure-Kunkel MN, Teitz-Tennenbaum S, et al. Anti-CD137 monoclonal antibody administration augments the antitumor efficacy of dendritic cell-based vaccines. *Cancer Res* 2004;**64**:8411–19.
78. Molckovsky A, Siu LL. First-in-class, first-in-human phase I results of targeted agents: highlights of the 2008 American society of clinical oncology meeting. *J Hematol Oncol* 2008;**1**:20.
79. Croft M. Co-stimulatory members of the TNFR family: keys to effective T-cell immunity? *Nat Rev Immunol* 2003;**3**:609–20.
80. Bansal-Pakala P, Halteman BS, Cheng MH, Croft M. Signaling through OX40 (CD134) breaks peripheral T-cell tolerance. *Nat Med* 2001;**7**:907–12.
81. Takeda I, Ine S, Killeen N, Ndhlovu LC, Murata K, Satomi S, et al. Distinct roles for the OX40-OX40 ligand interaction in regulatory and nonregulatory T cells. *J Immunol* 2004;**172**:3580–9.
82. So T, Croft M. Cutting edge: OX40 inhibits TGF-beta- and antigen-driven conversion of naïve CD4 T cells into CD25 + Foxp3 + T cells. *J Immunol* 2007;**179**:1427–30.
83. Weinberg AD, Rivera MM, Prell R, Morris A, Ramstad T, Vetto JT, et al. Engagement of the OX-40 receptor in vivo enhances antitumor immunity. *J Immunol* 2000;**164**:2160–9.
84. Lee SJ, Myers L, Muralimohan G, Dai J, Qiao Y, Li Z, et al. 4-1BB and OX40 dual costimulation synergistically stimulate primary specific CD8 T cells for robust effector function. *J Immunol* 2004;**173**:3002–12.
85. Gri G, Gallo E, Di Carlo E, Musiani P, Colombo MP. OX40 ligand-transduced tumor cell vaccine synergizes with GM-CSF and requires CD40-Apc signaling to boost the host T cell antitumor response. *J Immunol* 2003;**170**:99–106.
86. McHugh RS, Whitters MJ, Piccirillo CA, Young DA, Shevach EM, Collins M, et al. CD4(+)CD25(+) immunoregulatory T cells: gene expression analysis reveals a functional role for the glucocorticoid-induced TNF receptor. *Immunity* 2002;**16**:311–23.
87. Kanamaru F, Youngnak P, Hashiguchi M, Nishioka T, Takahashi T, Sakaguchi S, et al. Costimulation via glucocorticoid-induced TNF receptor in both conventional and CD25 + regulatory CD4+ T cells. *J Immunol* 2004;**172**:7306–14.
88. Shimizu J, Yamazaki S, Takahashi T, Ishida Y, Sakaguchi S. Stimulation of CD25(+)CD4(+) regulatory T cells through GITR breaks immunological self-tolerance. *Nat Immunol* 2002;**3**:135–42.
89. Stephens GL, McHugh RS, Whitters MJ, Young DA, Luxenberg D, Carreno BM, et al. Engagement of glucocorticoid-induced TNFR family-related receptor on effector T cells by its ligand mediates resistance to suppression by CD4+ CD25 + T cells. *J Immunol* 2004;**173**:5008–20.

90. Cohen AD, Schaer DA, Liu C, Li Y, Hirschhorn-Cymmerman D, Kim SC, et al. Agonist anti-GITR monoclonal antibody induces melanoma tumor immunity in mice by altering regulatory T cell stability and intra-tumor accumulation. *PLoS One* 2010;**5**:e10436.
91. Mitsui J, Nishikawa H, Muraoka D, Wang L, Noguchi T, Sato E, et al. Two distinct mechanisms of augmented antitumor activity by modulation of immunostimulatory/inhibitory signals. *Clin Cancer Res* 2010;**16**:2781–91.
92. Beatty GL, Chiorean EG, Fishman MP, Saboury B, Teitelbaum UR, Sun W, et al. CD40 agonists alter tumor stroma and show efficacy against pancreatic carcinoma in mice and humans. *Science* 2011;**331**:1612–16.
93. Vonderheide RH, Flaherty KT, Khalil M, Stumacher MS, Bajor DL, Hutnick NA, et al. Clinical activity and immune modulation in cancer patients treated with CP-870,893, a novel CD40 agonist monoclonal antibody. *J Clin Oncol* 2007;**25**:876–83.
94. Liakou CI, Kamat A, Tang DN, Chen H, Sun J, Troncoso P, et al. CTLA-4 blockade increases IFNgamma-producing CD4+ ICOShi cells to shift the ratio of effector to regulatory T cells in cancer patients. *Proc Natl Acad Sci USA* 2008;**105**:14987–92.
95. Yuan J, Gnjatic S, Li H, Powel S, Gallardo HF, Ritter E, et al. CTLA-4 blockade enhances polyfunctional NY-ESO-1 specific T cell responses in metastatic melanoma patients with clinical benefit. *Proc Natl Acad Sci USA* 2008;**105**:20410–15.
96. Korman AJ, Peggs KS, Allison JP. Checkpoint blockade in cancer immunotherapy. *Adv Immunol* 2006;**90**:297–339.
97. Peggs KS, Quezada SA, Allison JP. Cell intrinsic mechanisms of T-cell inhibition and application to cancer therapy. *Immunol Rev* 2008;**224**:141–65.
98. Callahan MK, Wolchok JD, Allison JP. Anti-CTLA-4 antibody therapy: immune monitoring during clinical development of a novel immunotherapy. *Semin Oncol* 2010;**37**:473–84.
99. Wolchok JD, Neyns B, Linette G, Negrier S, Lutzky J, Thomas L, et al. Ipilimumab monotherapy in patients with pretreated advanced melanoma: a randomised, double-blind, multicentre, phase 2, dose-ranging study. *Lancet Oncol* 2010;**11**:155–64.
100. Hodi FS, O'Day SJ, McDermott DF, Weber RW, Sosman JA, Haanen JB, et al. Improved survival with ipilimumab in patients with metastatic melanoma. *N Engl J Med* 2010;**363**:711–23.
101. Robert C, Thomas L, Bondarenko I, O'Day S, Weber J, Garbe C, et al. Ipilimumab plus dacarbazine for previously untreated metastatic melanoma. *N Engl J Med* 2011;**64**:2517–26.
102. Keir ME, Butte MJ, Freeman GJ, Sharpe AH. PD-1 and its ligands in tolerance and immunity. *Annu Rev Immunol* 2008;**26**:677–704.
103. Nishimura H, Nose M, Hiai H, Minato N, Honjo T. Development of lupus-like autoimmune diseases by disruption of the PD-1 gene encoding an ITIM motif-carrying immunoreceptor. *Immunity* 1999;**11**:141–51.
104. Nishimura H, Okazaki T, Tanaka Y, Nakatani K, Hara M, Matsumori A, et al. Autoimmune dilated cardiomyopathy in PD-1 receptor-deficient mice. *Science* 2001;**291**:319–22.
105. Iwai Y, Terawaki S, Honjo T. PD-1 blockade inhibits hematogenous spread of poorly immunogenic tumor cells by enhanced recruitment of effector T cells. *Int Immunol* 2005;**17**:133–44.
106. Nomi T, Sho M, Akahori T, Hamada K, Kubo A, Kanehiro H. Clinical significance and therapeutic potential of the programmed death-1 ligand/programmed death-1 pathway in human pancreatic cancer. *Clin Cancer Res* 2007;**13**:2151–7.

107. Iwai Y, Ishida M, Tanaka Y, Okazaki T, Honjo T, Minato N. Involvement of PD-L1 on tumor cells in the escape from host immune system and tumor immunotherapy by PD-L1 blockade. *Proc Natl Acad Sci USA* 2002;**99**:12293–7.
108. Brahmer JR, Drake CG, Wollner I, Powderly JD, Picus J, Sharfman WH, et al. Phase I study of single-agent anti-programmed death-1 (MDX-1106) in refractory solid tumors: safety, clinical activity, pharmacodynamics, and immunologic correlates. *J Clin Oncol* 2010;**28**:3167–75.
109. Topalian SL, Hodi FS, Brahmer JR, Gettinger SN, Smith DC, McDermott DF, et al. Safety, activity, and immune correlates of anti-PD-1 antibody in cancer. *N Engl J Med* 2012;**366**(26):2443–54.
110. Brahmer JR, Tykodi SS, Chow LQ, Hwu WJ, Topalian SL, Hwu P, et al. Safety and activity of anti-PD-L1 antibody in patients with advanced cancer. *N Engl J Med* 2012;**366** (26):2455–65.
111. Rosenberg SA, Terry WD. Passive immunotherapy of cancer in animals and man. *Adv Cancer Res* 1977;**25**:323–88.
112. Greenberg PD. Adoptive T cell therapy of tumors: mechanisms operative in the recognition and elimination of tumor cells. *Adv Immunol* 1991;**49**:281–355.
113. Melief CJ. Tumor eradication by adoptive transfer of cytotoxic T lymphocytes. *Adv Cancer Res* 1992;**58**:143–75.
114. Southam CM, Brunschwig A, Levin AG, Dizon QS. Effect of leukocytes on transplantability of human cancer. *Cancer* 1966;**19**:1743–53.
115. Jamieson BD, Ahmed R. T cell memory. Long-term persistence of virus-specific cytotoxic T cells. *J Exp Med* 1989;**169**:1993–2005.
116. Michie CA, McLean A, Alcock C, Beverley PC. Lifespan of human lymphocyte subsets defined by CD45 isoforms. *Nature* 1992;**360**:264–5.
117. Kaech SM, Ahmed R. Memory CD8 + T cell differentiation: initial antigen encounter triggers a developmental program in naive cells. *Nat Immunol* 2001;**2**:415–22.
118. Sallusto F, Geginat J, Lanzavecchia A. Central memory and effector memory T cell subsets: function, generation, and maintenance. *Annu Rev Immunol* 2004;**22**:745–63.
119. Sallusto F, Lenig D, Forster R, Lipp M, Lanzavecchia A. Two subsets of memory T lymphocytes with distinct homing potentials and effector functions. *Nature* 1999;**401**:708–12.
120. Stagg J, Johnstone RW, Smyth MJ. From cancer immunosurveillance to cancer immunotherapy. *Immunol Rev* 2007;**220**:82–101.
121. Zou W. Immunosuppressive networks in the tumour environment and their therapeutic relevance. *Nat Rev Cancer* 2005;**5**:263–74.
122. Gimmi CD, Freeman GJ, Gribben JG, Gray G, Nadler LM. Human T-cell clonal energy is induced by antigen presentation in the absence of B7 costimulation. *Proc Natl Acad Sci USA* 1993;**90**:6586–90.
123. Rossig C, Bollard CM, Nuchtern JG, Merchant DA, Brenner MK. Targeting of G(D2)-positive tumor cells by human T lymphocytes engineered to express chimeric T-cell receptor genes. *Int J Cancer* 2001;**94**:228–36.
124. Pule MA, Savoldo B, Myers GD, Rossig C, Russell HV, Dotti G, et al. Virus-specific T cells engineered to coexpress tumor-specific receptors: persistence and antitumor activity in individuals with neuroblastoma. *Nat Med* 2008;**14**:1264–70.
125. Stephan MT, Ponomarev V, Brentjens RJ, et al. T cell-encoded CD80 and 4-1BBL induce auto- and transcostimulation, resulting in potent tumor rejection. *Nat Med* 2007;**13**:1440–9.

126. Barrett DM, Zhao Y, Liu X, Jiang S, Carpenito C, Kalos M, et al. Treatment of advanced leukemia in mice with mRNA engineered T cells. *Hum Gene Ther* 2011;**22**(12): 1575–86.
127. Eshhar Z, Waks T, Gross G, Schindler DG. Specific activation and targeting of cytotoxic lymphocytes through chimeric single chains consisting of antibody-binding domains and the γ or ζ subunits of the immunoglobulin and T-cell receptors. *Proc Natl Acad Sci USA* 1993;**90**:720–4.
128. Deeks SG, Wagner B, Anton PA, et al. A phase II randomized study of HIV-specific T-cell gene therapy in subjects with undetectable plasma viremia on combination antiretroviral therapy. *Mol Ther* 2002;**5**:788–97.
129. Kershaw MH, Westwood JA, Parker LL, et al. A phase I study on adoptive immunotherapy using gene-modified T cells for ovarian cancer. *Clin Cancer Res* 2006;**12** (20 Pt 1):6106–15.
130. Till BG, Jensen MC, Wang J, et al. Adoptive immunotherapy for indolent non-Hodgkin lymphoma and mantle cell lymphoma using genetically modified autologous CD20-specific T cells. *Blood* 2008;**112**:2261–71.
131. Pinthus JH, Waks T, Malina V, et al. Adoptive immunotherapy of prostate cancer bone lesions using redirected effector lymphocytes. *J Clin Invest* 2004;**114**:1774–81.
132. Milone MC, Fish JD, Carpenita C, et al. Chimeric receptors containing CD137 signal transduction domains mediate enhanced survival of T cells and increased antileukemic efficacy in vivo. *Mol Ther* 2009;**17**(8):1453–64.
133. Sadelain M, Brentjens R, Rivière I. The promise and potential pitfalls of chimeric antigen receptors. *Curr Opin Immunol* 2009;**21**:215–23.
134. Park JR, Digiusto DL, Slovak M, et al. Adoptive transfer of chimeric antigen receptor re-directed cytolytic T lymphocyte clones in patients with neuroblastoma. *Mol Ther* 2007;**15**:825–33.
135. Pule MA, Straathof KC, Dotti G, Heslop HE, Rooney CM, Brenner MK. A chimeric T cell antigen receptor that augments cytokine release and supports clonal expansion of primary human T cells. *Mol Ther* 2005;**12**:933–41.
136. Vera J, Savoldo B, Vigouroux S, Biagi E, Pule M, Rossig C, et al. T lymphocytes redirected against the kappa light chain of human immunoglobulin efficiently kill mature B lymphocyte-derived malignant cells. *Blood* 2006;**108**(12):3890–7.
137. Imai C, Mihara K, Andreansky M, Nicholson IC, Pui CH, Geiger TL, et al. Chimeric receptors with 4-1BB signaling capacity provoke potent cytotoxicity against acute lymphoblastic leukemia. *Leukemia* 2004;**18**.
138. Finney HM, Lawson AD, Bebbington CR, Weir AN. Chimeric receptors providing both primary and costimulatory signaling in T cells from a single gene product. *J Immunol* 1998;**161**:2791–7.
139. Maher J, Brentjens RJ, Gunset G, Riviere I, Sadelain M. Human T-lymphocyte cytotoxicity and proliferation directed by a single chimeric TCRzeta/CD28 receptor. *Nat Biotechnol* 2002;**20**:70–5.
140. Finney HM, Akbar AN, Lawson AD. Activation of resting human primary T cells with chimeric receptors: costimulation from CD28, inducible costimulator, CD134, and CD137 in series with signals from the TCR zeta chain. *J Immunol* 2004;**172**:104–13.
141. Loskog A, Giandomenico V, Rossig C, Pule M, Dotti G, Brenner MK. Addition of the CD28 signaling domain to chimeric T-cell receptors enhances chimeric T-cell resistance to T regulatory cells. *Leukemia* 2006;**20**:1819–28.

142. Song DG, Ye Q, Carpenito C, et al. In vivo persistence, tumor localization, and antitumor activity of CAR-engineered T cells is enhanced by costimulatory signaling through CD137 (4−1BB). *Cancer Res* 2011;**71**:4617−27.
143. Porter DL, Levine BL, Kalos M, Bagg A, June CH. Chimeric antigen receptor-modified T cells in chronic lymphoid leukemia. *N Engl J Med* 2011;**365**:725−33.
144. Song DG, Ye Q, Poussin M, Harms GM, Figini M, Powell Jr. DJ. CD27 costimulation augments the survival and antitumor activity of redirected human T cells in vivo. *Blood* 2012;**119**:696−706.
145. Carpenito C, Milone MC, Hassan R, Simonet JC, Lakhal M, Suhoski MM, et al. Control of large, established tumor xenografts with genetically retargeted human T cells containing CD28 and CD137 domains. *Proc Natl Acad Sci USA* 2009;**106**(9):3360−5.
146. Zhao Y, Wang QJ, Yang S, et al. A herceptin-based chimeric antigen receptor with modified signaling domains leads to enhanced survival of transduced T lymphocytes and antitumor activity. *J Immunol* 2009;**183**:5563−74.
147. Kalos M, Levine BL, Porter DL, Katz S, Grupp SA, Bagg A, et al. T cells with chimeric antigen receptors have potent antitumor effects and can establish memory in patients with advanced leukemia. *Sci Transl Med* 2011;**3**(95):95ra73.
148. Savoldo B, Ramos CA, Liu E, Mims MP, Keating MJ, Carrum G, et al. CD28 costimulation improves expansion and persistence of chimeric antigen receptor-modified T cells in lymphoma patients. *J Clin Invest* 2011;**121**(5):1822−6.
149. Kochenderfer JN, Dudley ME, Feldman SA, Wilson WH, Spaner DE, Maric I, et al. B-cell depletion and remissions of malignancy along with cytokine-associated toxicity in a clinical trial of anti-CD19 chimeric-antigen-receptortransduced T cells. *Blood* 2012;**119** (12):2709−20.
150. Morgan RA, Yang JC, Kitano M, Dudley ME, Laurencot CM, Rosenberg SA. Case report of a serious adverse event following the administration of T cells transduced with a chimeric antigen receptor recognizing ERBB2. *Mol Ther* 2010;**18**(4):843−51.
151. Till BG, Jensen MC, Wang J, Qian X, Gopal AK, Maloney DG, et al. CD20-specific adoptive immunotherapy for lymphoma using a chimeric antigen receptor with both CD28 and 4-1BB domains: pilot clinical trial results. *Blood* 2012;**119**(17):3940−50.
152. Van Gool SW, Vandenberghe P, de Boer M, Ceuppens JL. CD80, CD86 and CD40 provide accessory signals in a multiple-step T-cell activation model. *Immunol Rev* 1996;**153**:47−83.
153. Gade PF, Hassen W, Santos E, et al. Targeted elimination of prostate cancer by genetically directed human T lymphocytes. *Cancer Res* 2005;**65**(19):9080−8.
154. Alvarez-Vallina L, Hawkins RE. Antigen-specific targeting of CD28-mediated T cell co-stimulation using chimeric single-chain antibody variable fragment-CD28 receptors. *Eur J Immunol* 1996;**26**(10):2304−9.
155. Krause A, Guo H-F, Latouche J-B, Tan C, Cheung N-KV, Sadelain M. Antigen-dependent CD28 signaling selectively enhances survival and proliferation in genetically modified activated human primary T lymphocytes. *J Exp Med* 1998;**188**(4):619−26.
156. Geiger TL, Nguyen P, Leitenberg D, Flavell RA. Integrated src kinase and costimulatory activity enhances signal transduction through single-chain chimeric receptors in T lymphocytes. *Blood* 2001;**98**(8):2364−71.
157. Hombach A, Sent D, Schneider C, et al. T-cell activation by recombinant receptors: CD28 costimulation is required for interleukin 2 secretion and receptor-mediated T-cell proliferation but does not affect receptor-mediated target cell lysis. *Cancer Res* 2001;**61** (5):1976−82.

158. Hombach A, Wieczarkowiecz A, Marquardt T, et al. Tumor-specific T cell activation by recombinant immunoreceptors: CD3ζ signaling and CD28 costimulation are simultaneously required for efficient IL-2 secretion and can be integrated into one combined CD28/CD3ζ signaling receptor molecule. *J Immunol* 2001;**167**(11):6123–31.
159. Kowolik CM, Topp MS, Gonzalez S, et al. CD28 costimulation provided through a CD19-specific chimeric antigen receptor enhances in vivo persistence and antitumor efficacy of adoptively transferred T cells. *Cancer Res* 2006;**66**(22):10995–1004.
160. Haynes NH, Trapani JA, Teng MWL, et al. Singlechain antigen recognition receptors that costimulate potent rejection of established experimental tumors. *Blood* 2002;**100**(9):3155–63.
161. Brentjens RJ, Santos E, Nikhamin Y, et al. Genetically targeted T cells eradicate systemic acute lymphoblastic leukemia xenografts. *Clin Cancer Res* 2007;**13**(18):5426–35.
162. Friedmann-Morvinski D, Bendavid A, Waks T, Schindler D, Eshhar Z. Redirected primary T cells harboring a chimeric receptor require costimulation for their antigen-specific activation. *Blood* 2005;**105**(8):3087–93.
163. Rabinovich GA, Gabrilovich D, Sotomayor EM. Immunosuppressive strategies that are mediated by tumor cells. *Annu Rev Immunol* 2007;**25**:267–96.
164. Koehler H, Kofler D, Hombach A, Abken H. CD28 costimulation overcomes transforming growth factor-β-mediated repression of proliferation of redirected human CD4+ and CD8 + T cells in an antitumor cell attack. *Cancer Res* 2007;**67**(5):2265–73.
165. Zou W. Regulatory T cells, tumour immunity and immunotherapy. *Nat Rev Immunol* 2006;**6**(4):295–307.
166. Croft M. The role of TNF superfamily members in T-cell function and diseases. *Nat Rev Immunol* 2009;**9**(4):271–85.
167. Greenwald RJ, Freeman GJ, Sharpe AH. The B7 family revisited. *Annu Rev Immunol* 2005;**23**:515–48.
168. Hombach A, Abken H. Costimulation tunes tumorspecific activation of redirected T cells in adoptive immunotherapy. *Cancer Immunol Immunother* 2007;**56**(5):731–7.
169. Smith-Garvin JE, Koretzky GA, Jordan MS. T cell activation. *Annu Rev Immunol* 2009;**27**:591–619.
170. Redmond WL, Ruby CE, Weinberg AD. The role of OX40-mediated co-stimulation in T-cell activation and survival. *Crit Rev Immunol* 2009;**29**(3):187–201.
171. Melero I, Murillo O, Dubrot J, Hervás-Stubbs S, Perez-Gracia JL. Multi-layered action mechanisms of CD137 (4-1BB)-targeted immunotherapies. *Trends Pharmacol Sci* 2008;**29**(8):383–90.
172. Zhang H, Snyder KM, Suhoski MM, et al. 4-1BB is superior to CD28 costimulation for generating CD8 + cytotoxic lymphocytes for adoptive immunotherapy. *J Immunol* 2007;**179**(7):4910–18.
173. Wang J, Jensen M, Lin Y, et al. Optimizing adoptive polyclonal T cell immunotherapy of lymphomas, using a chimeric T cell receptor possessing CD28 and CD137 costimulatory domains. *Human Gene Ther* 2007;**18**(8):712–25.
174. Jena B, Moyes JS, Huls H, et al. Driving CAR-based T-cell therapy to success. *Curr Hematol Malig Rep* 2014;**9**:50–6.
175. Brown CE, Starr R, Aguilar B, et al. Stem-like tumor-initiating cells isolated from IL13Rα2 expressing gliomas are targeted and killed by IL13-zetakine-redirected T cells. *Clin Cancer Res* 2012;**18**:2199–209.

176. Kumaresan PR, Manuri PR, Albert ND, et al. Bioengineering T cells to target carbohydrate to treat opportunistic fungal infection. *Proc Natl Acad Sci USA* 2014;**111**:10660–5.
177. Shaffer DR, Savoldo B, Yi Z, et al. T cells redirected against CD70 for the immunotherapy of CD70-positive malignancies. *Blood* 2011;**117**:4304–14.
178. James SE, Greenberg PD, Jensen MC, et al. Antigen sensitivity of CD22-specific chimeric TCR is modulated by target epitope distance from the cell membrane. *J Immunol* 2008;**180**:7028–38.
179. Hudecek M, Lupo-Stanghellini MT, Kosasih PL, et al. Receptor affinity and extracellular domain modifications affect tumor recognition by ROR1-specific chimeric antigen receptor T cells. *Clin Cancer Res* 2013;**19**:3153–64.
180. Hombach A, Hombach AA, Abken H. Adoptive immunotherapy with genetically engineered T cells: modification of the IgG1 Fc 'spacer' domain in the extracellular moiety of chimeric antigen receptors avoids 'off-target' activation and unintended initiation of an innate immune response. *Gene Ther* 2010;**17**:1206–13.
181. Bridgeman JS, Hawkins RE, Bagley S, et al. The optimal antigen response of chimeric antigen receptors harboring the CD3zeta transmembrane domain is dependent upon incorporation of the receptor into the endogenous TCR/CD3 complex. *J Immunol* 2010;**184**:6938–49.
182. Sadelain M, Brentjens R, Riviere I. The basic principles of chimeric antigen receptor design. *Cancer Discov* 2013;**3**:388–98.
183. Hackett PB, Largaespada DA, Switzer KC, et al. Evaluating risks of insertional mutagenesis by DNA transposons in gene therapy. *Transl Res* 2013;**161**:265–83.
184. Jensen MC, Popplewell L, Cooper LJ, et al. Antitransgene rejection responses contribute to attenuated persistence of adoptively transferred CD20/CD19-specific chimeric antigen receptor redirected T cells in humans. *Biol Blood Marrow Transplant* 2010;**16**:1245–56.
185. Singh H, Figliola MJ, Dawson MJ, et al. Manufacture of clinical-grade CD19-specific T cells stably expressing chimeric antigen receptor using Sleeping Beauty system and artificial antigen presenting cells. *PLoS One* 2013;**8**:e64138.
186. Maiti SN, Huls H, Singh H, et al. Sleeping beauty system to redirect T-cell specificity for human applications. *J Immunother* 2013;**36**:112–23.
187. Singh H, Huls H, Kebriaei P, et al. A new approach to gene therapy using sleeping beauty to genetically modify clinical-grade T cells to target CD19. *Immunol Rev* 2014;**257**:181–90.
188. Zhang M, Maiti S, Bernatchez C, et al. A new approach to simultaneously quantify both TCR alpha- and beta-chain diversity after adoptive immunotherapy. *Clin Cancer Res* 2012;**18**:4733–42.
189. Kochenderfer JN, Wilson WH, Janik JE, et al. Eradication of B-lineage cells and regression of lymphoma in a patient treated with autologous T cells genetically engineered to recognize CD19. *Blood* 2010;**116**:4099–102.
190. Kim YG, Cha J, Chandrasegaran S. Hybrid restriction enzymes: zinc finger fusions to Fok I cleavage domain. *Proc Natl Acad Sci USA* 1996;**93**:1156–60.
191. Miller JC, Tan SY, Qiao GJ, et al. A TALE nuclease architecture for efficient genome editing. *Nat Biotechnol* 2011;**29**:143–149.
192. Mali P, Aach J, Stranges PB, et al. CAS9 transcriptional activators for target specificity screening and paired nickases for cooperative genome engineering. *Nat Biotechnol* 2013;**31**:833–8.

193. Mali P, Esvelt KM, Church GM. Cas9 as a versatile tool for engineering biology. *Nat Methods* 2013;**10**:957–63.
194. Cong L, Ran FA, Cox D, et al. Multiplex genome engineering using CRISPR/Cas systems. *Science* 2013;**339**:819–23.
195. Phan GQ, Yang JC, Sherry RM, et al. Cancer regression and autoimmunity induced by cytotoxic T lymphocyte-associated antigen 4 blockade in patients with metastatic melanoma. *Proc Natl Acad Sci USA* 2003;**100**:8372–7.
196. Torikai H, Reik A, Liu PQ, et al. A foundation for universal T-cell based immunotherapy: T cells engineered to express a CD19-specific chimeric-antigen-receptor and eliminate expression of endogenous TCR. *Blood* 2012;**119**:5697–705.
197. Fearon DT, Manders P, Wagner SD. Arrested differentiation, the self-renewing memory lymphocyte, and vaccination. *Science* 2001;**293**:248–50.
198. Zhang Y, Joe G, Hexner E, Zhu J, Emerson SG. Host-reactive CD8 + memory stem cells in graft-versus-host disease. *Nat Med* 2005;**11**:1299–305.

Index

Note: Page numbers followed by "*f*" and "*t*" refer to figures and tables, respectively.

C

D

E

F

G

H

I

K

L

M

N

V

W

Y

Z

Kolibri 360 GmbH
Ferdinand-Jühlke-Straße 7
99095 Erfurt, Deutschland
produktsicherheit@kolibri360.de